T0324204

A Mathematical Modeling Approach to Infectious Diseases

Cross Diffusion PDE Models for Epidemiology

A Mathematical Modeling Approach to Infectious Diseases

Cross Diffusion PDE Models for Epidemiology

William E Schiesser

Lehigh University, USA

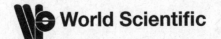
World Scientific

NEW JERSEY · LONDON · SINGAPORE · BEIJING · SHANGHAI · HONG KONG · TAIPEI · CHENNAI · TOKYO

Published by

World Scientific Publishing Co. Pte. Ltd.

5 Toh Tuck Link, Singapore 596224

USA office: 27 Warren Street, Suite 401-402, Hackensack, NJ 07601

UK office: 57 Shelton Street, Covent Garden, London WC2H 9HE

British Library Cataloguing-in-Publication Data
A catalogue record for this book is available from the British Library.

A MATHEMATICAL MODELING APPROACH TO INFECTIOUS DISEASES
Cross Diffusion PDE Models for Epidemiology

ISBN 978-981-3238-78-7

For any available supplementary material, please visit
http://www.worldscientific.com/worldscibooks/10.1142/10954#t=suppl

Typeset by Stallion Press
Email: enquiries@stallionpress.com

Printed in Singapore

To the authors of R, for their generous contribution of time and knowledge to provide an outstanding, open-source scientific computing system.

Contents

Preface   xi

Chapter 1.   Introduction to Spatiotemporal Models   1
(1.1)   Introduction   1
(1.2)   A Basic PDE Model   2
         (1.2.1)   Main program   6
         (1.2.2)   ODE/MOL routine   14
         (1.2.3)   Model output   19
(1.3)   H Refinement   32
(1.4)   P Refinement   37
(1.5)   R Refinement   43
(1.6)   Direct Differentiation   56
(1.7)   Summary and Conclusions   75
References   76

Chapter 2.   SIR Models   77
(2.1)   Introduction   77
(2.2)   Basic Model   77
         (2.2.1)   Main program   78
         (2.2.2)   ODE/MOL routine   86
         (2.2.3)   Model output   91
(2.3)   SEIR Model   97
         (2.3.1)   Main program   101
         (2.3.2)   ODE/MOL routine   110

	(2.3.3) Model output	116
(2.4)	Summary and Conclusions	133
References		133
Chapter 3.	Cross Diffusion	135
(3.1)	Introduction	135
(3.2)	Cross Diffusion Model	135
	(3.2.1) Main program	137
	(3.2.2) ODE/MOL routine	146
	(3.2.3) Model output	151
(3.3)	Detailed Analysis of the Cross Diffusion PDEs	160
	(3.3.1) Main program	160
	(3.3.2) ODE/MOL routine	170
	(3.3.3) Model output	170
(3.4)	Summary and Conclusions	180
References		181
Chapter 4.	Alternative Coordinate Systems	183
(4.1)	Introduction	183
(4.2)	Model in Radial Coordinates	183
	(4.2.1) Main program	185
	(4.2.2) ODE/MOL routine	194
	(4.2.3) Model output	201
(4.3)	Model in Polar Coordinates	210
(4.4)	3D Plotting	211
	(4.4.1) Main program	211
	(4.4.2) ODE/MOL routine	219
	(4.4.3) Model output	219
(4.5)	Summary and Conclusions	233
Reference		234
Chapter 5.	Vector-Borne Diseases, Malaria	235
(5.1)	Introduction	235
(5.2)	ODE Malaria Model, Low Transmission	235

(5.2.1)   Main program   239
(5.2.2)   ODE/MOL routine   252
(5.2.3)   Model output   256
(5.3)   ODE Malaria Model, High Transmission   269
(5.3.1)   Main program   269
(5.3.2)   ODE/MOL routine   276
(5.3.3)   Model output   278
(5.4)   PDE Malaria Model, Linear Diffusion   288
(5.4.1)   Main program   290
(5.4.2)   ODE/MOL routine   303
(5.4.3)   Model output   313
(5.5)   PDE Malaria Model, Cross Diffusion   325
(5.5.1)   Main program   326
(5.5.2)   ODE/MOL routine   336
(5.5.3)   Model output   344
(5.6)   Summary and Conclusions   350
References   352

Chapter 6.   Vector-Borne Diseases, Zika Virus   353
(6.1)   Introduction   353
(6.2)   ODE Zika Model   353
(6.2.1)   Main program   359
(6.2.2)   ODE/MOL routine   372
(6.2.3)   Model output   380
(6.3)   PDE Zika Model   385
(6.3.1)   Main program   391
(6.3.2)   ODE/MOL routine   407
(6.3.3)   Model output   426
(6.4)   Summary and Conclusions   432
References   432

Appendix A1: Function dss004   433

Appendix A2: Function dss044   437

Index   441

Preface

The intent of this book is to provide a methodology for the analysis of infectious diseases by computer-based mathematical models. The starting point is a basic SIR (Susceptible Infected Recovered) model that defines the S,I,R, populations as a function of time, t. The model therefore is a 3×3 (3 equations in 3 unknowns) system of ordinary differential equations (ODEs). Since the ODE model includes only temporal variations, it is then extended to include spatial effects (a spatiotemporal model) based on partial differential equations (PDEs).

Initially, the PDE models are 1D (one dimensional) in the Cartesian coordinate x ((x, y, z) in 3D). These x models are then extended to a radial coordinate, r, that can be considered as a 1D version in polar coordinates (r, θ), and that geometrically is a better fit to the physical system, e.g., a geographical area. The result are numerical solutions of the ODE/PDE models which demonstrate the spatiotemporal evolution of the infectious disease.

The radial models with independent variables (r, t) are approximated by the method of lines (MOL), a procedure for converting PDEs to approximating ODEs. The latter can then be solved numerically with a library initial-value ODE integrator. The programming is in R, an open-source scientific computing system that has an extensive ODE integrator library.

For each application, the model equations are stated first, including the initial conditions (ICs), boundary conditions (BCs) and model parameters. The coding (programming) of the application is then discussed in terms of documented R routines that are explained in detail. These routines are also available from a download so that the reader/analyst/researcher can use them to confirm the solutions presented in the book, then extend the routines to include additional effects and/or application to alternate models of interest.

The computer-based analysis of the SIR model is extended to SEIRS (Susceptible Exposed Infected Recovered Susceptible), and SIRC (Susceptible Infected Recovered Cross diffusion) models. The cross diffusion is a nonlinear effect that can be readily accommodated with the numerical methods implemented in R.

In conclusion, the ODE/PDE MOL methodology is applied to a malaria model and a Zika virus model. The ODE models are from the literature, then extended to PDE models. Both examples are for vector-borne diseases and include human and mosquito dynamics.

The author would welcome comments about the reported methodology and how it might be applied, and possibly extended, for an enhanced quantitative understanding of infectious diseases.

W. E. Schiesser
Bethlehem, PA USA
June 8, 2018

Chapter 1
Introduction to Spatiotemporal Models

(1.1) Introduction

The threat of infectious diseases continues as an urgent, worldwide health problem. The monitoring and treatment of infectious diseases on large spatial scales, e.g., epidemics in geographical regions, is therefore an on-going requirement.

To better understand this requirement, particularly the evolution of epidemics in space and time, mathematical models based on partial differential equations (PDEs) are the logical choice for quantitative analysis[1]

Several SIR PDE-based models have been reported in the literature. Generally the equations are sufficiently complicated that the solution of the PDEs requires a computer implementation. The PDEs are coded (programmed) to execute within an established scientific computing system (termed a *language*). Several languages are available. Here we select R, an open-source (no cost), quality scientific computing system that can be easily downloaded from the Internet[2].

---

[1]PDEs give the spatial and temporal (spatiotemporal) variations of key variables such as the susceptible (S), infected (I) and recovered (R) populations in an epidemic, so-called SIR models.

[2]R is available from the Internet in Linux, Mac, Windows formats: `http://cran.fhcrc.org/`. Also, the ODE/DAE library `deSolve` [2] can be downloaded for use with R.

Of the various PDE-SIR models that have been reported, a class of models is considered here which includes interactions with infected populations that are nonlinear[3], e.g., [1]. These interaction terms represent *cross diffusion*. This book focuses on cross diffusion PDE-based SIR models.

The presentation is in terms of example applications, presented at an introductory level[4]. Formal mathematics, e.g., theorems and proofs, is largely avoided. The model output is displayed in terms of numerical solutions presented in graphical format (2D, 3D plots) produced by the R graphics utilities.

We next consider a series of PDE-based models in order of increasing details. R coding for these models is presented as a series of routines with output presented for each model.

(1.2) A Basic PDE Model

To start, a PDE model is derived for two components, $S(x,t)$ (susceptibles) and $I(x,t)$ (infecteds). x is the first dimenion in the three dimensional Cartesian coordinate system (x, y, z). t is time.

A statement of a *dynamic conservation principle* is the starting point for the development of the model. A population balance for $S(x,t)$ on an incremental area $L\Delta x$ gives

---

The editor Rstudio is recommended for use in working with R and for facilitating graphical output in established formats (e.g., eps, png, pdf): http://rstudio.org/. deSolve can be conveniently downloaded via Rstudio.

[3]Nonlinear terms in a PDE are to other than the first power or degree. Nonlinearities are an important extension of linear terms, but generally they require computer implementation.

[4]Extensions of the basic SIR model are also considered, e.g.

SIRS: Susceptible → Infected → Recovered → Susceptible

SEIRS: Susceptible → Exposed → Infected → Recovered → Susceptible

$$LΔx\frac{∂S}{∂t} = -LD_s\frac{∂S}{∂x}|_x-\left(-LD_s\frac{∂S}{∂x}|_{x+Δx}\right)+LΔxr_{p1}S-LΔxr_iSI$$

(1.1a)

where (in SI (MKS) units)

$S(x,t)$ S population density (susceptibles/m^2)

$I(x,t)$ I population density (infecteds/m^2)

   x distance (m)

   t time (s = seconds)

   L cross sectional length of incremental area (m)

   D_s effective diffusivity for the susceptibles (m^2/s)

   r_{p1} net S population growth rate (birth rate - death rate) (1/s)

   r_i grow rate from S and I interactions ((m^2/infecteds) (1/s))

Eq. (1.1a) is based on partial derivatives, e.g., $\frac{∂S}{∂t}$, since the dependent variable $S(x,t)$ is a function of two independent variables, (x,t). Therefore, the independent variable must be identified in each of the derivatives (derivatives with respect to x and t appear in the following discussion).

The terms in eq. (1.1a) have the following interpretation:

- $LΔx\frac{∂S}{∂t}$: Accumulation (if > 0 or depletion if < 0)) of susceptibles in the incremental area $LΔx$ with units: (m)(m)(susceptibles/m^2)(1/s)=susceptibles/s

- $-LD_s\frac{\partial S}{\partial x}|_x$: Effective diffusion of susceptibles into the incremental area at x, with units: $(m)(m^2/s)$ (susceptibles/m^2)(1/m) = susceptibles/s. This term is based on the assumption that the spatial movement of the susceptibles is modeled as 1D diffusion which represents random motion. If the movement is more directed, this term can be supplemented by convection (a directed flow).

The net flux (random movement per unit length), q_x, is given by

$$q_x = -D_s\frac{\partial S}{\partial x} \tag{1.1b}$$

Eq. (1.1b) is generally termed *Fick's first law*. The minus is included so that the flux is in the positive x direction when the gradient $\frac{\partial S}{\partial x} < 0$, that is, the flux is in the direction of decreasing S in x.

- $-\left(-LD_s\frac{\partial S}{\partial x}|_{x+\Delta x}\right)$: Effective diffusion of susceptibles out of the incremental area at $x + \Delta x$. The net diffusive flux is the difference of the fluxes into and out of the incremental area (thus, the leading minus). Again, the units are susceptibles/s.

- $+L\Delta x r_{p1} S$: Net natural increase (with $r_{p1} > 0$) in susceptible population from birth rate > death rate, with units: $(m)(m)(1/s)$(susceptibles/m^2) = susceptibles/s. If $r_{p1} < 0$, from death rate > birth rate, this term is negative.

- $-L\Delta x r_i SI$: Rate of decrease of susceptibles from $S \to I$ (transmission of disease from susceptibles to infecteds), with units $(m)(m)(m^2/\text{infecteds})(1/s)$(susceptibles/$m^2$) (infecteds/$m^2$) = susceptibles/s. The minus corresponds to a decrease in S.

This term is nonlinear from the product SI. Also, a second dependent variable, I, is introduced which requires a second PDE in analogy with eq. (1.1a). In other words, the complete model consists of a 2×2 simultaneous (coupled) PDE system (two PDEs in two unknowns, $S(x,t)$ $I(x,t)$). This extension to include the PDE for $I(x,t)$ is discussed subsequently.

Note that all of terms in eq. (1.1a) have the net units of susceptibles/s, that is, the net change in the number of susceptibles in the incremental area $L\Delta x$ per second.

If eq. (1.1a) is rearranged to

$$\frac{\partial S}{\partial t} = \frac{D_s \frac{\partial S}{\partial x}|_{x+\Delta x} - D_s \frac{\partial S}{\partial x}|_x}{\Delta x} + r_{p1}S - r_i SI \qquad (1.1c)$$

The limiting case for eq. (1.1c) $\Delta x \to 0$ then gives a partial derivative in x (with D_s constant)

$$\frac{\partial S}{\partial t} = D_s \frac{\partial^2 S}{\partial x^2} + r_{p1}S - r_{si}SI \qquad (1.1d)$$

Eq. (1.1d) is the first of two PDEs that will be integrated (solved) numerically. The solution gives the dependent variable $S(x,t)$ as a function of the two independent variables, (x,t).

Since eq. (1.1d) has two unknown dependent variables, $S(x,t)$, $I(x,t)$, a second PDE is required. If a population balance for $I(x,t)$ is derived in the same way as for eq. (1.1d), the final result is

$$\frac{\partial I}{\partial t} = D_i \frac{\partial^2 I}{\partial x^2} + r_{p2}I + r_{si}SI \qquad (1.1e)$$

where now r_{p2} is a rate constant for eq. (1.1e). Note that the nonlinear interaction term is $-r_{si}SI$ which is the same as in eq. (1.1d) but opposite in sign indicating the rate of disappearance of susceptibles (eq. (1.1d)) equals the rate of appearance of infecteds (eq. (1.1e)) from the direct interaction of the two populations represented through the terms $\pm r_{si} S I$. D_i is the effective diffusivity for the infecteds. As with eq. (1.1d), each of the terms in eq. (1.1e) has the net units of infecteds/s.

Eqs. (1.1d,e) are each first order in t and second order in x. Therefore, each PDE requires one initial condition (IC) and two boundary conditions (BCs).

$$S(x, t = 0) = f_1(x); \ I(x, t = 0) = f_2(x) \qquad (1.2a,b)$$

$$\frac{\partial S(x = x_l, t)}{\partial x} = \frac{\partial S(x = x_u, t)}{\partial x} = 0 \qquad (1.2c,d)$$

$$\frac{\partial I(x = x_l, t)}{\partial x} = \frac{\partial I(x = x_u, t)}{\partial x} = 0 \qquad (1.2e,f)$$

$f_1(x), f_2(x)$ are functions to be specified. x_l, x_u are boundary values in x to be specified. Eqs. (1.2c,d,e,f) are homogeneous (zero) *Neumann* BCs[5].

Eqs. (1.1d,e), (1.2) constitute the 2×2 PDE system to be integrated numerically. The R routines for the integration are considered next.

(1.2.1) Main program

A main program for eqs. (1.1d,e), (1.2) follows.

```
#
#  Two PDE model
#
# Delete previous workspaces
  rm(list=ls(all=TRUE))
#
```

---

[5]Neumann BCs specify the derivatives in x while *Dirichlet* BCs specify the dependent variables $S(x = x_l, t)$, $S(x = x_u, t)$, $I(x = x_l, t)$, $I(x = x_u, t)$.

```
# Access ODE integrator
  library("deSolve");
#
# Access functions for numerical solution
  setwd("f:/infectious/chap1");
  source("pde1a.R");
  source("dss004.R");
#
# Select case
  ncase=1;
#
# Parameters
  if(ncase==1){
    f1=function(x)    1;
    f2=function(x)    0;
#   f2=function(x) 0.5;
    D_s=1;D_i=1;
    r_p1=0;r_p2=0;
    r_si=1;
  }
#
# Spatial grid (in x)
  nx=21;xl=-1;xu=1;
  x=seq(from=xl,to=xu,by=(xu-xl)/(nx-1));
#
# Independent variable for ODE integration
  t0=0;tf=0.1;nout=6;
  tout=seq(from=t0,to=tf,by=(tf-t0)/(nout-1));
#
# Initial condition (t=0)
  u0=rep(0,2*nx);
  for(i in 1:nx){
    u0[i]    =f1(x[i]);
    u0[i+nx]=f2(x[i]);
```

```
  }
  ncall=0;
#
# ODE integration
  out=lsodes(y=u0,times=tout,func=pde1a,
      sparsetype ="sparseint",rtol=1e-6,
      atol=1e-6,maxord=5);
  nrow(out)
  ncol(out)
#
# Arrays for plotting numerical solution
  S=matrix(0,nrow=nx,ncol=nout);
  I=matrix(0,nrow=nx,ncol=nout);
  for(it in 1:nout){
    for(i in 1:nx){
      S[i,it]=out[it,i+1];
      I[i,it]=out[it,i+1+nx];
    }
  }
#
# Display numerical solution
  for(it in 1:nout){
    cat(sprintf("\n        t       x       S(x,t)
                I(x,t)\n"));
    iv=seq(from=1,to=nx,by=2);
    for(i in iv){
      cat(sprintf("%6.2f%6.1f%12.3e%12.3e\n",
          tout[it],x[i],S[i,it],I[i,it]));
    }
  }
#
# Calls to ODE routine
  cat(sprintf("\n\n ncall = %5d\n\n",ncall));
#
```

```
# Plot PDE solutions
#
# S
  par(mfrow=c(1,1));
  matplot(x=x,y=S,type="l",xlab="x",
    ylab="S(x,t)",xlim=c(xl,xu),lty=1,
    main="",lwd=2,col="black");
#
# I
  par(mfrow=c(1,1));
  matplot(x=x,y=I,type="l",xlab="x",
    ylab="I(x,t)",xlim=c(xl,xu),lty=1,
    main="",lwd=2,col="black");
```

Listing 1.1: Main program for eqs. (1.1d,e), (1.2)

We can note the following details about Listing 1.1.

- Previous workspaces are deleted.

```
#
# Two PDE model
#
# Delete previous workspaces
  rm(list=ls(all=TRUE))
```

- The R ODE integrator library **deSolve** is accessed. Then the directory with the files for the solution of eqs. (1.1d,e), (1.2) is designated. Note that **setwd** (set working directory) uses / rather than the usual \.

```
#
# Access ODE integrator
  library("deSolve");
#
# Access functions for numerical solution
  setwd("f:/infectious/chap1");
```

```
source("pde1a.R");
source("dss004.R");
```

pde1a.R is the routine for the method of lines (MOL) approximation[6] of PDEs (1.1d,e) (discussed subsequently). dss004 (Differentiation in Space Subroutine) is a library routine for calculating a first derivative in x.

- A case is specified. For ncase=1 the functions in ICs (1.2a,b) are $f_1(x) = 1, f_2(x) = 0$ ($f_2(x) = 0.5$ is considered subsequently).

```
#
# Select case
  ncase=1;
#
# Parameters
  if(ncase==1){
    f1=function(x)   1;
    f2=function(x)   0;
#   f2=function(x) 0.5;
    D_s=1;D_i=1;
    r_p1=0;r_p2=0;
    r_si=1;
  }
```

---

[6]The method of lines is a general numerical procedure for the integration of PDEs in which the spatial (boundary value) derivatives are approximated algebraically, e.g., by finite differences (FDs), finite elements (FEs), weighted residuals, least squares, spectral methods. Then an initial value variable remains, usually time, and with one independent variable, the PDEs are approximated by a system of initial value ODEs that are integrated numerically, usually with a library ODE integrator. The present MOL analysis is based on FD approximations of the spatial derivatives.

The parameters D_s, D_i, r_{p1}, r_{p2}, r_{si} in eqs. (1.1d,e) are also defined numerically.

- A spatial grid of 21 points is defined for $x_l = -1 \leq x \leq x_u = 1$, so that x=-1,-0.9,...,1.

```
#
# Spatial grid (in x)
  nx=21;xl=-1;xu=1;
  x=seq(from=xl,to=xu,by=(xu-xl)/(nx-1));
```

- An interval in t of 6 points is defined for $0 \leq t \leq 0.1$ so that tout=0,0.02,...,0.1.

```
#
# Independent variable for ODE integration
  t0=0;tf=0.1;nout=6;
  tout=seq(from=t0,to=tf,by=(tf-t0)/(nout-1));
```

- ICs (1.2a,b) are defined.

```
#
# Initial condition (t=0)
  u0=rep(0,2*nx);
  for(i in 1:nx){
    u0[i]    =f1(x[i]);
    u0[i+nx]=f2(x[i]);
  }
  ncall=0;
```

The counter for the calls to the ODE/MOL routine pde1a is also initialized.

- The system of 42 MOL/ODEs is integrated by the library integrator lsodes[7] (available in deSolve). As expected, the inputs to lsode are the ODE function, pde1a, the IC vector u0, and the vector of output values of t, tout. The length of u0 (e.g., 42) informs lsodes how many ODEs are to be integrated. func,y,times are reserved names.

```
#
# ODE integration
out=lsodes(y=u0,times=tout,func=pde1a,
    sparsetype ="sparseint",rtol=1e-6,
    atol=1e-6,maxord=5);
nrow(out)
ncol(out)
```

The numerical solution to the ODEs is returned in matrix out. In this case, out has the dimensions $nout \times (2nx + 1) = 6 \times 2(21) + 1 = 42 + 1 = 43$, which are confirmed by the output from nrow(out),ncol(out) (included in the numerical output considered subsequently).

The offset $42 + 1$ is required since the first element of each column has the output t (also in tout), and the $2, ..., 2nx + 1 = 2, ..., 43$ column elements have the 42 ODE solutions.

- The solutions of the 42 ODEs returned in out by lsode are placed in arrays S,I.

```
#
# Arrays for plotting numerical solution
  S=matrix(0,nrow=nx,ncol=nout);
  I=matrix(0,nrow=nx,ncol=nout);
  for(it in 1:nout){
    for(i in 1:nx){
      S[i,it]=out[it,i+1];
      I[i,it]=out[it,i+1+nx];
```

---

[7] lsodes (Livermore Solver for Ordinary Differential Equations Sparse) is an initial value ODE integrator in deSolve that is based on sparse matrix processing of the ODE Jacobian matrix. Although lsodes requires added calculations internally for the sparse matrix algorithm, the additional calculations usually result in an efficient numerical solution of the ODE system, particularly as the size and stiffness of the ODE system increase.

```
    }
  }
```

Again, the offset i+1 is required since the first element
of each column of out has the value of t.

- $S(x, t), I(x, t)$ are displayed as a function of x and t, with
  every second value of x from by=2.

```
#
# Display numerical solution
  for(it in 1:nout){
    cat(sprintf("\n      t      x      S(x,t)
                I(x,t)\n"));
    iv=seq(from=1,to=nx,by=2);
    for(i in iv){
      cat(sprintf("%6.2f%6.1f%12.3e%12.3e\n",
          tout[it],x[i],S[i,it],I[i,it]));
    }
  }
```

- The number of calls to pde1a is displayed at the end of
  the solution.

```
#
# Calls to ODE routine
  cat(sprintf("\n\n ncall = %5d\n\n",ncall));
```

- $S(x, t)$ and $I(x, t)$ are plotted as a function of x with t as
  a parameter.

```
#
# Plot PDE solutions
#
# S
  par(mfrow=c(1,1));
  matplot(x=x,y=S,type="l",xlab="x",
```

```
        ylab="S(x,t)",xlim=c(xl,xu),lty=1,
        main="",lwd=2,col="black");
    #
    # I
      par(mfrow=c(1,1));
      matplot(x=x,y=I,type="l",xlab="x",
        ylab="I(x,t)",xlim=c(xl,xu),lty=1,
        main="",lwd=2,col="black");
```

This completes the main program. The ODE/MOL routine pde1a called by lsodes is considered next.

(1.2.2) ODE/MOL routine

Th ODE/MOL routine called by lsodes follows.

```
  pde1a=function(t,u,parms){
#
# Function pde1a computes the t derivative
# vectors of S(x,t),I(x,t)
#
# One vector to two vectors
  S=rep(0,nx);I=rep(0,nx);
  for(i in 1:nx){
    S[i]=u[i];
    I[i]=u[i+nx];
  }
#
# S*I
  SI=rep(0,nx);
  for(i in 1:nx){SI[i]=S[i]*I[i];}
#
# Sx,Ix
  Sx=dss004(xl,xu,nx,S);
  Ix=dss004(xl,xu,nx,I);
```

```
#
# BCs
  Sx[1]=0;Sx[nx]=0;
  Ix[1]=0;Ix[nx]=0;
#
# Sxx,Ixx
  Sxx=dss004(xl,xu,nx,Sx);
  Ixx=dss004(xl,xu,nx,Ix);
#
# PDEs
  St=rep(0,nx);It=rep(0,nx);
  for(i in 1:nx){
    St[i]=D_s*Sxx[i]+r_p1*S[i]-r_si*SI[i];
    It[i]=D_i*Ixx[i]+r_p2*I[i]+r_si*SI[i];
  }
#
# Two vectors to one vector
  ut=rep(0,2*nx);
  for(i in 1:nx){
    ut[i]    =St[i];
    ut[i+nx]=It[i];
  }
#
# Increment calls to pde1a
  ncall <<- ncall+1;
#
# Return derivative vector
  return(list(c(ut)));
  }
```

Listing 1.2: ODE/MOL routine for eqs. (1.1d,e), (1.2)

We can note the following details about Listing 1.2.

- The function is defined.

```
    pde1a=function(t,u,parms){
#
# Function pde1a computes the t derivative
# vectors of S(x,t),I(x,t)
```

t is the current value of t in eqs. (1.1d,e). u the 42-vector of ODE/MOL dependent variables. parm is an argument to pass parameters to pde1a (unused, but required in the argument list). The arguments must be listed in the order stated to properly interface with lsodes called in the main program of Listing 1.1. The derivative vector of the LHS of eqs. (1.1d,e) is calculated next and returned to lsodes.

- u is placed in two vectors, S,I, to facilitate the programming of eqs. (1.1d,e).

```
#
# One vector to two vectors
    S=rep(0,nx);I=rep(0,nx);
    for(i in 1:nx){
      S[i]=u[i];
      I[i]=u[i+nx];
    }
```

- The product of the two dependent variables of the terms $\pm r_{si} SI$ of eqs. (1.1d,e) is placed in SI.

```
#
# S*I
    SI=rep(0,nx);
    for(i in 1:nx){SI[i]=S[i]*I[i];}
```

SI introduces a nonlinearity into the PDE model.

- The derivatives $\dfrac{\partial S}{\partial x}, \dfrac{\partial I}{\partial x}$ are computed by dss004.

```
#
# Sx,Ix
  Sx=dss004(xl,xu,nx,S);
  Ix=dss004(xl,xu,nx,I);
```

Sx,Ix do not have to be allocated (with **rep**) since this is done by **dss004**.

- BCs (1.2c,d,e,f) are implemented (the subscripts 1,nx correspond to $x = x_l, x_u$).

```
#
# BCs
  Sx[1]=0;Sx[nx]=0;
  Ix[1]=0;Ix[nx]=0;
```

- The derivatives $\dfrac{\partial^2 S}{\partial x^2}, \dfrac{\partial^2 I}{\partial x^2}$ are computed by differentiating the first derivatives (*stagewise* or successive differentiation).

```
#
# Sxx,Ixx
  Sxx=dss004(xl,xu,nx,Sx);
  Ixx=dss004(xl,xu,nx,Ix);
```

Sxx,Ixx are allocated by **dss004** and therefore do not have to be declared before the calls to **dss004**, e.g., by **rep**. Additional details about **dss004** are available in Appendix A1.

- The PDEs are programmed. The similarity of eqs. (1.1d,e) and this coding is one of the advantages of the MOL.

```
#
# PDEs
  St=rep(0,nx);It=rep(0,nx);
  for(i in 1:nx){
```

```
St[i]=D_s*Sxx[i]+r_p1*S[i]-r_si*SI[i];
It[i]=D_i*Ixx[i]+r_p2*I[i]+r_si*SI[i];
}
```

The derivatives $\dfrac{\partial S}{\partial t}, \dfrac{\partial I}{\partial t}$ (LHSs of eqs. (1.1d,e)) are placed in St,It. The straightforward programming of the nonlinear terms $\pm r_{si}SI$ in eqs. (1.1d,e) is clear.

- The two vectors St,It are placed in a single derivative vector ut to return to lsodes.

```
#
# Two vectors to one vector
  ut=rep(0,2*nx);
  for(i in 1:nx){
    ut[i]   =St[i];
    ut[i+nx]=It[i];
  }
```

- The counter for the calls to pde1a is incremented and returned to the main program of Listing 1.1 with <<-.

```
#
# Increment calls to pde1a
  ncall <<- ncall+1;
```

- ut is returned to lsodes as a list (required by lsodes). c is the R vector utility.

```
#
# Return derivative vector
  return(list(c(ut)));
  }
```

The final } concludes pde1a.

The output from the main program and subordinate routine of Listings 1.1, 1.2 is considered next.

(1.2.3) Model output

Abbreviated numerical output is in Table 1.1

[1] 6

[1] 43

t	x	S(x,t)	I(x,t)
0.00	-1.0	1.000e+00	0.000e+00
0.00	-0.8	1.000e+00	0.000e+00
0.00	-0.6	1.000e+00	0.000e+00
0.00	-0.4	1.000e+00	0.000e+00
0.00	-0.2	1.000e+00	0.000e+00
0.00	0.0	1.000e+00	0.000e+00
0.00	0.2	1.000e+00	0.000e+00
0.00	0.4	1.000e+00	0.000e+00
0.00	0.6	1.000e+00	0.000e+00
0.00	0.8	1.000e+00	0.000e+00
0.00	1.0	1.000e+00	0.000e+00

.
.
.

Output for t = 0.02,..., 0.08 removed

.
.
.

t	x	S(x,t)	I(x,t)
0.10	-1.0	1.000e+00	0.000e+00
0.10	-0.8	1.000e+00	0.000e+00
0.10	-0.6	1.000e+00	0.000e+00
0.10	-0.4	1.000e+00	0.000e+00
0.10	-0.2	1.000e+00	0.000e+00
0.10	0.0	1.000e+00	0.000e+00
0.10	0.2	1.000e+00	0.000e+00

```
0.10    0.4    1.000e+00    0.000e+00
0.10    0.6    1.000e+00    0.000e+00
0.10    0.8    1.000e+00    0.000e+00
0.10    1.0    1.000e+00    0.000e+00


ncall =    70
```

Table 1.1: Abbreviated output for eqs. (1.1c,d) (1.2)

We can note the following details about this output.

- The dimensions of the solution matrix out are $nout \times 2n + 1 = 6 \times 2(21) + 1 = 43$. The offset $+1$ results from the value of t as the first element in each of the $nout = 6$ solution vectors. These same values of t are in tout,
- ICs (1.2a,b) $(t = 0)$ are verified for $f_1(x) = 1$, $f_2(x) = 0$. This is a worthwhile check since the ICs are the starting point for the solution.
- The output is for $x = -1, -0.8, ...1$ as programmed in Listing 1.1 (21 values at each value of t with every second value in x).
- The output is for $t = 0, 0.02, ..., 0.1$ as programmed in Listing 1.1.
- The solutions remain at $S(x,t) = 1$, $I(x,t) = 0$. The reason for this is that even though r_{si} in eqs. (1.1d,e) is not zero, all of the RHS terms of eqs. (1.1d,e) are zero. This includes the second derivatives $\dfrac{\partial^2 S}{\partial x^2}, \dfrac{\partial^2 I}{\partial x^2}$ which are zero since the solutions start at constant values in x and remain at constant values in x in accordance with BCs (1.2c,d,e,f)[8]. Also, $I(x,t) = 0$ gives zero values for the coupling terms $\pm r_{si} SI$.

---

[8]ICs (1.2a,b) and BCs (1.2c,d,e,f) are consistent. If they are not, a discontinuity would be introduced at $x = x_l, x = x_u$

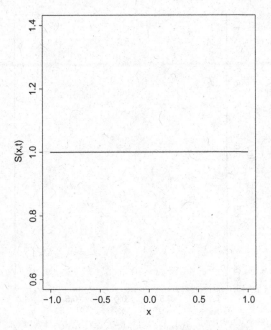

Figure 1.1a: Numerical solution $S(x, t)$ of eq. (1.1d)

- The computational effort by lsodes is low, ncall = 70, since the solution does not change with t.

The graphical output in Figs. 1.1a,b confirm the solutions in Table 1.1 (horizontal lines at $1, 0$).

This solution may seem trivial, but it is a worthwhile check since if the solutions did not remain invariant in x and t, a programming error would be indicated. This case also demonsrates the important property that the interaction (coupling) term $\pm r_{si} SI$ in eqs. (1.1d,e) has no effect (eqs. (1.1d,e) are uncoupled) if either $S(x, t)$ or $I(s, t)$ (or both) is zero. This suggests that the form of $\pm r_{si} SI$ might be modified so the term is not zero when either of the PDE variables is zero.

---

between $t = 0$ and $t > 1$ what could cause computational difficulties.

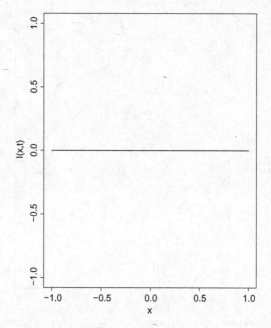

Figure 1.1b: Numerical solution $I(x,t)$ of eq. (1.1e)

We next consider another case that provides a test of the coding in Listings 1.1, 1.2. Specifically, $I(x, t = 0) = 0.5$ (rather than $I(x, t = 0) = 0$) so that the interaction terms $\pm r_{si}SI$ is now nonzero. This is accomplished with one change in f2 of Listing 1.1

```
#
# Parameters
  if(ncase==1){
    f1=function(x)    1;
#   f2=function(x)    0;
    f2=function(x) 0.5;
    D_s=1;D_i=1;
    r_p1=0;r_p2=0;
    r_si=1;
  }
```

Abbreviated numerical output for this case follows in Table 1.2.

[1] 6

[1] 43

t	x	S(x,t)	I(x,t)
0.00	-1.0	1.000e+00	5.000e-01
0.00	-0.8	1.000e+00	5.000e-01
0.00	-0.6	1.000e+00	5.000e-01
0.00	-0.4	1.000e+00	5.000e-01
0.00	-0.2	1.000e+00	5.000e-01
0.00	0.0	1.000e+00	5.000e-01
0.00	0.2	1.000e+00	5.000e-01
0.00	0.4	1.000e+00	5.000e-01
0.00	0.6	1.000e+00	5.000e-01
0.00	0.8	1.000e+00	5.000e-01
0.00	1.0	1.000e+00	5.000e-01

t	x	S(x,t)	I(x,t)
0.02	-1.0	9.900e-01	5.100e-01
0.02	-0.8	9.900e-01	5.100e-01
0.02	-0.6	9.900e-01	5.100e-01
0.02	-0.4	9.900e-01	5.100e-01
0.02	-0.2	9.900e-01	5.100e-01
0.02	0.0	9.900e-01	5.100e-01
0.02	0.2	9.900e-01	5.100e-01
0.02	0.4	9.900e-01	5.100e-01
0.02	0.6	9.900e-01	5.100e-01
0.02	0.8	9.900e-01	5.100e-01
0.02	1.0	9.900e-01	5.100e-01

.
.
.

```
Output for t = 0.04,..., 0.08 removed

       .                         .
       .                         .
       .                         .

     t     x       S(x,t)         I(x,t)
   0.10  -1.0    9.488e-01      5.512e-01
   0.10  -0.8    9.488e-01      5.512e-01
   0.10  -0.6    9.488e-01      5.512e-01
   0.10  -0.4    9.488e-01      5.512e-01
   0.10  -0.2    9.488e-01      5.512e-01
   0.10   0.0    9.488e-01      5.512e-01
   0.10   0.2    9.488e-01      5.512e-01
   0.10   0.4    9.488e-01      5.512e-01
   0.10   0.6    9.488e-01      5.512e-01
   0.10   0.8    9.488e-01      5.512e-01
   0.10   1.0    9.488e-01      5.512e-01


ncall =    72
```

Table 1.2: Abbreviated output for eqs. (1.1d,e) (1.2),
$$I(x, t = 0) = 0.5$$

We can note the following details about this output.

- The ICs $S(x, t = 0) = 1, I(x, t = 0) = 0.5$ are confirmed.
- There is no variation in the solutions with x since

  - Initially the solutions are uniform in x.
  - The second derivatives in eq. (1.1d,e) are zero from differentiating constants, $\dfrac{\partial^2 S}{\partial x^2} = \dfrac{\partial^2 I}{\partial x^2} = 0$. This, in effect, means that the solutions at adjacent points in x are unconnected.
  - BCs (1.2c,d,e,f) are consistent with constant solutions (no variation in x at the boundaries $x =$

x_l, x_u). This case illustrates the concept of consistency between the ICs and BCs. For example, if Dirichlet BCs are specified instead of Neumann BCs, and if the Dirichlet BCs are not $S(x = x_l = -1, t) = S(x = x_u = 1, t) = 1$, $I(x = x_l = -1, t) = I(x = x_u = 1, t) = 0.5$, a discontinuity between the ICs and BCs would be introduced (which might cause numerical difficulties).

• Since the solutions are constant in x, eqs. (1.1d,e) reduce to (with $r_{p1} = r_{p2} = 0, r_{si} = 1$ as defined in Listing 1.1)

$$\frac{\partial S}{\partial t} = 0 + 0 - r_{si}SI = -(1)(1)(0.5) = -0.5 \qquad (1.3a)$$

$$\frac{\partial I}{\partial t} = 0 + 0 + r_{si}SI = (1)(1)(0.5) = 0.5 \qquad (1.3b)$$

Therefore, $S(x, t)$ should decrease initially by -0.5 for each unit change in t, and $I(x, t)$ should increase by 0.5. This is observed in Table 1.2. For example, at $x = 0$

```
0.00    0.0    1.000e+00    5.000e-01
0.02    0.0    9.900e-01    5.100e-01
```

With a change in t of $0.02 - 0 = 0.02$, $S(x, t)$ changes by $0.9900 - 1.000 = -0.0100$ or $(0.02)(-0.5) = -0.01$, while $I(x, t)$ changes by $0.5100 - 0.5000 = 0.0100$ or $(0.02)(0.5) = 0.01$. The point of this calculation is to demonstrate how the terms in a PDE can be checked numerically for special cases, which provides confidence in the numerical solutions for more general cases, e.g., variations of the solutions with x as discussed subsequently (considering the derivatives from the differentiation routine dss004 have been verified previously). This type of numerical checking should be considered when an

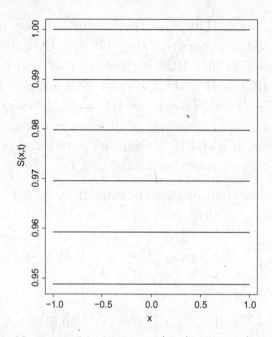

Figure 1.2a: Numerical solution $S(x,t)$ of eq. (1.1d), $I(x,t = 0) = 0.5$

analytical solution is not available, which is usually the case in realistic applications.

The numerical solution in Table 1.2 is also reflected in Figs. 1.2a,b.

Another case of eqs. (1.1d,e), (1.2) is now considered with variations of the solutions in x. If ICs (1.2a,b) are defined as

$$S(x, t = 0) = f_1(x) = e^{-100x^2} \qquad (1.4a)$$

$$I(x, t = 0) = f_2(x) = 0 \qquad (1.4b)$$

$f_1(x)$ defines an initial Gaussian function in $S(x,t)$, centered at $x = 0$. This distribution will decrease in x with increasing t. Also, $I(x,t)$ will not move away from the initial zero concentration through the interaction between eqs. (1.1d,e), $\pm r_{si}SI$ (as

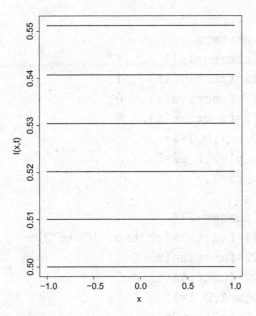

Figure 1.2b: Numerical solution $I(x, t)$ of eq. (1.1e), $I(x, t = 0) = 0.5$

discussed previously). This case can be programmed through the following changes in the main program of Listing 1.1.

- The ODE/MOL routine is now **pde1b** (which is the same as **pde1a** in Listing 1.2 except for the name change).

```
#
# Access functions for numerical solution
  setwd("f:/infectious/chap1");
  source("pde1b.R");
  source("dss004.R");
```

- For **ncase=2**, the Gaussian function is used as the IC for eq. (1.1d).

```
#
# Select case
  ncase=2;
```

```
#
# Parameters
  if(ncase==1){
    f1=function(x)    1;
    f2=function(x)    0;
#   f2=function(x) 0.5;
    D_s=1;D_i=1;
    r_p1=0;r_p2=0;
    r_si=1;
  }
  if(ncase==2){
    f1=function(x) exp(-100*x^2);
    f2=function(x) 0;
#   f2=function(x) 0.5;
    D_s=1;D_i=1;
    r_p1=0;r_p2=0;
    r_si=1;
  }
```

- For ncase=2, 51 points in x are used to improve the spatial resolution.

```
#
# Spatial grid (in x)
  if(ncase==1){nx=21;}
  if(ncase==2){nx=51;}
  xl=-1;xu=1;
  x=seq(from=xl,to=xu,by=(xu-xl)/(nx-1));
```

- pde1b is called by lsodes.

```
#
# ODE integration
  out=lsodes(y=u0,times=tout,func=pde1b,
      sparsetype ="sparseint",rtol=1e-6,
      atol=1e-6,maxord=5);
```

```
nrow(out)
ncol(out)
```

• For `ncase=2`, every fifth value of x is used in the output.

```
#
# Display numerical solution
for(it in 1:nout){
  cat(sprintf("\n      t      x        S(x,t)
              I(x,t)\n"));
  if(ncase==1){iv=seq(from=1,to=nx,by=2);}
  if(ncase==2){iv=seq(from=1,to=nx,by=5);}
  for(i in iv){
    cat(sprintf("%6.2f%6.1f%12.3e%12.3e\n",
        tout[it],x[i],S[i,it],I[i,it]));
  }
}
```

Abbreviated output for `ncase=2` is in Table 1.3.

[1] 6

[1] 103

t	x	S(x,t)	I(x,t)
0.00	-1.0	3.720e-44	0.000e+00
0.00	-0.8	1.604e-28	0.000e+00
0.00	-0.6	2.320e-16	0.000e+00
0.00	-0.4	1.125e-07	0.000e+00
0.00	-0.2	1.832e-02	0.000e+00
0.00	0.0	1.000e+00	0.000e+00
0.00	0.2	1.832e-02	0.000e+00
0.00	0.4	1.125e-07	0.000e+00
0.00	0.6	2.320e-16	0.000e+00
0.00	0.8	1.604e-28	0.000e+00
0.00	1.0	3.720e-44	0.000e+00

```
         .              .  .
         .
 0.02   0.0   3.335e-01   0.000e+00
         .              .
 0.04   0.0   2.426e-01   0.000e+00
         .              .
         .
 0.06   0.0   2.000e-01   0.000e+00
        .:             .
         .              .
 0.08   0.0   1.741e-01   0.000e+00
         .
         .              .
         .              .
   t     x      S(x,t)      I(x,t)
 0.10  -1.0   2.725e-02   0.000e+00
 0.10  -0.8   3.745e-02   0.000e+00
 0.10  -0.6   6.621e-02   0.000e+00
 0.10  -0.4   1.060e-01   0.000e+00
 0.10  -0.2   1.417e-01   0.000e+00
 0.10   0.0   1.562e-01   0.000e+00
 0.10   0.2   1.417e-01   0.000e+00
 0.10   0.4   1.060e-01   0.000e+00
 0.10   0.6   6.621e-02   0.000e+00
 0.10   0.8   3.745e-02   0.000e+00
 0.10   1.0   2.725e-02   0.000e+00

 ncall =    252
```

Table 1.3: Abbreviated output for eqs. (1.1d,e), ICs (1.4a,b), ncase=2

We can note the following details about this output.

- The dimensions of out are $6 \times 2(51) + 1 = 103$.

  [1] 6

  [1] 103

- The initial Gaussian distribution for $S(x,t)$, centered at $x = 0$, is clear. At $x = x_l = -1, x = x_u = 1$, the Gaussian is effectively zero.

t	x	S(x,t)	I(x,t)
0.00	-1.0	3.720e-44	0.000e+00
0.00	1.0	3.720e-44	0.000e+00

- The Gaussian remains centered at $x = 0$ with a diminshing value resulting from the dispersion in x. This can be observed in the successive values of $S(x = 0, t)$, starting at $S(x = 0, t = 0) = 1$ and ending at the final value $S(x = 0, t = 0.1) = 0.1562$

- The computational effort for the solution is modest, ncall= 252. That is, lsodes efficiently computes a complete solution to the $2(51) = 102$ ODEs.

These features of the solution are demonstrated in Figs. 1.3a,b.

Fig. 3.1a indicates the dispersion of the Gaussian with increasing t. Since only diffusion is active in eq. (1.1d) ($r_{p1} = 0$ and $-r_{si}SI = 0$ from $I(x,t) = 0$), the area under the successive solution curves remains constant (from mass conservation and the zero (no-flux) Neumann BCs); this could be checked by the reader by performing a quadrature (integration) in x on each solution curve.

Fig. 1.3b indicates $I(x,t)$ from eq. (1.1e) remains at zero.

We can now proceed with additional numerical experiments to demonstrate various concepts pertaining to the formulation

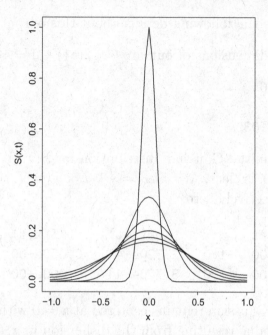

Figure 1.3a: Numerical solution $S(x,t)$ of eq. (1.1d), Gaussian IC

and computer implemention of spatiotemporal models, e.g., eqs. (1.1d,e).

(1.3) H Refinement

An essential consideration in the development of a numerical solution to a PDE model is the numerical accuracy of the solution. This might be ascertained by comparison with an analytical solution, but numerical methods are used when analytical solutions are precluded by the number and complexity of the PDEs. Therefore, methods to assess the accuracy of a numerical solution that no not require an analytical solution are essential. The following discussion pertains to *h refinement*[9].

---

[9]FD approximations of derivatives are based on polynomials from truncated Taylor series. For example, the FDs in

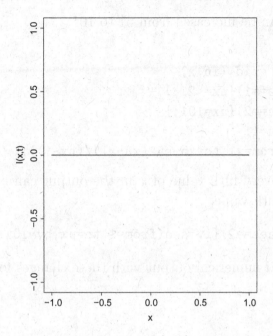

Figure 1.3b: Numerical solution $I(x,t)$ of eq. (1.1e), $I(x,t = 0) = 0$

A change in the number of grid points in x is easily accomplished in Listing 1.1. For example, with `ncase=2`, the number

---

`dss004` called in `pde1a` of Listing 1.2 are based on fourth order polynomials.

The error that results from truncating the Taylor series is termed *truncation error*, which has the form $err = c\Delta x^h$ where c is a constant for a particular FD approximation, Δx is the FD grid spacing and h is the order of the approximation. Thus, as Δx is varied by changing the number of points (e.g., $nx = 51$ in the preceding example), the error varies. Observing the effect on the numerical solution of changes in the number of FD grid points (and therefore changes in Δx) is h refinement (from the term Δx^h). $h = 4$ for the FDs in `dss004` so that these FDs are termed *fourth order correct*.

of points can be increased from 51 to 101

```
#
# Spatial grid (in x)
  if(ncase==1){nx= 21;}
  if(ncase==2){nx=101;}
  xl=-1;xu=1;
  x=seq(from=xl,to=xu,by=(xu-xl)/(nx-1));
```

Also, every fifth value of x in the output can be increased to every tenth value.

```
  if(ncase==2){iv=seq(from=1,to=nx,by=10);}
```

Abbreviated numerical output with these changes follows.

```
[1] 6

[1] 203
```

t	x	S(x,t)	I(x,t)
0.00	-1.0	3.720e-44	0.000e+00
0.00	-0.8	1.604e-28	0.000e+00
0.00	-0.6	2.320e-16	0.000e+00
0.00	-0.4	1.125e-07	0.000e+00
0.00	-0.2	1.832e-02	0.000e+00
0.00	0.0	1.000e+00	0.000e+00
0.00	0.2	1.832e-02	0.000e+00
0.00	0.4	1.125e-07	0.000e+00
0.00	0.6	2.320e-16	0.000e+00
0.00	0.8	1.604e-28	0.000e+00
0.00	1.0	3.720e-44	0.000e+00
.	.	.	.
0.02	0.0	3.333e-01	0.000e+00

```
     .                    .
     .                    .
     .                    .
0.04    0.0    2.425e-01    0.000e+00
     .                    .
     .                    .
     .                    .
0.06    0.0    2.000e-01    0.000e+00
     .                    .
     .                    .
     .                    .
0.08    0.0    1.741e-01    0.000e+00
     .                    .
     .                    .
     .                    .

   t     x     S(x,t)       I(x,t)
0.10   -1.0    2.725e-02    0.000e+00
0.10   -0.8    3.744e-02    0.000e+00
0.10   -0.6    6.622e-02    0.000e+00
0.10   -0.4    1.060e-01    0.000e+00
0.10   -0.2    1.417e-01    0.000e+00
0.10    0.0    1.562e-01    0.000e+00
0.10    0.2    1.417e-01    0.000e+00
0.10    0.4    1.060e-01    0.000e+00
0.10    0.6    6.622e-02    0.000e+00
0.10    0.8    3.744e-02    0.000e+00
0.10    1.0    2.725e-02    0.000e+00

ncall =    358
```

Table 1.4: Abbreviated output for eqs. (1.1d,e), ICs (1.4a,b),
$nx = 101$

We can note the following details about the solution in Table 1.4.

- The dimensions of the output matrix `out` from `lsodes` are $6 \times 2(101) + 1 = 203$ as expected.

```
[1] 6
```

```
[1] 203
```

- The solutions in Tables 1.3 and 1.4 are essentially the same. For example, at $x = 0$,

```
Table 1.3, nx=51
```

```
[1] 6
```

```
[1] 103
```

```
   t      x      S(x,t)        I(x,t)
 0.00    0.0    1.000e+00     0.000e+00
 0.02    0.0    3.335e-01     0.000e+00
 0.04    0.0    2.426e-01     0.000e+00
 0.06    0.0    2.000e-01     0.000e+00
 0.08    0.0    1.741e-01     0.000e+00
 0.10    0.0    1.562e-01     0.000e+00
```

```
 ncall =    252
```

```
Table 1.4, nx=101
```

```
[1] 6
```

```
[1] 203
```

t	x	S(x,t)	I(x,t)
0.00	0.0	1.000e+00	0.000e+00
0.02	0.0	3.333e-01	0.000e+00
0.04	0.0	2.425e-01	0.000e+00
0.06	0.0	2.000e-01	0.000e+00
0.08	0.0	1.741e-01	0.000e+00
0.10	0.0	1.562e-01	0.000e+00

```
ncall =    358
```

- The computational effort remains modest, `ncall` = 358.

The agreement between the solutions for $nx = 51$ and $nx = 101$ implies that the solution for $nx = 51$ is accurate to about four figures which is usually more than adequate for applications. If the apparent agreement is not adequate, larger numbers of grid points can be used to try to resolve the accuracy. An important point is that an analytical solution is not required for this assessment of accuracy. Some form of h refinement should therefore be considered for a new application.

Since the plots for $nx = 101$ are identical to Figs. 1.3a,b, they are not included here.

(1.4) P Refinement

Changes in the order of the FD approximation are easily implemented. For example, the calls to dss004 in pde1a of Listing 1.2 can be changed to calls to dss006 which is based on sixth order FDs[10]. All that is required to make this change is to replace dss004 with dss006 in Listing 1.2 (the calling sequence for the two routines is the same). Also, in the main program of Listing 1.1, dss006 has to be accessed.

---

[10]The error that results from changing the order of the FD approximation has the form $err = c\Delta x^p$ where p is the order

```
#
# Access functions for numerical solution
  setwd("f:/infectious/chap1");
  source("pde1b.R");
  source("dss004.R");
  source("dss006.R");
```

Abbreviated numerical output for **dss006** follows in Table 1.5.

[1] 6

[1] 103

t	x	S(x,t)	I(x,t)
0.00	-1.0	3.720e-44	0.000e+00
0.00	-0.8	1.604e-28	0.000e+00
0.00	-0.6	2.320e-16	0.000e+00
0.00	-0.4	1.125e-07	0.000e+00
0.00	-0.2	1.832e-02	0.000e+00
0.00	0.0	1.000e+00	0.000e+00
0.00	0.2	1.832e-02	0.000e+00
0.00	0.4	1.125e-07	0.000e+00
0.00	0.6	2.320e-16	0.000e+00
0.00	0.8	1.604e-28	0.000e+00
0.00	1.0	3.720e-44	0.000e+00
.	.	.	.
.	.	.	.
.	.	.	.
0.02	0.0	3.333e-01	0.000e+00
.	.		.
.	.		.
.	.		.

of the approximation. Thus, changing the order is termed *p refinement*.

```
0.04    0.0    2.425e-01    0.000e+00
         .                   .

         .                   .

0.06    0.0    2.000e-01    0.000e+00
         .
         .                   .

0.08    0.0    1.741e-01    0.000e+00
         .
         .                   .
```

t	x	S(x,t)	I(x,t)
0.10	-1.0	2.725e-02	0.000e+00
0.10	-0.8	3.744e-02	0.000e+00
0.10	-0.6	6.622e-02	0.000e+00
0.10	-0.4	1.060e-01	0.000e+00
0.10	-0.2	1.417e-01	0.000e+00
0.10	0.0	1.562e-01	0.000e+00
0.10	0.2	1.417e-01	0.000e+00
0.10	0.4	1.060e-01	0.000e+00
0.10	0.6	6.622e-02	0.000e+00
0.10	0.8	3.744e-02	0.000e+00
0.10	1.0	2.725e-02	0.000e+00

```
ncall =    276
```

Table 1.5: Abbreviated output for eqs. (1.1d,e), ICs (1.4a,b), $nx = 51$, dss006

We can note the following details about the solution in Table 1.5.

- The solutions in Table 1.3 and 1.5, for dss004 and dss006, respectively, are essentially the same, again implying that the fourth order FDs in dss004 are adequate.

Table 1.3, nx=51, dss004

[1] 6

[1] 103

t	x	S(x,t)	I(x,t)
0.00	0.0	1.000e+00	0.000e+00
0.02	0.0	3.335e-01	0.000e+00
0.04	0.0	2.426e-01	0.000e+00
0.06	0.0	2.000e-01	0.000e+00
0.08	0.0	1.741e-01	0.000e+00
0.10	0.0	1.562e-01	0.000e+00

ncall =   252

Table 1.5, nx=51, dss006

[1] 6

[1] 103

t	x	S(x,t)	I(x,t)
0.00	0.0	1.000e+00	0.000e+00
0.02	0.0	3.333e-01	0.000e+00
0.04	0.0	2.425e-01	0.000e+00
0.06	0.0	2.000e-01	0.000e+00
0.08	0.0	1.741e-01	0.000e+00
0.10	0.0	1.562e-01	0.000e+00

ncall =   276

- The computational effort is modest, ncall = 276.

Again, when computing a numerical solution in a new application, p refinement should be considered to assess the accuracy of the solution.

To conclude this discussion of the FD solution of eqs. (1.1d,e), (1.2), we consider `ncase=2` in the main program of Listing 1.1 with $I(x, t = 0) = 0.5$.

```
#
# Select case
  ncase=2;
#
# Parameters
  if(ncase==1){
    f1=function(x)    1;
    f2=function(x)    0;
#   f2=function(x)  0.5;
    D_s=1;D_i=1;
    r_p1=0;r_p2=0;
    r_si=1;
  }
  if(ncase==2){
    f1=function(x)  exp(-100*x^2);
#   f2=function(x)  0;
    f2=function(x)  0.5;
    D_s=1;D_i=1;
    r_p1=0;r_p2=0;
    r_si=10;
  }
```

Now eqs. (1.1d) and (1.1e) can interact through $\pm r_{si}SI$ since $S(x,t), I(x,t)$ are nonzero at $t = 0$ (r_{si} was increased from 1 to 10 to increase the interaction). Again, the ODE/PDE routine `pde1a` is in Listing 1.2.

Abbreviated numerical output is given in Table 1.6.

[1] 6

[1] 103

t	x	S(x,t)	I(x,t)
0.00	-1.0	3.720e-44	5.000e-01
0.00	-0.8	1.604e-28	5.000e-01
0.00	-0.6	2.320e-16	5.000e-01
0.00	-0.4	1.125e-07	5.000e-01
0.00	-0.2	1.832e-02	5.000e-01
0.00	0.0	1.000e+00	5.000e-01
0.00	0.2	1.832e-02	5.000e-01
0.00	0.4	1.125e-07	5.000e-01
0.00	0.6	2.320e-16	5.000e-01
0.00	0.8	1.604e-28	5.000e-01
0.00	1.0	3.720e-44	5.000e-01

.
.
.

Output for t = 0.02,..., 0.08 removed

.
.
.

t	x	S(x,t)	I(x,t)
0.10	-1.0	1.629e-02	5.110e-01
0.10	-0.8	2.229e-02	5.152e-01
0.10	-0.6	3.914e-02	5.271e-01
0.10	-0.4	6.224e-02	5.438e-01
0.10	-0.2	8.277e-02	5.589e-01
0.10	0.0	9.106e-02	5.651e-01
0.10	0.2	8.277e-02	5.589e-01
0.10	0.4	6.224e-02	5.438e-01

```
0.10    0.6    3.914e-02    5.271e-01
0.10    0.8    2.229e-02    5.152e-01
0.10    1.0    1.629e-02    5.110e-01


ncall =    253
```

Table 1.6: Abbreviated output for eqs. (1.1d,e), (1.2), $nx = 51$,
$$I(x, t = 0) = 0.5$$

We can note the following details about the solution in Table 1.6.

- The solution matrix **out** again has the dimensions 6×103 corresponding to $nx = 51$.

  [1] 6

  [1] 103

- The ICs $S(x, t = 0), I(x, t = 0)$ are confirmed.
- Significant transfer from eq. (1.1d) to eq (1.1e) occurs so that $I(x, t)$ departs from 0.5 (e.g., at $t = 0.1$).
- The computational effort is modest, **ncall = 253**.

These features of the solutions of eqs. (1.1d,e) are confirmed in Figs. 1.4a,b.

(1.5) R Refinement

Another approach to assess the accuracy of a numerical solution is to compute the solution with a different approximation for the spatial derivatives. This approach is termed *r refinement*. In the following discussion, splines are used in place of FDs. The spline analysis is based on the R utility **splinefun** which is part of the basic R system.

The programming of the ODE/MOL routines with splines is illustrated by the following **pde1a_sp**.

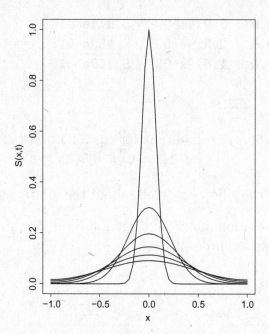

Figure 1.4a: Numerical solution $S(x,t)$ of eq. (1.1d), Gaussian IC

```
pde1a_sp=function(t,u,parms){
#
# Function pde1a_sp computes the t derivative
# vectors of S(x,t),I(x,t)
#
# One vector to two vectors
  S=rep(0,nx);I=rep(0,nx);
  for(i in 1:nx){
    S[i]=u[i];
    I[i]=u[i+nx];
  }
#
# S*I
  SI=rep(0,nx);
  for(i in 1:nx){SI[i]=S[i]*I[i];}
```

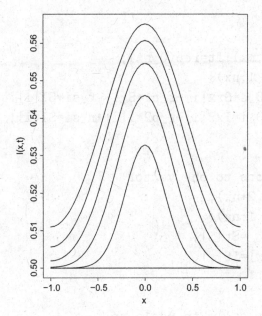

Figure 1.4b: Numerical solution $I(x,t)$ of eq. (1.1e), $I(x,t = 0) = 0.5$

```
#
# Sx,Ix
  tableSx=splinefun(x,S);
  Sx=tableSx(x,deriv=1);
  tableIx=splinefun(x,I);
  Ix=tableIx(x,deriv=1);
#
# BCs
  Sx[1]=0;Sx[nx]=0;
  Ix[1]=0;Ix[nx]=0;
#
# Sxx,Ixx
  tableSxx=splinefun(x,Sx);
  Sxx=tableSxx(x,deriv=1);
  tableIxx=splinefun(x,Ix);
  Ixx=tableIxx(x,deriv=1);
```

```
#
# PDEs
  St=rep(0,nx);It=rep(0,nx);
  for(i in 1:nx){
    St[i]=D_s*Sxx[i]+r_p1*S[i]-r_si*SI[i];
    It[i]=D_i*Ixx[i]+r_p2*I[i]+r_si*SI[i];
  }
#
# Two vectors to one vector
  ut=rep(0,2*nx);
  for(i in 1:nx){
    ut[i]    =St[i];
    ut[i+nx]=It[i];
  }
#
# Increment calls to pde1a_sp
  ncall <<- ncall+1;
#
# Return derivative vector
  return(list(c(ut)));
  }
```

Listing 1.3: ODE/MOL routine for eqs. (1.1d,e), (1.2),
$nx = 51$, splines

We can note the following details about Listing 1.3.

- The function is defined.

```
    pde1a_sp=function(t,u,parms){
#
# Function pde1a_sp computes the t derivative
# vectors of S(x,t),I(x,t)
```

The arguments of pde1a_sp are explained after Listing 1.2.

- The 102-vector u is placed in two vectors S,I to facilitate the programming of eqs. (1.1d,e).

```
#
# One vector to two vectors
  S=rep(0,nx);I=rep(0,nx);
  for(i in 1:nx){
    S[i]=u[i];
    I[i]=u[i+nx];
  }
```

- The product function SI in eqs. (1.1d,e) is defined.

```
#
# S*I
  SI=rep(0,nx);
  for(i in 1:nx){SI[i]=S[i]*I[i];}
```

- The derivatives $\frac{\partial S}{\partial x}, \frac{\partial I}{\partial x}$ are computed by the spline utility splinefun.

```
#
# Sx,Ix
  tableSx=splinefun(x,S);
  Sx=tableSx(x,deriv=1);
  tableIx=splinefun(x,I);
  Ix=tableIx(x,deriv=1);
```

The grid x defined in the main program of Listing 1.1 is passed to splinefun. Two steps are required in using splinefun: (1) A table of spline coefficients is computed, e.g., tableSx=splinefun(x,S) and (2) The table is used to compute the derivative, e.g., Sx=tableSx(x,deriv=1). deriv=1 specifies a first order numerical derivative.

- BCs (1.2c,d,e,f) are implemented (as in Listing 1.2).

```
#
# BCs
  Sx[1]=0;Sx[nx]=0;
  Ix[1]=0;Ix[nx]=0;
```

- The derivatives $\dfrac{\partial^2 S}{\partial x^2}, \dfrac{\partial^2 I}{\partial x^2}$ are computed as the derivatives of the first derivatives (stagewise or successive differentiation).

```
#
# Sxx,Ixx
  tableSxx=splinefun(x,Sx);
  Sxx=tableSxx(x,deriv=1);
  tableIxx=splinefun(x,Ix);
  Ixx=tableIxx(x,deriv=1);
```

- Eqs. (1.1d,e) are programmed (as in Listing 1.2).

```
#
# PDEs
  St=rep(0,nx);It=rep(0,nx);
  for(i in 1:nx){
    St[i]=D_s*Sxx[i]+r_p1*S[i]-r_si*SI[i];
    It[i]=D_i*Ixx[i]+r_p2*I[i]+r_si*SI[i];
  }
```

- The derivatives $\dfrac{\partial S}{\partial t}, \dfrac{\partial I}{\partial t}$ are placed in a single vector ut to return to lsodes.

```
#
# Two vectors to one vector
  ut=rep(0,2*nx);
  for(i in 1:nx){
    ut[i]    =St[i];
```

```
    ut[i+nx]=It[i];
  }
```

- The number of calls to `pde1a_sp` is incremented and returned to the main program with `<<-`.

```
#
# Increment calls to pde1a_sp
  ncall <<- ncall+1;
```

- The derivative vector is returned to `lsodes` as a list. `c` is the R vector operator.

```
#
# Return derivative vector
  return(list(c(ut)));
  }
```

The final `}` concludes `pde1a_sp`.

This concludes the programming of eqs. (1.1d,e), (1.2). Abbreviated output follows.

```
[1] 6
```

```
[1] 103
```

t	x	S(x,t)	I(x,t)
0.00	-1.0	3.720e-44	0.000e+00
0.00	-0.8	1.604e-28	0.000e+00
0.00	-0.6	2.320e-16	0.000e+00
0.00	-0.4	1.125e-07	0.000e+00
0.00	-0.2	1.832e-02	0.000e+00
0.00	0.0	1.000e+00	0.000e+00
0.00	0.2	1.832e-02	0.000e+00
0.00	0.4	1.125e-07	0.000e+00
0.00	0.6	2.320e-16	0.000e+00

```
0.00   0.8   1.604e-28   0.000e+00
0.00   1.0   3.720e-44   0.000e+00
        .                  .
        .                  .
        .                  .

Output for t = 0.02,..., 0.08 removed
        .                  .
        .                  .
        .                  .

   t     x      S(x,t)       I(x,t)
 0.10  -1.0   2.725e-02   -6.167e-29
 0.10  -0.8   3.744e-02   -1.374e-29
 0.10  -0.6   6.622e-02   -1.991e-29
 0.10  -0.4   1.060e-01   -5.832e-30
 0.10  -0.2   1.417e-01   -8.104e-30
 0.10   0.0   1.562e-01    1.048e-30
 0.10   0.2   1.417e-01   -4.089e-30
 0.10   0.4   1.060e-01    6.797e-31
 0.10   0.6   6.622e-02   -4.783e-30
 0.10   0.8   3.744e-02   -1.839e-30
 0.10   1.0   2.725e-02   -1.778e-29


ncall =    464
```

Table 1.7: Abbreviated output for eqs. (1.1d,e), ICs (1.4a,b), splines

We can note the following details about the abbreviated output.

- The solution matrix out again has the dimensions 6×103 corresponding to $nx = 51$.
- ICs (1.2a,b) are confirmed for $S(x, t = 0) = e^{-100x^2}$, $I(x, t = 0) = 0$.
- $I(x, t)$ does not remain at zero as in Table 1.3, but has small nonzero values. In other words, the splines do not

differentiate a constant to zero exactly as FDs, but the approximation to the derivative is accurate[11].

- The computational effort is modest, `ncall = 464`. Therefore the splines efficiently provide a numerical solution.

The solution is close to the FD solution in Table 1.3.

Table 1.3, FD, dss004

[1] 6

[1] 103

t	x	S(x,t)	I(x,t)
0.10	-1.0	2.725e-02	0.000e+00
0.10	-0.8	3.745e-02	0.000e+00
0.10	-0.6	6.621e-02	0.000e+00
0.10	-0.4	1.060e-01	0.000e+00
0.10	-0.2	1.417e-01	0.000e+00
0.10	0.0	1.562e-01	0.000e+00
0.10	0.2	1.417e-01	0.000e+00
0.10	0.4	1.060e-01	0.000e+00
0.10	0.6	6.621e-02	0.000e+00
0.10	0.8	3.745e-02	0.000e+00
0.10	1.0	2.725e-02	0.000e+00

ncall = 252

---

[11]The weighting coefficients of the FDs sum to zero so the derivative of a constant is zero (Table 1.3). The splines differentiate a constant to a small value that is well below the machine epsilon (unit roundoff) of approximately 10^{-15}, and therefore, for the purposes of numerical calculations, the value is effectively zero.

Table 1.7, splines, splinefun

[1] 6

[1] 103

t	x	S(x,t)	I(x,t)
0.10	-1.0	2.725e-02	-6.167e-29
0.10	-0.8	3.744e-02	-1.374e-29
0.10	-0.6	6.622e-02	-1.991e-29
0.10	-0.4	1.060e-01	-5.832e-30
0.10	-0.2	1.417e-01	-8.104e-30
0.10	0.0	1.562e-01	1.048e-30
0.10	0.2	1.417e-01	-4.089e-30
0.10	0.4	1.060e-01	6.797e-31
0.10	0.6	6.622e-02	-4.783e-30
0.10	0.8	3.744e-02	-1.839e-30
0.10	1.0	2.725e-02	-1.778e-29

ncall =   464

Therefore, the r refinement (splines in place of FDs) gives asurance that the numerical solution is correct. Of course, this comparison of solutions does not guarantee that the solution is correct (this is not a proof), but is offered as a way to infer accuracy (without an analytical solution).

The solutions in Table 1.7 are plotted in Figs (1.5a,b).

Fig. 1.5a indicates a smooth solution that is essentially the same as Fig 1.3a (since the solutions for FDs and splines are the same). Fig 1.5b indicates that $I(x,t)$ has small nonzero values (note the vertical scale) as expected from Table 1.7.

If the IC $I(x, t = 0) = 0.5$ is used, the splinefunc solution is essentially the same as in Table 1.6 (with FDs).

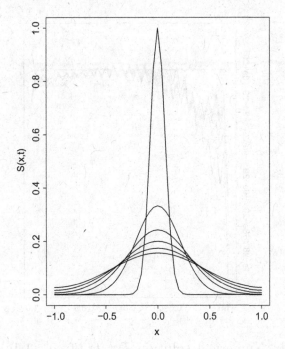

Figure 1.5a: Numerical solution $S(x,t)$ of eq. (1.1d), Gaussian IC, splines

[1] 6

[1] 103

t	x	S(x,t)	I(x,t)
0.00	-1.0	3.720e-44	5.000e-01
0.00	-0.8	1.604e-28	5.000e-01
0.00	-0.6	2.320e-16	5.000e-01
0.00	-0.4	1.125e-07	5.000e-01
0.00	-0.2	1.832e-02	5.000e-01
0.00	0.0	1.000e+00	5.000e-01
0.00	0.2	1.832e-02	5.000e-01
0.00	0.4	1.125e-07	5.000e-01
0.00	0.6	2.320e-16	5.000e-01

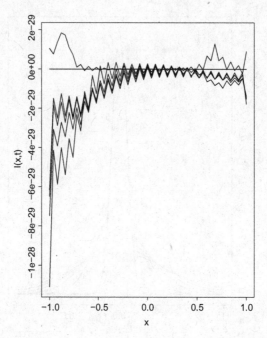

Figure 1.5b: Numerical solution $I(x,t)$ of eq. (1.1e), $I(x,t = 0) = 0$, splines

```
0.00    0.8    1.604e-28    5.000e-01
0.00    1.0    3.720e-44    5.000e-01
                  .                .

                  .                .

                  .                .

Output for t = 0.02,..., 0.08 removed

                  .                .

                  .                .

                  .                .

   t      x      S(x,t)        I(x,t)
0.10    -1.0    1.629e-02    5.110e-01
0.10    -0.8    2.229e-02    5.152e-01
0.10    -0.6    3.914e-02    5.271e-01
0.10    -0.4    6.224e-02    5.438e-01
```

```
0.10   -0.2    8.277e-02    5.589e-01
0.10    0.0    9.105e-02    5.651e-01
0.10    0.2    8.277e-02    5.589e-01
0.10    0.4    6.224e-02    5.438e-01
0.10    0.6    3.914e-02    5.271e-01
0.10    0.8    2.229e-02    5.152e-01
0.10    1.0    1.629e-02    5.110e-01


ncall =    441
```

Table 1.8: Abbreviated output for eqs. (1.1d,e),
$I(x, t = 0) = 0.5$, splines

A comparison of the FD and spline solutions follows.

```
Table 1.6, FDs, dss004

[1] 6

[1] 103
      t      x       S(x,t)        I(x,t)
   0.10   -1.0    1.629e-02    5.110e-01
   0.10   -0.8    2.229e-02    5.152e-01
   0.10   -0.6    3.914e-02    5.271e-01
   0.10   -0.4    6.224e-02    5.438e-01
   0.10   -0.2    8.277e-02    5.589e-01
   0.10    0.0    9.106e-02    5.651e-01
   0.10    0.2    8.277e-02    5.589e-01
   0.10    0.4    6.224e-02    5.438e-01
   0.10    0.6    3.914e-02    5.271e-01
   0.10    0.8    2.229e-02    5.152e-01
   0.10    1.0    1.629e-02    5.110e-01


ncall =    253
```

```
Table 1.8, splines, splinefun
```

[1] 6

[1] 103

t	x	S(x,t)	I(x,t)
0.10	-1.0	1.629e-02	5.110e-01
0.10	-0.8	2.229e-02	5.152e-01
0.10	-0.6	3.914e-02	5.271e-01
0.10	-0.4	6.224e-02	5.438e-01
0.10	-0.2	8.277e-02	5.589e-01
0.10	0.0	9.105e-02	5.651e-01
0.10	0.2	8.277e-02	5.589e-01
0.10	0.4	6.224e-02	5.438e-01
0.10	0.6	3.914e-02	5.271e-01
0.10	0.8	2.229e-02	5.152e-01
0.10	1.0	1.629e-02	5.110e-01

```
ncall =    441
```

The graphical output is not included here since it essentially the same in Figs. 1.4a,b.

As a next case, direct differentiation to compute the second derivatives in eqs. (1.1d,e) is used in place of the stagewise differentiation used previously, e.g., in Listing 1.2.

(1.6) Direct Differentiation

ODE/MOL routine pde1a is modified in pde1b for direct differentiation.

```
  pde1b=function(t,u,parms){
#
# Function pde1b computes the t derivative
# vectors of S(x,t),I(x,t)
#
```

```
# One vector to two vectors
  S=rep(0,nx);I=rep(0,nx);
  for(i in 1:nx){
    S[i]=u[i];
    I[i]=u[i+nx];
  }
#
# S*I
  SI=rep(0,nx);
  for(i in 1:nx){SI[i]=S[i]*I[i];}
#
# BCs
  Sx=rep(0,nx);Ix=rep(0,nx);
  nl=2;nu=2
  Sx[1]=0;Sx[nx]=0;
  Ix[1]=0;Ix[nx]=0;
#
# Sxx,Ixx
  Sxx=dss044(xl,xu,nx,S,Sx,nl,nu);
  Ixx=dss044(xl,xu,nx,I,Ix,nl,nu);
#
# PDEs
  St=rep(0,nx);It=rep(0,nx);
  for(i in 1:nx){
    St[i]=D_s*Sxx[i]+r_p1*S[i]-r_si*SI[i];
    It[i]=D_i*Ixx[i]+r_p2*I[i]+r_si*SI[i];
  }
#
# Two vectors to one vector
  ut=rep(0,2*nx);
  for(i in 1:nx){
    ut[i]   =St[i];
    ut[i+nx]=It[i];
  }
```

```
#
# Increment calls to pde1b
  ncall <<- ncall+1;
#
# Return derivative vector
  return(list(c(ut)));
  }
```

Listing 1.4: ODE/MOL routine for eqs. (1.1d,e), (1.2), direct differentiation

We can note the following details about pde1b.

- The function is defined, and the ODE dependent vector u is placed in two vectors, S,I, to facilitate the programming of eqs. (1.1d,e).

```
pde1b=function(t,u,parms){
#
# Function pde1b computes the t derivative
# vectors of S(x,t),I(x,t)
#
# One vector to two vectors
  S=rep(0,nx);I=rep(0,nx);
  for(i in 1:nx){
    S[i]=u[i];
    I[i]=u[i+nx];
  }
```

- The product funtion SI in eqs. (1.1d,e) is placed in vector SI as a function of x.

```
#
# S*I
  SI=rep(0,nx);
  for(i in 1:nx){SI[i]=S[i]*I[i];}
```

- BCs (1.2c,d,e,f) are programmed (subscripts 1,nx correspond to $x_l = -1, x_u = 1$). nl=nu=2 specify Neumann BCs in the following calls to dss044.

```
#
# BCs
  Sx=rep(0,nx);Ix=rep(0,nx);
  nl=2;nu=2
  Sx[1]=0;Sx[nx]=0;
  Ix[1]=0;Ix[nx]=0;
```

- $\dfrac{\partial^2 S}{\partial x^2}, \dfrac{\partial^2 I}{\partial x^2}$ are computed by dss044 directly from $S(x,t), I(x,t)$. The first derivative vectors Sx,Ix are inputs for the BCs (only the boundary values of Sx,Ix are used by dss044).

```
#
# Sxx,Ixx
  Sxx=dss044(xl,xu,nx,S,Sx,nl,nu);
  Ixx=dss044(xl,xu,nx,I,Ix,nl,nu);
```

Additional details about dss044 are given in Appendix A2.

- $\dfrac{\partial S}{\partial t}, \dfrac{\partial I}{\partial t}$ are computed from eqs. (1.1d,e) (as in Listing 1.2).

```
#
# PDEs
  St=rep(0,nx);It=rep(0,nx);
  for(i in 1:nx){
    St[i]=D_s*Sxx[i]+r_p1*S[i]-r_si*SI[i];
    It[i]=D_i*Ixx[i]+r_p2*I[i]+r_si*SI[i];
  }
```

- The two derivative vectors in t are placed in a single vector ut for use by lsodes in taking the next step in t along the solution.

```
#
# Two vectors to one vector
  ut=rep(0,2*nx);
  for(i in 1:nx){
    ut[i]   =St[i];
    ut[i+nx]=It[i];
  }
```

- The number of calls to pde1b is incremented and returned to the main program via <<-.

```
#
# Increment calls to pde1b
  ncall <<- ncall+1;
```

- The derivative vector is returned to lsodes as a list. c is the R vector utility.

```
#
# Return derivative vector
  return(list(c(ut)));
  }
```

The final } concludes pde1b.

The changes in the main program of Listing 1.1 for the use of pde1b follow.

- pde1b (Listing 1.4) is used in place of pde1a (Listing 1.2), and dss044 (direct differentiation) is used in place of dss004 (stagewise differentiation).

```
#
# Access functions for numerical solution
  setwd("f:/infectious/chap1");
  source("pde1b.R");
  source("dss044.R");
```

- For ncase=2, $I(x, t = 0) = 0.5$ is the IC for $I(x, t)$. Also, $r_{si} = 10$ is used to increase the interaction between eqs. (1.1d) and (1.1e).

```
#
# Select case
  ncase=2;
#
# Parameters
  if(ncase==1){
    f1=function(x)    1;
    f2=function(x)    0;
#   f2=function(x) 0.5;
    D_s=1;D_i=1;
    r_p1=0;r_p2=0;
    r_si=1;
  }
  if(ncase==2){
    f1=function(x) exp(-100*x^2);
#   f2=function(x) 0;
    f2=function(x) 0.5;
    D_s=1;D_i=1;
    r_p1=0;r_p2=0;
    r_si=10;
  }
```

- $nx = 51$ is used for ncase=2.

```
#
# Spatial grid (in x)
```

```
   if(ncase==1){nx=21;}
   if(ncase==2){nx=51;}
   xl=-1;xu=1;
   x=seq(from=xl,to=xu,by=(xu-xl)/(nx-1));
```

- lsodes calls pde1b (Listing 1.4) to integrate the 51
  MOL/ODEs.

```
   #
   # ODE integration
   out=lsodes(y=u0,times=tout,func=pde1b,
      sparsetype ="sparseint",rtol=1e-6,
      atol=1e-6,maxord=5);
   nrow(out)
   ncol(out)
```

Abbreviated numerical output is in Table 1.9

```
[1]  6
```

```
[1]  103
```

t	x	S(x,t)	I(x,t)
0.00	-1.0	3.720e-44	5.000e-01
0.00	-0.8	1.604e-28	5.000e-01
0.00	-0.6	2.320e-16	5.000e-01
0.00	-0.4	1.125e-07	5.000e-01
0.00	-0.2	1.832e-02	5.000e-01
0.00	0.0	1.000e+00	5.000e-01
0.00	0.2	1.832e-02	5.000e-01
0.00	0.4	1.125e-07	5.000e-01
0.00	0.6	2.320e-16	5.000e-01
0.00	0.8	1.604e-28	5.000e-01
0.00	1.0	3.720e-44	5.000e-01

.
.
.

```
Output for t = 0.02,..., 0.08 removed

        .           .
        .           .
        .           .

    t     x      S(x,t)        I(x,t)
  0.10  -1.0   1.628e-02     5.110e-01
  0.10  -0.8   2.229e-02     5.152e-01
  0.10  -0.6   3.914e-02     5.271e-01
  0.10  -0.4   6.224e-02     5.438e-01
  0.10  -0.2   8.277e-02     5.589e-01
  0.10   0.0   9.105e-02     5.651e-01
  0.10   0.2   8.277e-02     5.589e-01
  0.10   0.4   6.224e-02     5.438e-01
  0.10   0.6   3.914e-02     5.271e-01
  0.10   0.8   2.229e-02     5.152e-01
  0.10   1.0   1.628e-02     5.110e-01

ncall =    236
```

Table 1.9: Abbreviated output for eqs. (1.1d,e),
$I(x, t = 0) = 0.5$, dss044

The output in Table 1.6 (stagewise differentiaion) and Table 1.9 (direct differentiation) is essentially the same.

```
Table 1.6, stagewise differentiation, dss004

[1] 6

[1] 103

    t     x      S(x,t)        I(x,t)
  0.10  -1.0   1.629e-02     5.110e-01
  0.10  -0.8   2.229e-02     5.152e-01
  0.10  -0.6   3.914e-02     5.271e-01
```

```
0.10   -0.4   6.224e-02   5.438e-01
0.10   -0.2   8.277e-02   5.589e-01
0.10    0.0   9.106e-02   5.651e-01
0.10    0.2   8.277e-02   5.589e-01
0.10    0.4   6.224e-02   5.438e-01
0.10    0.6   3.914e-02   5.271e-01
0.10    0.8   2.229e-02   5.152e-01
0.10    1.0   1.629e-02   5.110e-01

ncall =   253
```

Table 1.9, direct differentiation, dss044

[1] 6

[1] 103

```
   t      x       S(x,t)       I(x,t)
 0.10   -1.0   1.628e-02   5.110e-01
 0.10   -0.8   2.229e-02   5.152e-01
 0.10   -0.6   3.914e-02   5.271e-01
 0.10   -0.4   6.224e-02   5.438e-01
 0.10   -0.2   8.277e-02   5.589e-01
 0.10    0.0   9.105e-02   5.651e-01
 0.10    0.2   8.277e-02   5.589e-01
 0.10    0.4   6.224e-02   5.438e-01
 0.10    0.6   3.914e-02   5.271e-01
 0.10    0.8   2.229e-02   5.152e-01
 0.10    1.0   1.628e-02   5.110e-01

ncall =   236
```

The graphical output is not included here since it is the same as in Figs. 1.4a,b.

   Direct differentiation can also be used with splines. The
ODE/MOL routine is listed next.

```
  pde1b_sp=function(t,u,parms){
#
# Function pde1b_sp computes the t derivative
# vectors of S(x,t),I(x,t)
#
# One vector to two vectors
  S=rep(0,nx);I=rep(0,nx);
  for(i in 1:nx){
    S[i]=u[i];
    I[i]=u[i+nx];
  }
#
# S*I
  SI=rep(0,nx);
  for(i in 1:nx){SI[i]=S[i]*I[i];}
#
# BCs
  S[1]=S[2];S[nx]=S[nx-1];
  I[1]=I[2];I[nx]=I[nx-1];
#
# Sxx,Ixx
  tableSxx=splinefun(x,S);
  Sxx=tableSxx(x,deriv=2);
  tableIxx=splinefun(x,I);
  Ixx=tableIxx(x,deriv=2);
#
# PDEs
  St=rep(0,nx);It=rep(0,nx);
  for(i in 1:nx){
    St[i]=D_s*Sxx[i]+r_p1*S[i]-r_si*SI[i];
    It[i]=D_i*Ixx[i]+r_p2*I[i]+r_si*SI[i];
  }
```

```
#
# Two vectors to one vector
  ut=rep(0,2*nx);
  for(i in 1:nx){
    ut[i]    =St[i];
    ut[i+nx]=It[i];
  }
#
# Increment calls to pde1b_sp
  ncall <<- ncall+1;
#
# Return derivative vector
  return(list(c(ut)));
  }
```

Listing 1.5: ODE/MOL routine for eqs. (1.1d,e), (1.2), splines, direct differentiation

We can note the following points about Listing 1.5.

- The function is defined and the ODE dependent vactor u is placed in two vectors to facilitate the programming of eqs. (1.1d,e).

```
pde1b_sp=function(t,u,parms){
#
# Function pde1b_sp computes the t derivative
# vectors of S(x,t),I(x,t)
#
# One vector to two vectors
  S=rep(0,nx);I=rep(0,nx);
  for(i in 1:nx){
    S[i]=u[i];
    I[i]=u[i+nx];
  }
```

- The nonlinear product funtion SI in eqs. (1.1d,e) is placed in vector SI.

```
#
# S*I
  SI=rep(0,nx);
  for(i in 1:nx){SI[i]=S[i]*I[i];}
```

- BCs (1.2c,d,e,f) are approximated.

```
#
# BCs
  S[1]=S[2];S[nx]=S[nx-1];
  I[1]=I[2];I[nx]=I[nx-1];
```

These approximations require some additional explanation.

– The derivative $\dfrac{\partial S}{\partial x}$ is approximated with a first order FD at $x =_l= -1$

$$\frac{\partial S(x = x_l = -1, t)}{\partial x} \approx \frac{S(2) - S(1)}{\Delta x} = 0$$

or

$$S(1) = S(2)$$

which is programmed as

```
S[1]=S[2]
```

– Similarly

$$\frac{\partial S(x = x_u = 1, t)}{\partial x} \approx \frac{S(nx) - S(nx - 1)}{\Delta x} = 0$$

or

$$S(nx) = S(nx - 1)$$

which is programmed as

```
S[nx]=S[nx-1]
```

– Similar programming is used for $I(x, t)$.

```
I[1] =I[2]
I[nx]=I[nx-1]
```

– Since these first order FDs have limited accuracy, they could be replaced by more accurate (high order) FDs. For example

$$\frac{\partial S(x = x_l = -1, t)}{\partial x} \approx$$
$$\frac{1}{12\Delta x}[-25S(1) + 48S(2) - 36S(3)$$
$$+16S(4) - 3S(5)] = 0 \qquad (1.5a)$$

which could be programmed as

```
ux[1]=(1/25)*(48*u[2]-36*u[3]+16*u[4]-3*u[5])
```

This FD is fourth order correct, but uses only the interior values $S(1), S(2), S(3), S(4), S(5)$. Eq. (1.5a) is taken from dss004. Similarly, for $x = x_u = 1$,

$$\frac{\partial S(x = x_u = 1, t)}{\partial x} \approx$$
$$\frac{1}{12\Delta x}[25S(nx) - 48S(nx - 1) + 36S(nx - 2)$$
$$-16S(nx - 3) + 3S(nx - 4)] = 0$$
$$\qquad (1.5b)$$

which can be used to calculate S[nx].

– In effect, this approach is a hybrid FD-spline method.

• The derivatives $\frac{\partial^2 S}{\partial x^2}, \frac{\partial^2 I}{\partial x^2}$ are computed directly from $S(x, t), I(x, t)$. The boundary values computed previously are used in this calculation.

```
#
# Sxx,Ixx
  tableSxx=splinefun(x,S);
  Sxx=tableSxx(x,deriv=2);
  tableIxx=splinefun(x,I);
  Ixx=tableIxx(x,deriv=2);
```

`deriv=2` indicates that a second order derivative is calculated.

- Eqs. (1.1d,e) are programmed in a MOL format.

```
#
# PDEs
  St=rep(0,nx);It=rep(0,nx);
  for(i in 1:nx){
    St[i]=D_s*Sxx[i]+r_p1*S[i]-r_si*SI[i];
    It[i]=D_i*Ixx[i]+r_p2*I[i]+r_si*SI[i];
  }
```

- The MOL/ODE vectors are placed in a single vector `ut`

```
#
# Two vectors to one vector
  ut=rep(0,2*nx);
  for(i in 1:nx){
    ut[i]   =St[i];
    ut[i+nx]=It[i];
  }
```

- The counter for the calls to `pde1b_sp` is incremented and returned to the main program with `<<-`.

```
#
# Increment calls to pde1b_sp
  ncall <<- ncall+1;
```

- The derivative vector `ut` is returned to `lsodes` as a list.

```
#
# Return derivative vector
  return(list(c(ut)));
  }
```

The final } concludes pde1b_sp.

The statements in the main program to accommodate pde1b_sp follow.

- Function pde1b_sp is accessed.

```
#
# Access functions for numerical solution
  setwd("f:/infectious/chap1");
  source("pde1b_sp.R");
```

- For `ncase=2`, the IC functions of eqs. (1.2a,b) are programmed and $r_{si} = 10$ to increase the interaction between eqs. (1.1d,e).

```
#
# Select case
  ncase=2;
#
# Parameters
  if(ncase==1){
    f1=function(x)    1;
    f2=function(x)    0;
#   f2=function(x)  0.5;
    D_s=1;D_i=1;
    r_p1=0;r_p2=0;
    r_si=1;
  }
```

```
    if(ncase==2){
      f1=function(x) exp(-100*x^2);
#     f2=function(x) 0;
      f2=function(x) 0.5;
      D_s=1;D_i=1;
      r_p1=0;r_p2=0;
      r_si=10;
    }
```

- pde1b_sp is called by lsodes.

```
    #
    # ODE integration
    out=lsodes(y=u0,times=tout,func=pde1b_sp,
        sparsetype ="sparseint",rtol=1e-6,
        atol=1e-6,maxord=5);
    nrow(out)
```

Otherwise, the main program is the same as in Listing 1.1.
    Abbreviated numerical output follows.

[1] 6

[1] 103

t	x	S(x,t)	I(x,t)
0.00	-1.0	3.720e-44	5.000e-01
0.00	-0.8	1.604e-28	5.000e-01
0.00	-0.6	2.320e-16	5.000e-01
0.00	-0.4	1.125e-07	5.000e-01
0.00	-0.2	1.832e-02	5.000e-01
0.00	0.0	1.000e+00	5.000e-01
0.00	0.2	1.832e-02	5.000e-01
0.00	0.4	1.125e-07	5.000e-01
0.00	0.6	2.320e-16	5.000e-01
0.00	0.8	1.604e-28	5.000e-01

```
0.00   1.0   3.720e-44   5.000e-01
         .                  .

         .                  .

         .                  .

Output for t = 0.02,..., 0.08 removed

         .                  .

         .                  .

         .                  .

   t     x      S(x,t)       I(x,t)
 0.10  -1.0   1.741e-02   5.117e-01
 0.10  -0.8   2.305e-02   5.157e-01
 0.10  -0.6   3.943e-02   5.273e-01
 0.10  -0.4   6.232e-02   5.438e-01
 0.10  -0.2   8.274e-02   5.589e-01
 0.10   0.0   9.097e-02   5.651e-01
 0.10   0.2   8.274e-02   5.589e-01
 0.10   0.4   6.232e-02   5.438e-01
 0.10   0.6   3.943e-02   5.273e-01
 0.10   0.8   2.305e-02   5.157e-01
 0.10   1.0   1.741e-02   5.117e-01

ncall =   440
```

Table 1.10: Abbreviated output for eqs. (1.1d,e), splines, direct differentiation

The output in Table 1.10 (direct differentiation) is similar to the output in Table 1.8 (stagewise differentation).

```
Table 1.8, splines, stagewise differentiation

[1] 6

[1] 103
```

t	x	S(x,t)	I(x,t)
0.10	-1.0	1.629e-02	5.110e-01
0.10	-0.8	2.229e-02	5.152e-01
0.10	-0.6	3.914e-02	5.271e-01
0.10	-0.4	6.224e-02	5.438e-01
0.10	-0.2	8.277e-02	5.589e-01
0.10	0.0	9.105e-02	5.651e-01
0.10	0.2	8.277e-02	5.589e-01
0.10	0.4	6.224e-02	5.438e-01
0.10	0.6	3.914e-02	5.271e-01
0.10	0.8	2.229e-02	5.152e-01
0.10	1.0	1.629e-02	5.110e-01

```
ncall =   441
```

Table 1.10, splines, direct differentiation

```
[1] 6
```

```
[1] 103
```

t	x	S(x,t)	I(x,t)
0.10	-1.0	1.741e-02	5.117e-01
0.10	-0.8	2.305e-02	5.157e-01
0.10	-0.6	3.943e-02	5.273e-01
0.10	-0.4	6.232e-02	5.438e-01
0.10	-0.2	8.274e-02	5.589e-01
0.10	0.0	9.097e-02	5.651e-01
0.10	0.2	8.274e-02	5.589e-01
0.10	0.4	6.232e-02	5.438e-01
0.10	0.6	3.943e-02	5.273e-01
0.10	0.8	2.305e-02	5.157e-01
0.10	1.0	1.741e-02	5.117e-01

```
ncall =   440
```

The solution in Table 1.8 is probably more accurate because of the limited accuracy of the BC approximations in `pde1b_sp`. The use of a more accurate approximation of the BCs in `pde1b_sp` is left as an exercise for the reader (e.g., using the fourth order FDs discussed previously).

The graphical output is in Figs. 1.6a,b, which is similar to Figs. 1.4a,b.

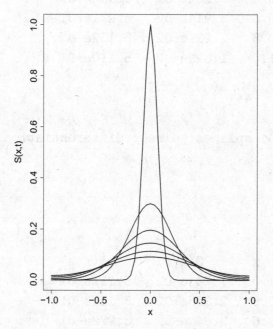

Figure 1.6a: Numerical solution $S(x,t)$ of eq. (1.1d), Gaussian IC

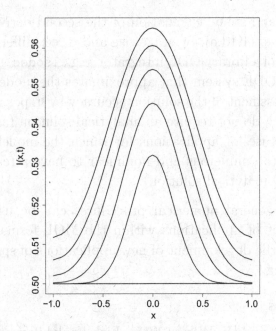

Figure 1.6b: Numerical solution $I(x,t)$ of eq. (1.1e), $I(x,t = 0) = 0.5$

(1.7) Summary and Conclusions

This chapter is intended as an introduction to spatiotemporal modeling that can then be extended in subsequent chapters to the modeling of infectious disease epidemiology. The features of spatiotemporal models discussed in this chapter include:

- A 2×2 PDE model, eqs. (1.d,e), that includes nonlinear coupling of the PDEs (through $\pm r_{si}SI$).
- Implmentation of ICs (1.2a,b) and Neumann BCs (1.2c,d,e,f).

- FD and spline calculation of the second derivatives in x in eqs. (1.1d,e), by stagewise and direct differentiation.
- Use of a library ODE integrator, e.g., `lsodes`, to integrate the ODE system that approximates the model PDEs.
- Assessment of the solution accuracy by h, p, r refinement, which do not require an analytical solution (as is usually the case for applications for which the model equations are too numerous and nonlinear to have a readily available analytical solution).

These general numerical procedures can be used for the development of applications within the MOL format. We now proceed to the development of new applications of spatiotemporal modeling.

References

[1] Cai, Y., and W. Wang (2015), Fish-hook bifurcation branch in a spatial heterogeneous epidemic model with cross-diffusion, *Nonlinear Analysis: Real World Applications*, **30**, 99-125

[2] Soetaert, K., J. Cash, and F. Mazzia (2012), *Solving Differential Equations in R*, Springer-Verlag, Heidelberg, Germany.

Chapter 2

SIR Models

(2.1) Introduction

In Chapter 2, basic 3×3 (3 PDEs in 3 unknowns) models are considered that can be used as a starting point for the development of spatiotemporal models of infectious disease. This development is formulated in this chapter within a 1D Cartiesian coordinate system. In Chapter 3, this development is extended to other spatial coordinate systems.

(2.2) Basic Model

A basic 3×3 SIR (Susceptibles Infecteds Recovereds) model follows [2], p271.

$$\frac{\partial S}{\partial t} = D_s \frac{\partial^2 S}{\partial x^2} + r_{p1}S - r_{si}SI \qquad (2.1a)$$

$$\frac{\partial I}{\partial t} = D_i \frac{\partial^2 I}{\partial x^2} + r_{p2}I + r_{si}SI - r_iI \qquad (2.1b)$$

$$\frac{\partial R}{\partial t} = D_r \frac{\partial^2 R}{\partial x^2} + r_{p3}I + r_iI \qquad (2.1c)$$

Eq. (2.1a) is eq. (1.1d) restated to facilitate this discussion of the SIR model. Eq. (2.1b) is eq. (1.1e) with the term $-r_iI$ added to reflect the transition from infecteds to recovereds[1]. Eq. (2.1c) is the added PDE for the recovereds, with terms that follow from eqs. (2.1a,b). $r_i I$ appears in eqs. (2.1b,c) with opposite signs to reflect that the rate of disappearance of infecteds is the rate of appearance of recovereds.

Eqs. (2.1) are first order in t and each requires an initial condition (IC).

$$S(x, t = 0) = f_1(x); \quad I(x, t = 0) = f_2(x); \quad R(x, t = 0) = f_3(x)$$
$$(2.2a,b,c)$$

Eqs. (2.1) are second order in x and each requires two boundary conditions (BCs).

$$\frac{\partial S(x = x_l, t)}{\partial x} = \frac{\partial S(x = x_u, t)}{\partial x} = 0 \qquad (2.3a,b)$$

$$\frac{\partial I(x = x_l, t)}{\partial x} = \frac{\partial I(x = x_u, t)}{\partial x} = 0 \qquad (2.3c,d)$$

$$\frac{\partial R(x = x_l, t)}{\partial x} = \frac{\partial R(x = x_u, t)}{\partial x} = 0 \qquad (2.3e,f)$$

$f_1(x), f_2(x), f_3(x)$ are functions to be specified. x_l, x_u are boundary values in x to be specified. Eqs. (2.3) are homogeneous (zero) *Neumann* BCs.

Eqs. (2.1), (2.2), (2.3) constitute the first SIR model to be considered. Routines for these equations follow.

(2.2.1) Main program

```
#
# Three PDE model
#
# Delete previous workspaces
```

---

[1]A nonlinear term of the form $r_{ri} RI$ could be included using the methods developed in Chapter 1 for the term $r_{si} SI$.

```
  rm(list=ls(all=TRUE))
#
# Access ODE integrator
  library("deSolve");
#
# Access functions for numerical solution
  setwd("f:/infectious/chap2");
  source("pde1a.R");
  source("dss004.R");
#
# Parameters
  f1=function(x) 1;
  f2=function(x) exp(-100*x^2);
  f3=function(x) 0;
  D_s=0.25;D_i=0.25;D_r=0.25;
  r_p1=0.02;r_p2=0.02;r_p3=0.02;
  r_si=10;r_i=10;
#
# Spatial grid (in x)
  nx=51;
  xl=-1;xu=1;
  x=seq(from=xl,to=xu,by=(xu-xl)/(nx-1));
#
# Independent variable for ODE integration
  t0=0;tf=0.1;nout=6;
  tout=seq(from=t0,to=tf,by=(tf-t0)/(nout-1));
#
# Initial condition (t=0)
  u0=rep(0,3*nx);
  for(i in 1:nx){
    u0[i]     =f1(x[i]);
    u0[i+nx]  =f2(x[i]);
    u0[i+2*nx]=f3(x[i]);
  }
```

```
  ncall=0;
#
# ODE integration
  out=lsodes(y=u0,times=tout,func=pde1a,
      sparsetype="sparseint",rtol=1e-6,
      atol=1e-6,maxord=5);
  nrow(out)
  ncol(out)
#
# Arrays for plotting numerical solution
  S=matrix(0,nrow=nx,ncol=nout);
  I=matrix(0,nrow=nx,ncol=nout);
  R=matrix(0,nrow=nx,ncol=nout);
  for(it in 1:nout){
    for(i in 1:nx){
      S[i,it]=out[it,i+1];
      I[i,it]=out[it,i+1+nx];
      R[i,it]=out[it,i+1+2*nx];
    }
  }
#
# Display numerical solution
  for(it in 1:nout){
    cat(sprintf("\n      t      x       S(x,t)
                I(x,t)       R(x,t)\n"));
    iv=seq(from=1,to=nx,by=5);
    for(i in iv){
      cat(sprintf("%6.2f%6.1f%12.3e%12.3e%12.3e\n",
          tout[it],x[i],S[i,it],I[i,it],R[i,it]));
    }
  }
#
# Calls to ODE routine
  cat(sprintf("\n\n ncall = %5d\n\n",ncall));
```

```
#
# Plot PDE solutions
#
# S
  par(mfrow=c(1,1));
  matplot(x=x,y=S,type="l",xlab="x",ylab="S(x,t)",
    xlim=c(xl,xu),lty=1,main="",lwd=2,col="black");
# I
  par(mfrow=c(1,1));
  matplot(x=x,y=I,type="l",xlab="x",ylab="I(x,t)",
    xlim=c(xl,xu),lty=1,main="",lwd=2,col="black");
# R
  par(mfrow=c(1,1));
  matplot(x=x,y=R,type="l",xlab="x",ylab="R(x,t)",
    xlim=c(xl,xu),lty=1,main="",lwd=2,col="black");
```

Listing 2.1: Main program for eqs. (2.1), (2.2), (2.3)

We can note the following details about Listing 2.1.

- Previous workspaces are deleted.

  ```
  #
  # Three PDE model
  #
  # Delete previous workspaces
    rm(list=ls(all=TRUE))
  ```

- The R ODE integrator library deSolve is accessed. Then
  the directory with the files for the solution of eqs. (2.1),
  (2.2), (2.3) is designated. Note that setwd (set working
  directory) uses / rather than the usual \.

  ```
  #
  # Access functions for numerical solution
    setwd("f:/infectious/chap2");
    source("pde1a.R");
  ```

```
source("dss004.R");
```

pde1a.R is the routine for the method of lines (MOL) approximation of PDEs (2.1) (discussed subsequently). dss004 (Differentiation in Space Subroutine) is a library routine for calculating a first derivative in x.

- The model parameters are defined numerically.

```
#
# Parameters
  f1=function(x) 1;
  f2=function(x) exp(-100*x^2);
  f3=function(x) 0;
  D_s=0.25;D_i=0.25;D_r=0.25;
  r_p1=1;r_p2=1;r_p3=1;
  r_si=10;r_i=10;
```

These parameters require some additonal explanation.

– The IC functions of eqs. (2.2) are defined.

```
    f1=function(x) 1;
    f2=function(x) exp(-100*x^2);
    f3=function(x) 0;
```

f_1 defines a uniform initial susceptible population that is then subjected to an infectious disease. f_2 defines a Gaussian centered at $x = 0$ that represents the infected population (an epidemic centered at $x = 0$). f_3 is zero to reflect no recovereds initally.

– The three diffusivities of eqs. (2.1) are defined. These values are the same suggesting there is no basic difference in the rate of diffusion (dispersion) of the three populations.

```
    D_s=0.25;D_i=0.25;D_r=0.25;
```

The units are 1/yr so that the time scale of the solutions is in yrs (x is normalized to the interval $-1 \le x \le 1$ as explained next).
- The natural increase in the three populations (births greater than deaths) is set at 0.02/yr (2%/yr).

```
r_p1=0.02;r_p2=0.02;r_p3=0.02;
```

- r_{si}, r_i in eqs. (2.1) are defined with the time units of yrs.

```
r_si=10;r_i=10;
```

- A normalized (nondimensional) spatial grid of 51 points is defined for $x_l = -1 \le x \le x_u = 1$, so that x=-1,-(1-1/50)=-0.98,...,1.

```
#
# Spatial grid (in x)
  nx=51;
  xl=-1;xu=1;
  x=seq(from=xl,to=xu,by=(xu-xl)/(nx-1));
```

- An interval in t of 6 points is defined for $0 \le t \le 0.1$ yr so that tout=0,0.02,...,0.1.

```
#
# Independent variable for ODE integration
  t0=0;tf=0.1;nout=6;
  tout=seq(from=t0,to=tf,by=(tf-t0)/(nout-1));
```

- ICs (2.2) are defined.

```
#
# Initial condition (t=0)
  u0=rep(0,3*nx);
  for(i in 1:nx){
    u0[i]      =f1(x[i]);
    u0[i+nx]   =f2(x[i]);
```

```
    u0[i+2*nx]=f3(x[i]);
  }
  ncall=0;
```

u0 therefore has $(3)(51) = 153$ elements. The counter for the calls to the ODE/MOL routine pde1a is also initialized.

- The system of 153 MOL/ODEs is integrated by the library integrator lsodes (available in deSolve). As expected, the inputs to lsodes are the ODE function, pde1a, the IC vector u0, and the vector of output values of t, tout. The length of u0 (153) informs lsodes how many ODEs are to be integrated. func,y,times are reserved names.

```
#
# ODE integration
  out=lsodes(y=u0,times=tout,func=pde1a,
      sparsetype="sparseint",rtol=1e-6,
      atol=1e-6,maxord=5);
  nrow(out)
  ncol(out)
```

The numerical solution to the ODEs is returned in matrix out. In this case, out has the dimensions $nout \times (3nx + 1) = 6 \times 3(51) + 1 = 153 + 1 = 154$, which are confirmed by the output from nrow(out),ncol(out) (included in the numerical output considered subsequently).

The offset $153 + 1$ is required since the first element of each column has the output t (also in tout), and the $2, ..., 3nx + 1 = 2, ..., 154$ column elements have the 153 ODE solutions.

- The solutions of the 153 ODEs returned in out by lsodes are placed in arrays S,I,R.

```
#
# Arrays for plotting numerical solution
```

```
S=matrix(0,nrow=nx,ncol=nout);
I=matrix(0,nrow=nx,ncol=nout);
R=matrix(0,nrow=nx,ncol=nout);
for(it in 1:nout){
  for(i in 1:nx){
    S[i,it]=out[it,i+1];
    I[i,it]=out[it,i+1+nx];
    R[i,it]=out[it,i+1+2*nx];
  }
}
```

Again, the offset i+1 is required since the first element of each column of out has the value of t.

- $S(x,t), I(x,t), R(x,t)$ are displayed as a function of x and t, with every fifth value of x from by=5.

```
#
# Display numerical solution
  for(it in 1:nout){
    cat(sprintf("\n      t      x       S(x,t)
                  I(x,t)        R(x,t)\n"));
    iv=seq(from=1,to=nx,by=5);
    for(i in iv){
      cat(sprintf(
        "%6.2f%6.1f%12.3e%12.3e%12.3e\n",
        tout[it],x[i],S[i,it],I[i,it],R[i,it]));
    }
  }
```

- The number of calls to pde1a is displayed at the end of the solution.

```
#
# Calls to ODE routine
  cat(sprintf("\n\n ncall = %5d\n\n",ncall));
```

- $S(x,t)$, $I(x,t)$, $R(x,t)$ are plotted as a function of x with t as a parameter.

```
#
# Plot PDE solutions
#
# S
  par(mfrow=c(1,1));
  matplot(
    x=x,y=S,type="l",xlab="x",ylab="S(x,t)",
    xlim=c(xl,xu),lty=1,main="",lwd=2,
    col="black");
# I
  par(mfrow=c(1,1));
  matplot(
    x=x,y=I,type="l",xlab="x",ylab="I(x,t)",
    xlim=c(xl,xu),lty=1,main="",lwd=2,
    col="black");
# R
  par(mfrow=c(1,1));
  matplot(
    x=x,y=R,type="l",xlab="x",ylab="R(x,t)",
    xlim=c(xl,xu),lty=1,main="",lwd=2,
    col="black");
```

This completes the main program. The ODE/MOL routine pde1a called by lsodes is considered next.

(2.2.2) ODE/MOL routine

The ODE/MOL routine called by lsodes follows.

```
  pde1a=function(t,u,parms){
#
# Function pde1a computes the t derivative
# vectors of S(x,t),I(x,t),R(x,t)
```

```
#
# One vector to three vectors
  S=rep(0,nx);I=rep(0,nx);R=rep(0,nx);
  for(i in 1:nx){
    S[i]=u[i];
    I[i]=u[i+nx];
    R[i]=u[i+2*nx];
  }
#
# S*I
  SI=rep(0,nx);
  for(i in 1:nx){SI[i]=S[i]*I[i];}
#
# Sx,Ix,Rx
  Sx=dss004(xl,xu,nx,S);
  Ix=dss004(xl,xu,nx,I);
  Rx=dss004(xl,xu,nx,R);
#
# BCs
  Sx[1]=0;Sx[nx]=0;
  Ix[1]=0;Ix[nx]=0;
  Rx[1]=0;Rx[nx]=0;
#
# Sxx,Ixx,Rxx
  Sxx=dss004(xl,xu,nx,Sx);
  Ixx=dss004(xl,xu,nx,Ix);
  Rxx=dss004(xl,xu,nx,Rx);
#
# PDEs
  St=rep(0,nx);It=rep(0,nx);Rt=rep(0,nx);
  for(i in 1:nx){
    St[i]=D_s*Sxx[i]+r_p1*S[i]-r_si*SI[i];
    It[i]=D_i*Ixx[i]+r_p2*I[i]+r_si*SI[i]-
          r_i*I[i];
```

```
    Rt[i]=D_r*Rxx[i]+r_p3*R[i]+r_i*I[i];
  }
#
# Three vectors to one vector
  ut=rep(0,3*nx);
  for(i in 1:nx){
    ut[i]      =St[i];
    ut[i+nx]   =It[i];
    ut[i+2*nx]=Rt[i];
  }
#
# Increment calls to pde1a
  ncall <<- ncall+1;
#
# Return derivative vector
  return(list(c(ut)));
  }
```

Listing 2.2: ODE/MOL routine for eqs. (2.1), (2.2), (2.3)

We can note the following details about Listing 2.2.

- The function is defined.

  ```
    pde1a=function(t,u,parms){
  #
  # Function pde1a computes the t derivative
  # vectors of S(x,t),I(x,t),R(x,t)
  ```

  t is the current value of t in eqs. (2.1). u the 153-vector of ODE/MOL dependent variables. parm is an argument to pass parameters to pde1a (unused, but required in the argument list). The arguments must be listed in the order stated to properly interface with lsodes called in the main program of Listing 2.1. The derivative vector of

the LHS of eqs. (2.1) is calculated next and returned to
lsodes.

- u is placed in three vectors, S,I,R, to facilitate the programming of eqs. (2.1).

```
#
# One vector to three vectors
  S=rep(0,nx);I=rep(0,nx);R=rep(0,nx);
  for(i in 1:nx){
    S[i]=u[i];
    I[i]=u[i+nx];
    R[i]=u[i+2*nx];
  }
```

- The product of the two dependent variables of the terms
  $\pm r_{si}SI$ of eqs. (2.1a,b) is placed in SI.

```
#
# S*I
  SI=rep(0,nx);
  for(i in 1:nx){SI[i]=S[i]*I[i];}
```

- The derivatives $\dfrac{\partial S}{\partial x}, \dfrac{\partial I}{\partial x}, \dfrac{\partial R}{\partial x}$ are computed by dss004.

```
#
# Sx,Ix
  Sx=dss004(xl,xu,nx,S);
  Ix=dss004(xl,xu,nx,I);
  Rx=dss004(xl,xu,nx,R);
```

Sx,Ix,Rx do not have to be allocated (with rep) since
this is done by dss004. Additional details about dss004
are available in Appendix A1.

- BCs (2.3) are implemented (the subscripts 1,nx correspond to $x = x_l, x_u$).

```
#
# BCs
  Sx[1]=0;Sx[nx]=0;
  Ix[1]=0;Ix[nx]=0;
  Rx[1]=0;Rx[nx]=0;
```

- The derivatives $\dfrac{\partial^2 S}{\partial x^2}$, $\dfrac{\partial^2 I}{\partial x^2}$, $\dfrac{\partial^2 I}{\partial x^2}$ are computed by differentiating the first derivatives (stagewise or successive differentiation).

```
#
# Sxx,Ixx
  Sxx=dss004(xl,xu,nx,Sx);
  Ixx=dss004(xl,xu,nx,Ix);
  Rxx=dss004(xl,xu,nx,Rx);
```

- Eqs. (2.1) are programmed.

```
#
# PDEs
  St=rep(0,nx);It=rep(0,nx);Rt=rep(0,nx);
  for(i in 1:nx){
    St[i]=D_s*Sxx[i]+r_p1*S[i]-r_si*SI[i];
    It[i]=D_i*Ixx[i]+r_p2*I[i]+r_si*SI[i]-
          r_i*I[i];
    Rt[i]=D_r*Rxx[i]+r_p3*R[i]+r_i*I[i];
  }
```

The derivatives $\dfrac{\partial S}{\partial t}$, $\dfrac{\partial I}{\partial t}$, $\dfrac{\partial R}{\partial t}$, (LHSs of eqs. (2.1)) are placed in St,It,Rt. The programming of the nonlinear terms $\pm r_{si}SI$ in eqs. (2.1a,b) and the linear terms $\pm r_i I$ in eqs. (2.1b,c) is clear.

- The three vectors St,It,Rt are placed in a single derivative vector ut to return to lsodes.

```
#
# Three vectors to one vector
  ut=rep(0,3*nx);
  for(i in 1:nx){
    ut[i]      =St[i];
    ut[i+nx]   =It[i];
    ut[i+2*nx]=Rt[i];
  }
```

- The counter for the calls to pde1a is incremented and returned to the main program of Listing 2.1 with <<-.

```
#
# Increment calls to pde1a
  ncall <<- ncall+1;
```

- ut is returned to lsodes as a list (required by lsodes). c is the R vector utility.

```
#
# Return derivative vector
  return(list(c(ut)));
  }
```

The final } concludes pde1a.

The output from the main program and subordinate routine of Listings 2.1, 2.2 is considered next.

(2.2.3) Model output

Abbreviated numerical output is in Table 2.1.

[1] 6

[1] 154

t	x	S(x,t)	I(x,t)	R(x,t)
0.00	-1.0	1.000e+00	3.720e-44	0.000e+00
0.00	-0.8	1.000e+00	1.604e-28	0.000e+00
0.00	-0.6	1.000e+00	2.320e-16	0.000e+00
0.00	-0.4	1.000e+00	1.125e-07	0.000e+00
0.00	-0.2	1.000e+00	1.832e-02	0.000e+00
0.00	0.0	1.000e+00	1.000e+00	0.000e+00
0.00	0.2	1.000e+00	1.832e-02	0.000e+00
0.00	0.4	1.000e+00	1.125e-07	0.000e+00
0.00	0.6	1.000e+00	2.320e-16	0.000e+00
0.00	0.8	1.000e+00	1.604e-28	0.000e+00
0.00	1.0	1.000e+00	3.720e-44	0.000e+00

.
.
.

Output for t=0.02,..., 0.08 removed

.
.
.

t	x	S(x,t)	I(x,t)	R(x,t)
0.10	-1.0	1.002e+00	6.412e-05	6.423e-05
0.10	-0.8	1.001e+00	8.842e-04	8.882e-04
0.10	-0.6	9.911e-01	1.108e-02	1.125e-02
0.10	-0.4	9.386e-01	6.565e-02	6.825e-02
0.10	-0.2	8.252e-01	1.863e-01	2.004e-01
0.10	0.0	7.557e-01	2.618e-01	2.867e-01
0.10	0.2	8.252e-01	1.863e-01	2.004e-01
0.10	0.4	9.386e-01	6.565e-02	6.825e-02
0.10	0.6	9.911e-01	1.108e-02	1.125e-02
0.10	0.8	1.001e+00	8.842e-04	8.882e-04
0.10	1.0	1.002e+00	6.412e-05	6.423e-05

ncall =   255

Table 2.1: Abbreviated output for eqs. (2.1), (2.2), (2.3)

We can note the following details about this output.

- The dimensions of the solution matrix out are *nout* × $3nx + 1 = 6 \times 3(51) + 1 = 154$. The offset $+1$ results from the value of t as the first element in each of the *nout* $= 6$ solution vectors. These same values of t are in tout,
- ICs (2.2) ($t = 0$) are verified for $f_1(x)$, $f_2(x)$, $f_3(x)$.
- The output is for $x = -1, -0.8, ...1$ as programmed in Listing 2.1 (51 values at each value of t with every fifth value in x).
- The output is for $t = 0, 0.02, ..., 0.1$ as programmed in Listing 2.1.
- $S(x,t)$, $R(x,t)$ depart from their constant initial values as a consequence of the input from $I(x,t)$. The susceptibles decrease due to the increased infection and the recovereds increase in response to recovery from infection.
- The computational effort is modest, ncall = 255, indicating lsodes efficiently computes a solution to the 153 MOL/ODEs.

The graphical output in Figs. 2.1a,b,c confirm the solutions in Table 2.1. Generally, the solution indicates that the infecteds decrease with time as a consequence of eventual recovery.

The dimensionless distance interval $-1 \leq x \leq 1$ can be considered in dimensional terms, e.g., $-100 \leq x \leq 100$ in km (kilometers). The parameters with distance can then be converted to reflect dimensional distance, that is, D_s, D_i, D_r in eqs. (2.1).

As a variant of the preceding example, we note in Figs. 2.1a,b,c that S, I, R are symmetric with respect to $x = 0$. Therefore, an equivalent problem is to use a spatial interval $0 \leq x \leq 1$ with zero Neumann BCs at $x = 0$. This change requires only a minor change in the main program of Listing 2.1.

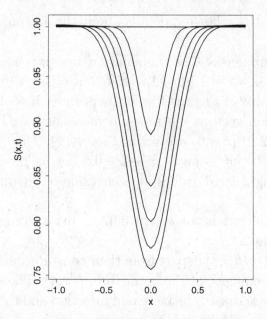

Figure 2.1a: Numerical solution $S(x,t)$ from eq. (2.1a)

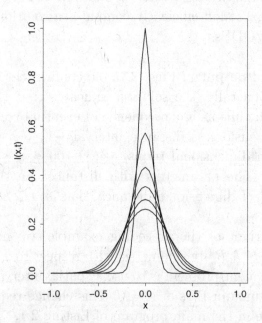

Figure 2.1b: Numerical solution $I(x,t)$ from eq. (2.1b)

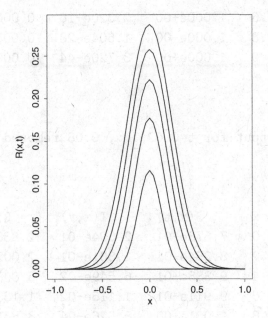

Figure 2.1c: Numerical solution $R(x,t)$ from eq. (2.1c)

```
#
# Spatial grid (in x)
  nx=26;
  xl=0;xu=1;
  x=seq(from=xl,to=xu,by=(xu-xl)/(nx-1));
```

The resulting solution is approximately equivalent to the solution in Table 2.1.

```
[1] 6

[1] 79
```

t	x	S(x,t)	I(x,t)	R(x,t)
0.00	0.0	1.000e+00	1.000e+00	0.000e+00
0.00	0.2	1.000e+00	1.832e-02	0.000e+00
0.00	0.4	1.000e+00	1.125e-07	0.000e+00

```
0.00    0.6    1.000e+00    2.320e-16    0.000e+00
0.00    0.8    1.000e+00    1.604e-28    0.000e+00
0.00    1.0    1.000e+00    3.720e-44    0.000e+00
          .                                    .
          .                                    .
          .                                    .

      Output for t=0.02,..., 0.08 removed
          .                                    .
          .                                    .
          .                                    .

    t      x        S(x,t)        I(x,t)        R(x,t)
  0.10    0.0    7.578e-01    2.594e-01    2.838e-01
  0.10    0.2    8.254e-01    1.861e-01    2.002e-01
  0.10    0.4    9.388e-01    6.549e-02    6.808e-02
  0.10    0.6    9.911e-01    1.116e-02    1.133e-02
  0.10    0.8    1.001e+00    8.526e-04    8.561e-04
  0.10    1.0    1.002e+00    2.203e-04    2.224e-04

  ncall =    187
```

Table 2.2: Abbreviated output for eqs. (2.1), (2.2), (2.3),
$$0 \leq x \leq 1$$

For example, at $x = 0, t = 0.1$,

Table 2.1

```
  0.10    0.0    7.557e-01    2.618e-01    2.867e-01
```

Table 2.2

```
  0.10    0.0    7.578e-01    2.594e-01    2.838e-01
```

Therefore, a solution can be computed with $3(26) = 78$ MOL/ODEs rather than $3(51) = 153$ MOL/ODEs. For large

MOL/ODE systems, this is a substantial reduction (and generally, symmetry should be used to reduce the total calculation of a solution).

S, I, R are plotted in Figs. 2.2a,b,c. The appearance of Figs. 2.2a,b,c is different than Figs. 2.1a,b,c, (note the horizontal axis intervals) but the solutions are essentially the same.

The preceding discussion of a basic SIR model is now extended to include other effects. The SEIR (Susceptible Exposed Infected Recovered) model has been studied extensively.

(2.3) SEIR Model

The following 4×4 SEIR model [3, 1] has a PDE added to the previous SIR model for an exposed population.

$$\frac{\partial S}{\partial t} = D_s \frac{\partial^2 S}{\partial x^2} = r_{ns}(N - S) - r_{si}SI/N - r_s S \qquad (2.4a)$$

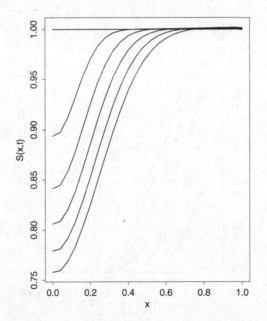

Figure 2.2a: Numerical solution $S(x, t)$, $0 \leq x \leq 1$

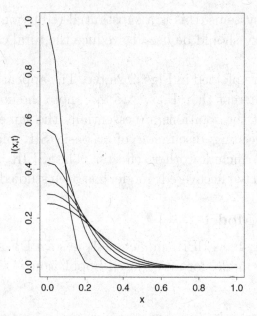

Figure 2.2b: Numerical solution $I(x,t)$, $0 \leq x \leq 1$

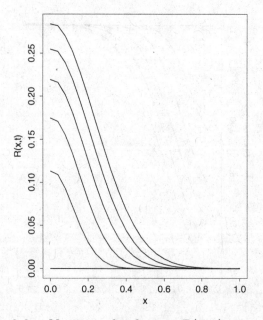

Figure 2.2c: Numerical solution $R(x,t)$, $0 \leq x \leq 1$

$$\frac{\partial E}{\partial t} = D_e \frac{\partial^2 E}{\partial x^2} + r_{si} SI/N - (r_{ns} + r_e)E \qquad (2.4b)$$

$$\frac{\partial I}{\partial t} = D_i \frac{\partial^2 I}{\partial x^2} + r_e E - (r_{ns} + r_i)I \qquad (2.4c)$$

$$\frac{\partial R}{\partial t} = D_r \frac{\partial^2 R}{\partial x^2} + r_i I - r_{ns}R + r_s S \qquad (2.4d)$$

$$N = S + E + I + R \qquad (2.4e)$$

N from eq. (2.5e) is used to normalize the SI interaction terms in eqs. 2.4a,b, $\pm r_{si} SI/N$.

Eqs. (2.4) have the following ICs.

$$S(x, t = 0) = f_1(x); \; E(x, t = 0) = f_2(x) \qquad (2.5a,b)$$

$$I(x, t = 0) = f_3(x); \; R(x, t = 0) = f_4(x) \qquad (2.5c,d)$$

The BCs are homogeneous Neumann.

$$\frac{\partial S(x = x_l, t)}{\partial x} = \frac{\partial S(x = x_u, t)}{\partial x} = 0 \qquad (2.6a,b)$$

$$\frac{\partial E(x = x_l, t)}{\partial x} = \frac{\partial E(x = x_u, t)}{\partial x} = 0 \qquad (2.6c,d)$$

$$\frac{\partial I(x = x_l, t)}{\partial x} = \frac{\partial I(x = x_u, t)}{\partial x} = 0 \qquad (2.6e,f)$$

$$\frac{\partial R(x = x_l, t)}{\partial x} = \frac{\partial R(x = x_u, t)}{\partial x} = 0 \qquad (2.6g,h)$$

If eqs. (2.4a,b,c,d) are added,

- LHSs:

$$\frac{\partial S}{\partial t} + \frac{\partial E}{\partial t} + \frac{\partial I}{\partial t} + \frac{\partial R}{\partial t} = \frac{\partial (S + E + I + R)}{\partial t} = \frac{\partial N}{\partial t}$$

(2.4f)

from eq. (2.4e).
- RHSs: With $D_s = D_e = D_i = D_r = D_{seir}$, eq. (2.4e),

$$D_{seir}\left(\frac{\partial^2 S}{\partial x^2} + \frac{\partial^2 E}{\partial x^2} + \frac{\partial^2 I}{\partial x^2} + \frac{\partial^2 R}{\partial x^2}\right) +$$

$$r_{ns}(S + E + I + R - S) - r_{si}SI/N - r_s S + r_{si}SI/N$$

$$-(r_{ns} + r_e)E + r_e E - (r_{ns} + r_i)I + r_i I - r_{ns}R + r_s S$$

$$= D_{seir}\left(\frac{\partial^2 N}{\partial x^2}\right)$$

Thus, from eqs. (2.4a,b,c,d) with equal diffusivities, N follows the 1D diffusion equation

$$\frac{\partial N}{\partial t} = D_{seir}\left(\frac{\partial^2 N}{\partial x^2}\right)$$

(2.4g)

and with no diffusion ($D_{seir} = 0$), N is constant (does not vary with t)

$$\frac{\partial N}{\partial t} = 0$$

(2.4h)

Eq. (2.4h) is tested with the routines and solutions that follow.

(2.3.1) Main program

A main program for eqs. (2.4), (2.5), (2.6) follows.

```
#
# SEIR model
#
# Delete previous workspaces
  rm(list=ls(all=TRUE))
#
# Access ODE integrator
  library("deSolve");
#
# Access functions for numerical solution
  setwd("f:/infectious/chap2");
  source("pde1b.R");
  source("dss004.R");
#
# Select case
  ncase=2;
#
# Parameters
  if(ncase==1){
    f1=function(x) 10;
    f2=function(x)  1;
    f3=function(x)  0;
    f4=function(x)  0;
    r_ns=0; r_si=0.9;
    r_s=0; r_e=0.5; r_i=0.2;
    D_s=0; D_e=0; D_i=0; D_r=0;
  }
  if(ncase==2){
    f1=function(x) 10;
    f2=function(x) exp(-100*x^2);
    f3=function(x) 0;
```

```
    f4=function(x) 0;
    r_ns=0; r_si=0.9;
    r_s=0; r_e=0.5; r_i=0.2;
    D_s=0.25/365; D_e=0.25/365;
    D_i=0.25/365; D_r=0.25/365;
  }
#
# Spatial grid (in x)
  nx=51;
  xl=-1;xu=1;
  x=seq(from=xl,to=xu,by=(xu-xl)/(nx-1));
#
# Independent variable for ODE integration
  t0=0;tf=15;nout=6;
  tout=seq(from=t0,to=tf,by=(tf-t0)/(nout-1));
#
# Initial condition (t=0)
  u0=rep(0,4*nx);
  for(i in 1:nx){
    u0[i]      =f1(x[i]);
    u0[i+nx]   =f2(x[i]);
    u0[i+2*nx]=f3(x[i]);
    u0[i+3*nx]=f4(x[i]);
  }
  ncall=0;
#
# ODE integration
  out=lsodes(y=u0,times=tout,func=pde1b,
      sparsetype="sparseint",rtol=1e-6,
      atol=1e-6,maxord=5);
  nrow(out)
  ncol(out)
#
# Arrays for plotting numerical solution
```

```
  S=matrix(0,nrow=nx,ncol=nout);
  E=matrix(0,nrow=nx,ncol=nout);
  I=matrix(0,nrow=nx,ncol=nout);
  R=matrix(0,nrow=nx,ncol=nout);
  N=matrix(0,nrow=nx,ncol=nout);
  for(it in 1:nout){
    for(i in 1:nx){
      S[i,it]=out[it,i+1];
      E[i,it]=out[it,i+1+nx];
      I[i,it]=out[it,i+1+2*nx];
      R[i,it]=out[it,i+1+3*nx];
      N[i,it]=S[i,it]+E[i,it]+
              I[i,it]+R[i,it];
    }
  }
#
# Display numerical solution
  for(it in 1:nout){
    cat(sprintf("\n        t       x       S(x,t)
                E(x,t)"));
    cat(sprintf("\n        I(x,t)        R(x,t)
                N(x,t)\n"));
    iv=seq(from=1,to=nx,by=5);
    for(i in iv){
      cat(sprintf("%6.2f%6.1f%12.3e%12.3e\n",
          tout[it],x[i],S[i,it],E[i,it]));
      cat(sprintf("%12.3e%12.3e%12.3e\n\n",
          I[i,it],R[i,it],N[i,it]));
    }
  }
#
# Calls to ODE routine
  cat(sprintf("\n\n ncall = %5d\n\n",ncall));
#
```

```
# Plot PDE solutions
#
# S
  par(mfrow=c(1,1));
  matplot(x=x,y=S,type="l",xlab="x",
    ylab="S(x,t)",xlim=c(xl,xu),lty=1,
    main="",lwd=2,col="black");
#
# E
  par(mfrow=c(1,1));
  matplot(x=x,y=E,type="l",xlab="x",
    ylab="E(x,t)",xlim=c(xl,xu),lty=1,
    main="",lwd=2,col="black");
#
# I
  par(mfrow=c(1,1));
  matplot(x=x,y=I,type="l",xlab="x",
    ylab="I(x,t)",xlim=c(xl,xu),lty=1,
    main="",lwd=2,col="black");
#
# R
  par(mfrow=c(1,1));
  matplot(x=x,y=R,type="l",xlab="x",
    ylab="R(x,t)",xlim=c(xl,xu),lty=1,
    main="",lwd=2,col="black");
#
# N
  par(mfrow=c(1,1));
  if(ncase==1){
    matplot(x=x,y=N,type="l",xlab="x",
      ylab="N(x,t)",xlim=c(xl,xu),lty=1,
      main="",lwd=2,col="black",
      ylim=c(10.5,11.5));}
  if(ncase==2){
```

```
matplot(x=x,y=N,type="l",xlab="x",
  ylab="N(x,t)",xlim=c(xl,xu),lty=1,
  main="",lwd=2,col="black");}
```

Listing 2.3: Main program for eqs. (2.4), (2.5), (2.6)

Listing 2.3 is similar to Listing 2.1 so the differences will be emphasized.

- Previous workspaces are removed.

```
#
# SEIR model
#
# Delete previous workspaces
  rm(list=ls(all=TRUE))
```

- The ODE/MOL routines is pde1b.

```
#
# Access ODE integrator
  library("deSolve");
#
# Access functions for numerical solution
  setwd("f:/infectious/chap2");
  source("pde1b.R");
  source("dss004.R");
```

- Two cases are programmed. For ncase=1, the ICs and parameters are taken from [3].

```
#
# Parameters
  if(ncase==1){
    f1=function(x) 10;
    f2=function(x)  1;
    f3=function(x)  0;
    f4=function(x)  0;
```

```
    r_ns=0; r_si=0.9;
    r_s=0; r_e=0.5; r_i=0.2;
    D_s=0; D_e=0; D_i=0; D_r=0;
}
```

Since the ICs are constant in x, and BCs (2.6) are consistent with these ICs, the solutions have no variation in x (as discussed in Chapter 1).

For `ncase=2`, the IC $E(x, t = 0)$ has a Gaussian variation in x symmetric around $x = 0$. Also, the diffusivities are nonzero (a conversion from yrs to days is made so that the model t scale is in days [3]).

```
if(ncase==2){
    f1=function(x) 10;
    f2=function(x) exp(-100*x^2);
    f3=function(x) 0;
    f4=function(x) 0;
    r_ns=0; r_si=0.9;
    r_s=0; r_e=0.5; r_i=0.2;
    D_s=0.25/365; D_e=0.25/365;
    D_i=0.25/365; D_r=0.25/365;
}
```

This case therefore demonstrates variations in x and t.

- A normalized spatial interval $-1 \leq x \leq 1$ of 51 points is defined (a total of $(4)(nx) = (4)(51) = 204$ MOL/ODEs).

```
#
# Spatial grid (in x)
    nx=51;
    xl=-1;xu=1;
    x=seq(from=xl,to=xu,by=(xu-xl)/(nx-1));
```

- A t interval of 15 days is defined with 6 output points.

```
#
# Independent variable for ODE integration
  t0=0;tf=15;nout=6;
  tout=seq(from=t0,to=tf,by=(tf-t0)/(nout-1));
```

- f_1, f_2, f_3, f_4 of eqs. (2.5) are used to define the 204 ICs.

```
#
# Initial condition (t=0)
  u0=rep(0,4*nx);
  for(i in 1:nx){
    u0[i]      =f1(x[i]);
    u0[i+nx]   =f2(x[i]);
    u0[i+2*nx]=f3(x[i]);
    u0[i+3*nx]=f4(x[i]);
  }
  ncall=0;
```

The counter for the calls to pde1b is also initialzed.
- The 204 ODEs are integrated by lsodes (available in deSolve).

```
#
# ODE integration
  out=lsodes(y=u0,times=tout,func=pde1b,
      sparsetype="sparseint",rtol=1e-6,
      atol=1e-6,maxord=5);
  nrow(out)
  ncol(out)
```

The arguments of lsodes are explained in the discussion of Listing 2.1. The solution array out is $6 \times 204 + 1 = 205$ (+1 includes t) as confirmed in the subsequent output.
- S, E, I, R, N are placed in arrays for subsequent numerical and graphical output.

```
#
# Arrays for plotting numerical solution
  S=matrix(0,nrow=nx,ncol=nout);
  E=matrix(0,nrow=nx,ncol=nout);
  I=matrix(0,nrow=nx,ncol=nout);
  R=matrix(0,nrow=nx,ncol=nout);
  N=matrix(0,nrow=nx,ncol=nout);
  for(it in 1:nout){
    for(i in 1:nx){
      S[i,it]=out[it,i+1];
      E[i,it]=out[it,i+1+nx];
      I[i,it]=out[it,i+1+2*nx];
      R[i,it]=out[it,i+1+3*nx];
      N[i,it]=S[i,it]+E[i,it]+
              I[i,it]+R[i,it];
    }
  }
```

The subscripting for out is explained with Listing 2.1.

- The number of calls to pde1b is displayed at the end of the solution.

```
#
# Calls to ODE routine
  cat(sprintf("\n\n ncall = %5d\n\n",ncall));
```

- S, E, I, R are plotted as a function of x with parameterization in t.

```
#
# Plot PDE solutions
#
# S
  par(mfrow=c(1,1));
  matplot(x=x,y=S,type="l",xlab="x",
    ylab="S(x,t)",xlim=c(xl,xu),lty=1,
    main="",lwd=2,col="black");
```

```
#
# E
  par(mfrow=c(1,1));
  matplot(x=x,y=E,type="l",xlab="x",
    ylab="E(x,t)",xlim=c(xl,xu),lty=1,
    main="",lwd=2,col="black");
#
# I
  par(mfrow=c(1,1));
  matplot(x=x,y=I,type="l",xlab="x",
    ylab="I(x,t)",xlim=c(xl,xu),lty=1,
    main="",lwd=2,col="black");
#
# R
  par(mfrow=c(1,1));
  matplot(x=x,y=R,type="l",xlab="x",
    ylab="R(x,t)",xlim=c(xl,xu),lty=1,
    main="",lwd=2,col="black");
```

- N is plotted as a function of x with parameterization in t. Two different calls to matplot are used for ncase=1,2. For ncase=1, $N(x,t)$ is constant in x and t so explicit scaling of the vertical axis (ylim=c(10.5,11.5)) is used to improve the appearance of the plot. For ncase=2, automatic scaling of the vertical axis is used.

```
#
# N
  par(mfrow=c(1,1));
  if(ncase==1){
    matplot(x=x,y=N,type="l",xlab="x",
      ylab="N(x,t)",xlim=c(xl,xu),lty=1,
      main="",lwd=2,col="black",
      ylim=c(10.5,11.5));}
  if(ncase==2){
```

```
            matplot(x=x,y=N,type="l",xlab="x",
            ylab="N(x,t)",xlim=c(xl,xu),lty=1,
            main="",lwd=2,col="black");}
```

This completes the main program of Listing 2.3.

(2.3.2) ODE/MOL routine

pde1b is listed next.

```
    pde1b=function(t,u,parms){
#
# Function pde1b computes the t derivative
# vectors of S(x,t),E(x,t),I(x,t),R(x,t)
#
# One vector to four vectors
    S=rep(0,nx);E=rep(0,nx);
    I=rep(0,nx);R=rep(0,nx);
    N=rep(0,nx);
    for(i in 1:nx){
      S[i]=u[i];
      E[i]=u[i+nx];
      I[i]=u[i+2*nx];
      R[i]=u[i+3*nx];
      N[i]=S[i]+E[i]+I[i]+R[i];
    }
#
# S*I
    SI=rep(0,nx);
    for(i in 1:nx){SI[i]=S[i]*I[i];}
#
# Sx,Ex,Ix,Rx
    Sx=dss004(xl,xu,nx,S);
    Ex=dss004(xl,xu,nx,E);
    Ix=dss004(xl,xu,nx,I);
```

```
  Rx=dss004(xl,xu,nx,R);
#
# BCs
  Sx[1]=0;Sx[nx]=0;
  Ex[1]=0;Ex[nx]=0;
  Ix[1]=0;Ix[nx]=0;
  Rx[1]=0;Rx[nx]=0;
#
# Sxx,Exx,Ixx,Rxx
  Sxx=dss004(xl,xu,nx,Sx);
  Exx=dss004(xl,xu,nx,Ex);
  Ixx=dss004(xl,xu,nx,Ix);
  Rxx=dss004(xl,xu,nx,Rx);
#
# PDEs
  St=rep(0,nx);Et=rep(0,nx);
  It=rep(0,nx);Rt=rep(0,nx);
  for(i in 1:nx){
    St[i]=D_s*Sxx[i]+r_ns*(N[i]-S[i])-
          r_si*SI[i]/N[i]-r_s*S[i];
    Et[i]=D_e*Exx[i]+r_si*SI[i]/N[i]-
          (r_ns+r_e)*E[i];
    It[i]=D_i*Ixx[i]+r_e*E[i]-
          (r_ns+r_i)*I[i];
    Rt[i]=D_r*Rxx[i]+r_i*I[i]-
          r_ns*R[i]+r_s*S[i];
  }
#
# Four vectors to one vector
  ut=rep(0,4*nx);
  for(i in 1:nx){
    ut[i]     =St[i];
    ut[i+nx]  =Et[i];
    ut[i+2*nx]=It[i];
```

```
    ut[i+3*nx]=Rt[i];
  }
#
# Increment calls to pde1b
  ncall <<- ncall+1;
#
# Return derivative vector
  return(list(c(ut)));
  }
```

Listing 2.4: ODE/MOL routine for eqs. (2.4), (2.5), (2.6)

We can note the following details about pde1b. See also the discussion of Listing 2.2 for additional details.

- The function is defined,

```
    pde1b=function(t,u,parms){
    #
    # Function pde1b computes the t derivative
    # vectors of S(x,t),E(x,t),I(x,t),R(x,t)
```

- u is placed in four ODE dependent vectors, S, E, I, R, and a supplemental vector N to facilitate the programming of eqs. (2.4).

```
    #
    # One vector to four vectors
      S=rep(0,nx);E=rep(0,nx);
      I=rep(0,nx);R=rep(0,nx);
      N=rep(0,nx);
      for(i in 1:nx){
        S[i]=u[i];
        E[i]=u[i+nx];
        I[i]=u[i+2*nx];
        R[i]=u[i+3*nx];
        N[i]=S[i]+E[i]+I[i]+R[i];
      }
```

Eq. (2.4e) is algebraic and is added to the differential equations, eqs. (2.4a,b,c,d). Thus, the system is a basic form of a differential-algebraic equation (DAE) system[2].

- The nonlinear product function *SI* in eqs. (2.4a,b) is placed in vector SI.

```
#
# S*I
  SI=rep(0,nx);
  for(i in 1:nx){SI[i]=S[i]*I[i];}
```

- The first derivatives $\frac{\partial S}{\partial x}, \frac{\partial E}{\partial x}, \frac{\partial I}{\partial x}, \frac{\partial R}{\partial x}$ are computed.

```
#
# Sx,Ex,Ix,Rx
  Sx=dss004(xl,xu,nx,S);
  Ex=dss004(xl,xu,nx,E);
  Ix=dss004(xl,xu,nx,I);
  Rx=dss004(xl,xu,nx,R);
```

Additional details about dss004, which has fourth order FDs, are given in Appendix A1.

---

[2]More generally, DAE systems have algebraic equations that define additional variables as functions of the ODE dependent variables. The functions may be nonlinear, so that a solver, such as a variant of Newton's method, may be required. The calls to the solver can possibly be placed at the beginning of the ODE routine, depending on the *index* of the DAE system. Or the DAE system may have a higher index that requires more elaborate algorithms. DAE algorithms and their computer implementation have been studied extensively, but are not discussed here. The linear (defining) algebraic eq. (2.4e) for N is placed at the beginning of pde1b so that N can be used in the subsequent programming of the MOL/ODEs.

- BCs (2.6) are implemented. Subscripts 1,nx correspond to $x = x_l = -1, x = x_u = 1$.

```
#
# BCs
  Sx[1]=0;Sx[nx]=0;
  Ex[1]=0;Ex[nx]=0;
  Ix[1]=0;Ix[nx]=0;
  Rx[1]=0;Rx[nx]=0;
```

- The second derivatives $\dfrac{\partial^2 S}{\partial x^2}, \dfrac{\partial^2 E}{\partial x^2}, \dfrac{\partial^2 I}{\partial x^2}, \dfrac{\partial^2 R}{\partial x^2}$ are computed from the first derivatives (stagewise or sucessive differentiation).

```
#
# Sxx,Exx,Ixx,Rxx
  Sxx=dss004(xl,xu,nx,Sx);
  Exx=dss004(xl,xu,nx,Ex);
  Ixx=dss004(xl,xu,nx,Ix);
  Rxx=dss004(xl,xu,nx,Rx);
```

- The MOL/ODE approximations of eqs. (2.4a,b,c,d) are programmed (a total of $(4)(51) = 204$ ODEs).

```
#
# PDEs
  St=rep(0,nx);Et=rep(0,nx);
  It=rep(0,nx);Rt=rep(0,nx);
  for(i in 1:nx){
    St[i]=D_s*Sxx[i]+r_ns*(N[i]-S[i])-
          r_si*SI[i]/N[i]-r_s*S[i];
    Et[i]=D_e*Exx[i]+r_si*SI[i]/N[i]-
          (r_ns+r_e)*E[i];
    It[i]=D_i*Ixx[i]+r_e*E[i]-
          (r_ns+r_i)*I[i];
    Rt[i]=D_r*Rxx[i]+r_i*I[i]-
```

```
                    r_ns*R[i]+r_s*S[i];
    }
```

- The derivatives $\dfrac{\partial S}{\partial t}, \dfrac{\partial E}{\partial t}, \dfrac{\partial I}{\partial t}, \dfrac{\partial R}{\partial t}$ (LHSs of eqs. (2.4a,b, c,d)) are placed in a single vector, ut.

```
#
# Four vectors to one vector
  ut=rep(0,4*nx);
  for(i in 1:nx){
    ut[i]     =St[i];
    ut[i+nx]  =Et[i];
    ut[i+2*nx]=It[i];
    ut[i+3*nx]=Rt[i];
  }
```

- The counter for the calls to pde1b is incremented and returned to the main program of Listing 2.3 by <<-.

```
#
# Increment calls to pde1b
  ncall <<- ncall+1;
```

- The derivative vector ut is returned to lsodes as a list for the next step along the solution.

```
#
# Return derivative vector
  return(list(c(ut)));
  }
```

c is the R vector operator.

This completes the programming of eqs. (2.4). The output from the routines of Listings 2.3, 2.4 is discused next.

(2.3.3) Model output

Abbreviated numerical and graphical output from the main program of Listing 2.3 and pde1b of Listing 2.4 follows.

[1] 6

[1] 205

```
      t      x        S(x,t)        E(x,t)
         I(x,t)       R(x,t)        N(x,t)
    0.00  -1.0     1.000e+01     1.000e+00
     0.000e+00    0.000e+00     1.100e+01

    0.00  -0.8     1.000e+01     1.000e+00
     0.000e+00    0.000e+00     1.100e+01

    0.00  -0.6     1.000e+01     1.000e+00
     0.000e+00    0.000e+00     1.100e+01

    0.00  -0.4     1.000e+01     1.000e+00
     0.000e+00    0.000e+00     1.100e+01

    0.00  -0.2     1.000e+01     1.000e+00
     0.000e+00    0.000e+00     1.100e+01

    0.00   0.0     1.000e+01     1.000e+00
     0.000e+00    0.000e+00     1.100e+01

    0.00   0.2     1.000e+01     1.000e+00
     0.000e+00    0.000e+00     1.100e+01

    0.00   0.4     1.000e+01     1.000e+00
     0.000e+00    0.000e+00     1.100e+01
```

```
0.00    0.6   1.000e+01   1.000e+00
   0.000e+00   0.000e+00   1.100e+01


0.00    0.8   1.000e+01   1.000e+00
   0.000e+00   0.000e+00   1.100e+01


0.00    1.0   1.000e+01   1.000e+00
   0.000e+00   0.000e+00   1.100e+01
 .                            .
 ..                           .
 .                            .

Output for t = 3,...12 removed
 .                            .
 .                            .
 .                            .

 t     x      S(x,t)       E(x,t)
   I(x,t)     R(x,t)       N(x,t)
15.00  -1.0   6.359e-01   6.543e-01
   2.975e+00   6.735e+00   1.100e+01


15.00  -0.8   6.359e-01   6.543e-01
   2.975e+00   6.735e+00   1.100e+01


15.00  -0.6   6.359e-01   6.543e-01
   2.975e+00   6.735e+00   1.100e+01


15.00  -0.4   6.359e-01   6.543e-01
   2.975e+00   6.735e+00   1.100e+01


15.00  -0.2   6.359e-01   6.543e-01
   2.975e+00   6.735e+00   1.100e+01


15.00   0.0   6.359e-01   6.543e-01
   2.975e+00   6.735e+00   1.100e+01
```

```
15.00    0.2    6.359e-01    6.543e-01
         2.975e+00    6.735e+00    1.100e+01

15.00    0.4    6.359e-01    6.543e-01
         2.975e+00    6.735e+00    1.100e+01

15.00    0.6    6.359e-01    6.543e-01
         2.975e+00    6.735e+00    1.100e+01

15.00    0.8    6.359e-01    6.543e-01
         2.975e+00    6.735e+00    1.100e+01

15.00    1.0    6.359e-01    6.543e-01
         2.975e+00    6.735e+00    1.100e+01

ncall =    300
```

Table 2.3: Abbreviated output for eqs. (2.4), (2.5), (2.6), ncase=1

We can note the following details about this output.

- The solution matrix out has the dimensions $6 \times 4(51) + 1 = 205$.

  [1] 6

  [1] 205

- ICs (2.5) are confirmed. In particular, $N(x, t = 0) = 10 + 1 = 11$ which remains constant throughout the solution, i.e., $N(x, t = 15) = 11$.
- S, E, I, R, N do not vary with x since the ICs are constant in x and the homogeneous Neumann BCs are consistent with the constant solutions. In other words, the second

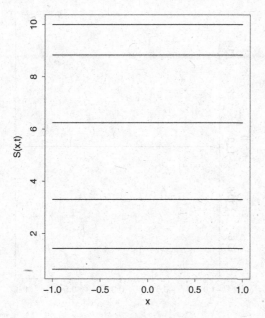

Figure 2.3a: Numerical solution $S(x, t)$, `ncase=1`

derivatives in eqs. (2.4a,b,c,d) are zero (this conclusion would not change if the diffusivities D_s, D_e, D_i, D_r are nonzero).

- The computational effort is modest, `ncall = 300`.

The solutions in Table 2.3 are confirmed in the graphical output (only $S(x, t)$, $N(x,t)$ follow in Figs. 2.3a,e to conserve space).

Fig. 2.3a indicates that $S(x, t)$ decays from the initial $S(x, t = 0) = 10$ to $S(x, t = 15) = 6.359e - 01$.

Fig. 2.3e indicates that $N(x, t)$ remains constant at the initial $N(x, t = 0) = 11$ according to eq. (2.4h).

For `ncase=2` the solutions vary in x and t due to the Gaussian IC for $E(x, t = 0)$. (Listing 2.3). Also, the diffusivities D_s, D_e, D_i, D_r are nonzero so that variations in x of S, E, I, R result. Abbreviated numerical and graphical output follows.

[1] 6

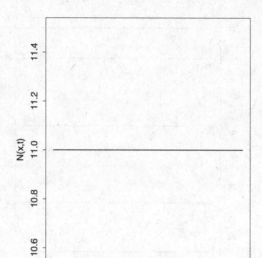

Figure 2.3e: $N(x,t)$, ncase=1

[1] 205

```
     t     x        S(x,t)        E(x,t)
        I(x,t)      R(x,t)        N(x,t)
  0.00  -1.0    1.000e+01     3.720e-44
     0.000e+00  0.000e+00     1.000e+01


  0.00  -0.8    1.000e+01     1.604e-28
     0.000e+00  0.000e+00     1.000e+01


  0.00  -0.6    1.000e+01     2.320e-16
     0.000e+00  0.000e+00     1.000e+01


  0.00  -0.4    1.000e+01     1.125e-07
     0.000e+00  0.000e+00     1.000e+01
```

```
0.00  -0.2   1.000e+01   1.832e-02
   0.000e+00   0.000e+00   1.002e+01

0.00   0.0   1.000e+01   1.000e+00
   0.000e+00   0.000e+00   1.100e+01

0.00   0.2   1.000e+01   1.832e-02
   0.000e+00   0.000e+00   1.002e+01

0.00   0.4   1.000e+01   1.125e-07
   0.000e+00   0.000e+00   1.000e+01

0.00   0.6   1.000e+01   2.320e-16
   0.000e+00   0.000e+00   1.000e+01

0.00   0.8   1.000e+01   1.604e-28
   0.000e+00   0.000e+00   1.000e+01

0.00   1.0   1.000e+01   3.720e-44
   0.000e+00   0.000e+00   1.000e+01
       .                      .
       .                      .
       .                      .
Output for t = 3,...12 removed
       .                      .
       .                      .
       .                      .
    t    x      S(x,t)      E(x,t)
       I(x,t)     R(x,t)      N(x,t)
15.00  -1.0   1.000e+01  -1.248e-06
  -1.161e-06  -6.830e-07   1.000e+01
```

```
15.00   -0.8    1.000e+01    1.677e-05
         1.560e-05    9.054e-06    1.000e+01


15.00   -0.6    9.948e+00    2.115e-02
         1.975e-02    1.171e-02    1.000e+01


15.00   -0.4    8.211e+00    6.565e-01
         6.853e-01    4.664e-01    1.002e+01


15.00   -0.2    3.064e+00    1.536e+00
         2.701e+00    2.901e+00    1.020e+01


15.00    0.0    1.311e+00    1.144e+00
         3.195e+00    4.793e+00    1.044e+01


15.00    0.2    3.064e+00    1.536e+00
         2.701e+00    2.901e+00    1.020e+01


15.00    0.4    8.211e+00    6.565e-01
         6.853e-01    4.664e-01    1.002e+01


15.00    0.6    9.948e+00    2.115e-02
         1.975e-02    1.171e-02    1.000e+01


15.00    0.8    1.000e+01    1.677e-05
         1.560e-05    9.054e-06    1.000e+01


15.00    1.0    1.000e+01   -1.248e-06
        -1.161e-06   -6.830e-07    1.000e+01


ncall =    352
```

Table 2.4: Abbreviated output for eqs. (2.4), (2.5), (2.6),
ncase=2

We can note the following details about this output.

- The solution matrix `out` again has the dimensions $6 \times 4(51) + 1 = 205$.

  ```
  [1] 6
  ```

  ```
  [1] 205
  ```

- ICs (2.5) are confirmed. In particular, $E(x, t = 0)$ is a Gaussian function.
- S, E, I, R, N do vary with x since the ICs are not constant in x. The homogeneous Neumann BCs are still consistent with the solutions as indicated in the graphical output Figs. 2.4a,b,c,d,e that follows.
- The computational effort is modest, `ncall = 352`.

The solutions in Table 2.4 are confirmed in the following graphical output.

Fig. 2.4a indicates $S(x, t = 0) = 10$ which then decays most rapidly at $x = 0$ in response to E, I, R.

Fig. 2.4b indicates $E(x, t = 0)$ undergoes a complicated transient through interactions with S, I, R according to eqs. (2.4).

Fig. 2.4c indicates $I(x, t)$ moves from the zero IC in response to $E(x, t)$

Fig. 2.4d indicates $R(x, t)$ moves from the zero IC in response to $E(x, t)$

Fig. 2.4e indicates that $N(x, t)$ does not remain constant according to eq. (2.4g).

The preceding graphical output of the SEIR model, eqs. (2.4), (2.5), (2.6), consisted of plots of the dependent variables S, E, I, R against x with t as a parameter. However, plots of S, E, I, R against t for a particular x can be easily produced to give a better indication of the variation of the solutions with t.

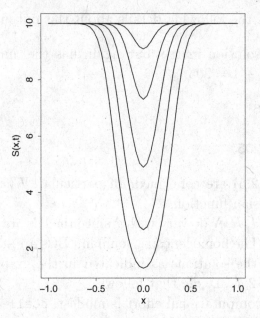

Figure 2.4a: Numerical solution $S(x, t)$, `ncase=2`

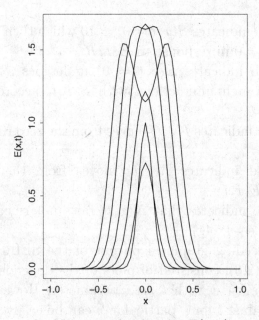

Figure 2.4b: Numerical solution $E(x, t)$, `ncase=2`

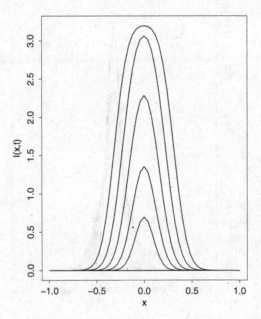

Figure 2.4c: Numerical solution $I(x,t)$, `ncase=2`

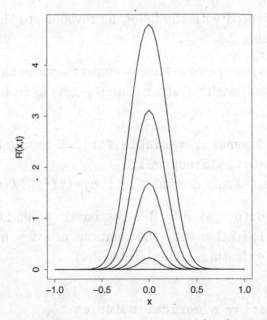

Figure 2.4d: Numerical solution $R(x,t)$, `ncase=2`

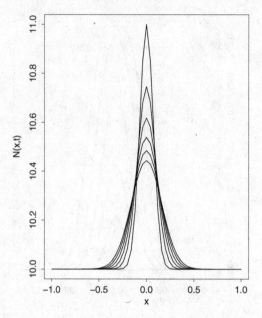

Figure 2.4e: $N(x, t)$, `ncase=2`

This is illustrated with the following revisions to the main program of Listing 2.3.

- 31 output points in t are specified to give sufficients points for plots with t (rather than 6 points as in Listing 2.3).

```
#
# Independent variable for ODE integration
  t0=0;tf=15;nout=31;
  tout=seq(from=t0,to=tf,by=(tf-t0)/(nout-1));
```

- The output at $x = 0$ is displayed (point 26 in x with `nx=51`) (rather than the solutions at every fifth point in x as in Listing 2.3 and Table 2.4).

```
#
# Display numerical solution
  for(it in 1:nout){
```

```
    if(it==1){
      cat(sprintf("\n          t        x      S(x=0,t)
                    E(x=0,t)"));
      cat(sprintf("\n      I(x=0,t)       R(x=0,t)
                    N(x=0,t)\n\n"));
    }
    cat(sprintf("%6.2f%6.1f%12.3e%12.3e\n",
          tout[it],x[26],S[26,it],E[26,it]));
    cat(sprintf("%12.3e%12.3e%12.3e\n\n",
          I[26,it],R[26,it],N[26,it]));
  }
```

- The solution at $x = 0$ is placed in five vectors of length nout=31 for plotting.

```
#
# Plot PDE solutions (x=0)
  Splot=rep(0,nout);Eplot=rep(0,nout);
  Iplot=rep(0,nout);Rplot=rep(0,nout);
  Nplot=rep(0,nout);
  for(it in 1:nout){
    Splot[it]=S[26,it];
    Eplot[it]=E[26,it];
    Iplot[it]=I[26,it];
    Rplot[it]=R[26,it];
    Nplot[it]=N[26,it];
  }
```

- The solution at $x = 0$ is plotted against t (rather than against x as in Listing 2.3).

```
#
# S
  par(mfrow=c(1,1));
  matplot(x=tout,y=Splot,type="l",xlab="t",
```

```
    ylab="S(x=0,t)",lty=1,main="",lwd=2,
    col="black");
#
# E
  par(mfrow=c(1,1));
  matplot(x=tout,y=Eplot,type="l",xlab="t",
    ylab="E(x=0,t)",lty=1,main="",lwd=2,
    col="black");
#
# I
  par(mfrow=c(1,1));
  matplot(x=tout,y=Iplot,type="l",xlab="t",
    ylab="I(x=0,t)",lty=1,main="",lwd=2,
    col="black");
#
# R
  par(mfrow=c(1,1));
  matplot(x=tout,y=Rplot,type="l",xlab="t",
    ylab="R(x=0,t)",lty=1,main="",lwd=2,
    col="black");
#
# N
  par(mfrow=c(1,1));
  if(ncase==1){
    matplot(x=tout,y=Nplot,type="l",xlab="t",
    ylab="N(x=0,t)",lty=1,main="",lwd=2,
    col="black",ylim=c(10.5,11.5));
  }
  if(ncase==2){
    matplot(x=tout,y=Nplot,type="l",xlab="t",
    ylab="N(x=0,t)",lty=1,main="",lwd=2,
    col="black");
  }
```

The output for these changes in Listing 2.3 follows for `ncase=2`.

[1] 31

[1] 205

```
     t      x     S(x=0,t)       E(x=0,t)
   I(x=0,t)      R(x=0,t)       N(x=0,t)


  0.00    0.0    1.000e+01      1.000e+00
  0.000e+00      0.000e+00      1.100e+01


  0.50    0.0    9.957e+00      7.730e-01
  2.011e-01      1.057e-02      1.094e+01


  1.00    0.0    9.850e+00      6.674e-01
  3.371e-01      3.664e-02      1.089e+01
   .                             .
   .                             .
   .                             .

     Output for t = 1.50,...,13.50
               removed

   .                             .
   .                             .
   .                             .

  14.00   0.0    1.664e+00      1.332e+00
  3.232e+00      4.227e+00      1.046e+01


  14.50   0.0    1.476e+00      1.239e+00
  3.223e+00      4.511e+00      1.045e+01


  15.00   0.0    1.311e+00      1.144e+00
  3.195e+00      4.793e+00      1.044e+01


  ncall =    351
```

Table 2.5: Abbreviated output for eqs. (2.4), (2.5), (2.6), $x = 0$,

ncase=2

The graphical output of the solutions is in Figs. 2.5a,b,c,d,e.

Fig. 2.5a indicates $S(x, t = 0) = 10$ which then decays to $S(x = 0, t = 15) = 1.311e + 00$.

Fig. 2.5b indicates $E(x = 0, t = 0) = 1$ (the Gaussian at $x = 0$) oscillates and ends at $E(x = 0, t = 15) = 1.144e + 00$.

Fig. 2.5c indicates $I(x, t)$ peaks near $t = 15$.

Fig. 2.5d indicates $R(x, t)$ increases throughout t.

Fig. 2.5e indicates that $N(x = 0, t = 0) = 11$ and does not remain constant, but decreases to $N(x = 0, t = 15) = 1.044e + 01$.

The complexity of these solutions suggests additional insight would be useful. One way this can be achieved is to examine the individual terms in the PDEs, e.g., eqs. (2.1a,b,c) and eqs. (2.4a,b,c,d), as a function of x and t. This can be accomplished by a straightforward extension of the output statements

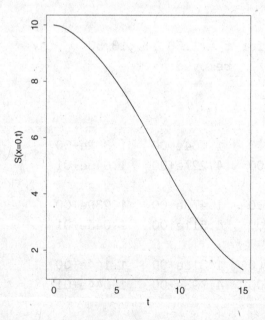

Figure 2.5a: Numerical solution $S(x, t)$, ncase=2

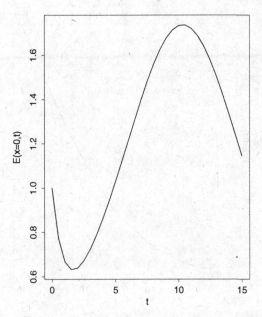

Figure 2.5b: Numerical solution $E(x,t)$, `ncase=2`

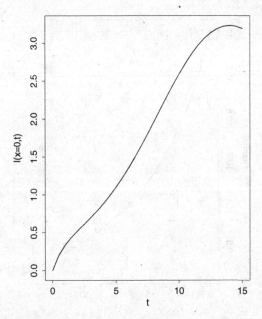

Figure 2.5c: Numerical solution $I(x,t)$, `ncase=2`

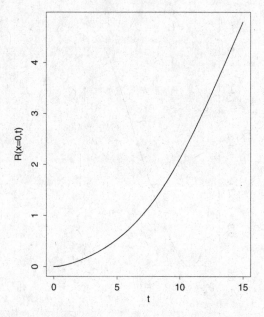

Figure 2.5d: Numerical solution $R(x, t)$, `ncase=2`

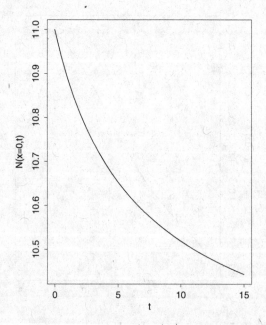

Figure 2.5e: $N(x, t)$, `ncase=2`

in the main programs. This procedure of a detailed examination of the terms in the PDEs is illustrated in the next chapter.

This completes the discussion of the PDE SEIR model, eqs. (2.4), (2.5), (2.6). The basic SIR model of eqs. (2.1), (2.2) and (2.3) will now be extended in Chapter 3 to include cross diffusion.

(2.4) Summary and Conclusions

The MOL analysis of the 3×3 SIR model and the 4×4 SEIR model is straightforward. The addition of a PDE is demonstrated with these examples so that the extension of models by adding PDEs is straightforward.

References

[1] Li, M.Y., H.L. Smith, and L. Wang (2001), Global Dynamics of an SEIR Epidemic Model with Vertical Transmission, *SIAM Journal Applied Mathematics*, **62**, no. 1, pp 58-59

[2] Mondaini, R.P. (2017), *Mathematical Biology and Biological Physics*, World Scientific, New Jersey, USA

[3] Nesse, H., http://www.public.asu.edu/~hnesse/; H. Nesse reported an SEIR ODE model, including an interesting interactive computer implementation

Chapter 3

Cross Diffusion

(3.1) Introduction

In Chapter 2, a basic SIR 3×3 (3 PDEs in 3 unknowns) model is discussed which can be used as a starting point for the development of spatiotemporal models of infectious disease that include cross diffusion.

(3.2) Cross Diffusion Model

If we again consider the SIR model of eqs. (2.1), (2.2) and (2.3), the product terms $\pm r_{si}SI$ in eqs. (2.1a,b) account for the interactions between the susceptible population and the infected population, which is an essential feature of an infectious disease epidemic model. However, if the model is spatiotemporal (based on PDEs), the interaction terms $\pm r_{si}SI$ pertain to only a particular point in x. But the SI interaction will be spatially distributed, and may not be accounted for by just the the individual S and I population diffusion terms

$$D_s \frac{\partial^2 S}{\partial x^2}; \; D_i \frac{\partial^2 I}{\partial x^2} \qquad (3.1a)$$

One approach to account for the spatially distributed $S + I$ interaction is through a term of the form

$$\frac{\partial}{\partial x}\left(D_{si}\frac{\partial SI}{\partial x}\right) \tag{3.1b}$$

where the diffusing species is SI and D_{si} is an effective diffusivity[1]. Function (3.1b) represents *cross diffusion*, which is considered next[2].

A SIR model with cross diffusion (SIRC[3]) can be formulated as an extension of eqs. (2.1), (2.2), (2.3).

$$\frac{\partial S}{\partial t} = D_{si}\frac{\partial^2 SI}{\partial x^2} + D_s\frac{\partial^2 S}{\partial x^2} + r_{p1}S - r_{si}SI \tag{3.2a}$$

$$\frac{\partial I}{\partial t} = D_{si}\frac{\partial^2 SI}{\partial x^2} + D_i\frac{\partial^2 I}{\partial x^2} + r_{p2}I + r_{si}SI - r_iI \tag{3.2b}$$

$$\frac{\partial R}{\partial t} = D_r\frac{\partial^2 R}{\partial x^2} + r_{p3}I + r_iI \tag{3.2c}$$

---

[1]For D_{si} constant, function (3.1b) reduces to

$$\frac{\partial}{\partial x}\left(D_{si}\frac{\partial SI}{\partial x}\right) = D_{si}\frac{\partial^2 SI}{\partial x^2} = D_{si}\left(S\frac{\partial I}{\partial x} + I\frac{\partial S}{\partial x}\right) \tag{3.1c}$$

Eq. (3.1c) is an alternate form of the cross diffusion term that can be implemented within the MOL format discussed subsequently.

[2]Cross diffusion has been described in a series of applications, both deterministic and stochastic [2, 5, 6]. For example, pattern formation can be generated by cross diffusion [4]. Other applications include epidemics [1] and predator-prey models [3, 7].

[3]SIRC $\Rightarrow$ Susceptibles Infecteds Recovereds Cross diffusion.

Eqs. (3.2) are first order in t and each requires an initial condition (IC).

$$S(x, t = 0) = f_1(x); \quad I(x, t = 0) = f_2(x); \quad R(x, t = 0) = f_3(x)$$
$$(3.3a,b,c)$$

Eqs. (3.2) are second order in x and each requires two boundary conditions (BCs).

$$\frac{\partial S(x = x_l, t)}{\partial x} = \frac{\partial S(x = x_u, t)}{\partial x} = 0 \qquad (3.4a,b)$$

$$\frac{\partial I(x = x_l, t)}{\partial x} = \frac{\partial I(x = x_u, t)}{\partial x} = 0 \qquad (3.4c,d)$$

$$\frac{\partial R(x = x_l, t)}{\partial x} = \frac{\partial R(x = x_u, t)}{\partial x} = 0 \qquad (3.4e,f)$$

Eqs. (3.2), (3.3) and (3.4) constitute the SIRC model to be solved numerically with the following routines, which are an extension of the SIR main program and ODE/MOL routines of Listings 2.1, 2.2.

(3.2.1) Main program

```
#
# SIRC model
#
# Delete previous workspaces
  rm(list=ls(all=TRUE))
#
# Access ODE integrator
  library("deSolve");
#
# Access functions for numerical solution
  setwd("f:/infectious/chap3");
  source("pde1a.R");
```

```
  source("dss004.R");
#
# Parameters
  f1=function(x) 1;
  f2=function(x) exp(-100*x^2);
  f3=function(x) 0;
  r_p1=0.02;r_p2=0.02;r_p3=0.02;
  r_si=10;r_i=10;
#
# Select case
  ncase=1;
  if(ncase==1){D_s=0.25;D_i=0.25;
               D_r=0.25;D_si=0    ;}
  if(ncase==2){D_s=0    ; D_i=0;
               D_r=0.25;D_si=0.25;}
  if(ncase==3){D_s=0.25; D_i=0.25;
               D_r=0.25;D_si=0.25;}
#
# Spatial grid (in x)
  nx=51;
  xl=-1;xu=1;
  x=seq(from=xl,to=xu,by=(xu-xl)/(nx-1));
#
# Independent variable for ODE integration
  t0=0;tf=0.1;nout=6;
  tout=seq(from=t0,to=tf,by=(tf-t0)/(nout-1));
#
# Initial condition (t=0)
  u0=rep(0,3*nx);
  for(i in 1:nx){
    u0[i]     =f1(x[i]);
    u0[i+nx]  =f2(x[i]);
    u0[i+2*nx]=f3(x[i]);
  }
```

```
  ncall=0;
#
# ODE integration
  out=lsodes(y=u0,times=tout,func=pde1a,
      sparsetype="sparseint",rtol=1e-6,
      atol=1e-6,maxord=5);
  nrow(out)
  ncol(out)
#
# Arrays for plotting numerical solution
  S=matrix(0,nrow=nx,ncol=nout);
  I=matrix(0,nrow=nx,ncol=nout);
  R=matrix(0,nrow=nx,ncol=nout);
  for(it in 1:nout){
    for(i in 1:nx){
      S[i,it]=out[it,i+1];
      I[i,it]=out[it,i+1+nx];
      R[i,it]=out[it,i+1+2*nx];
    }
  }
#
# Display numerical solution
  for(it in 1:nout){
    cat(sprintf("\n      t       x       S(x,t)
                 I(x,t)       R(x,t)\n"));
    iv=seq(from=1,to=nx,by=5);
    for(i in iv){
      cat(sprintf(
        "%6.2f%6.1f%12.3e%12.3e%12.3e\n",
         tout[it],x[i],S[i,it],I[i,it],R[i,it]));
    }
  }
#
# Calls to ODE routine
```

```
  cat(sprintf("\n\n ncall = %5d\n\n",ncall));
#
# Plot PDE solutions
#
# S
  par(mfrow=c(1,1));
  matplot(x=x,y=S,type="l",xlab="x",
    ylab="S(x,t)",xlim=c(xl,xu),lty=1,
    main="",lwd=2,col="black");
#
# I
  par(mfrow=c(1,1));
  matplot(x=x,y=I,type="l",xlab="x",
    ylab="I(x,t)",xlim=c(xl,xu),lty=1,
    main="",lwd=2,col="black");
#
# R
  par(mfrow=c(1,1));
  matplot(x=x,y=R,type="l",xlab="x",
    ylab="R(x,t)",xlim=c(xl,xu),lty=1,
    main="",lwd=2,col="black");
```

Listing 3.1: Main program for eqs. (3.2), (3.3), (3.4)

We can note the following details about Listing 3.1.

- Previous workspaces are deleted.

```
    #
    # SIRC model
    #
    # Delete previous workspaces
      rm(list=ls(all=TRUE))
```

- The R ODE integrator library deSolve is accessed. Then the directory with the files for the solution of eqs. (3.2),

(3.3), (3.4) is designated. Note that `setwd` (set working directory) uses / rather than the usual \.

```
#
# Access ODE integrator
  library("deSolve");
#
# Access functions for numerical solution
  setwd("f:/infectious/chap3");
  source("pde1a.R");
  source("dss004.R");
```

`pde1a.R` is the routine for the method of lines (MOL) approximation of PDEs (3.2) (discussed subsequently). `dss004` (Differentiation in Space Subroutine) is a library routine for calculating a first derivative in x. Additional details about `dss004` are given in Appendix A1.

- A subset of the model parameters is defined numerically.

```
#
# Parameters
  f1=function(x) 1;
  f2=function(x) exp(-100*x^2);
  f3=function(x) 0;
  r_p1=0.02;r_p2=0.02;r_p3=0.02;
  r_si=10;r_i=10;
```

These parameters require some additonal explanation.

- The IC functions of eqs. (3.3) are defined.

```
      f1=function(x) 1;
      f2=function(x) exp(-100*x^2);
      f3=function(x) 0;
```

f_1 defines a uniform initial susceptible population that is then subjected to an infectious disease. f_2

defines a Gaussian centered at $x = 0$ that represents the infected population (an epidemic centered at $x = 0$). f_3 is zero to reflect no recovereds initally.

- The natural increase in the three populations (births greater than deaths) is set at 0.02/yr (2%/yr). Therefore, these parameters set the model time scale units as yr.

```
r_p1=0.02;r_p2=0.02;r_p3=0.02;
```

- r_{si}, r_i in eqs. (3.2) are defined with the time units of 1/yr.

```
r_si=10;r_i=10;
```

• The four diffusivities of eqs. (3.2) are defined for three cases.

```
#
# Select case
  ncase=1;
  if(ncase==1){D_s=0.25;D_i=0.25;
               D_r=0.25;D_si=0   ;}
  if(ncase==2){D_s=0   ; D_i=0;
               D_r=0.25;D_si=0.25;}
  if(ncase==3){D_s=0.25; D_i=0.25;
               D_r=0.25;D_si=0.25;}
```

The units are 1/yr (x is normalized to the interval $-1 \leq x \leq 1$ as explained next).

For ncase=1, only linear (Fickian) diffusion is used with the diffusivities D_s, D_i, D_r.

For ncase=2, only cross diffusion is used with the diffusivity D_{si}.

For ncase=3, linear and cross diffusion are used with the diffusivities D_s, D_i, D_r, D_{si}.

- A normalized spatial grid of 51 points is defined for $x_l = -1 \leq x \leq x_u = 1$, so that x=-1,-0.96,...,1.

```
#
# Spatial grid (in x)
  nx=51;
  xl=-1;xu=1;
  x=seq(from=xl,to=xu,by=(xu-xl)/(nx-1));
```

- An interval in t of 6 points is defined for $0 \leq t \leq 0.1$ yr so that tout=0,0.02,...,0.1.

```
#
# Independent variable for ODE integration
  t0=0;tf=0.1;nout=6;
  tout=seq(from=t0,to=tf,by=(tf-t0)/(nout-1));
```

- ICs (3.3) are defined.

```
#
# Initial condition (t=0)
  u0=rep(0,3*nx);
  for(i in 1:nx){
    u0[i]      =f1(x[i]);
    u0[i+nx]   =f2(x[i]);
    u0[i+2*nx]=f3(x[i]);
  }
  ncall=0;
```

u0 therefore has $(3)(51) = 153$ elements. The counter for the calls to the ODE/MOL routine pde1a is also initialized.

- The system of 153 MOL/ODEs is integrated by the library integrator lsodes (available in deSolve). As expected, the inputs to lsodes are the ODE function, pde1a, the IC vector u0, and the vector of output values of t, tout. The length of u0 (153) informs lsodes how many ODEs are to be integrated. `func,y,times` are reserved names.

```
#
# ODE integration
  out=lsodes(y=u0,times=tout,func=pde1a,
    sparsetype="sparseint",rtol=1e-6,
    atol=1e-6,maxord=5);
  nrow(out)
  ncol(out)
```

The numerical solution to the ODEs is returned in matrix `out`. In this case, `out` has the dimensions $nout \times (3nx + 1) = 6 \times 3(51) + 1 = 153 + 1 = 154$, which are confirmed by the output from `nrow(out),ncol(out)` (included in the numerical output considered subsequently).

The offset $153 + 1$ is required since the first element of each column has the output t (also in `tout`), and the $2, ..., 3nx + 1 = 2, ..., 154$ column elements have the 153 ODE solutions.

• The solutions of the 153 ODEs returned in `out` by `lsodes` are placed in arrays `S,I,R`.

```
#
# Arrays for plotting numerical solution
  S=matrix(0,nrow=nx,ncol=nout);
  I=matrix(0,nrow=nx,ncol=nout);
  R=matrix(0,nrow=nx,ncol=nout);
  for(it in 1:nout){
    for(i in 1:nx){
      S[i,it]=out[it,i+1];
      I[i,it]=out[it,i+1+nx];
      R[i,it]=out[it,i+1+2*nx];
    }
  }
```

Again, the offset i+1 is required since the first element of each column of out has the value of t.

- $S(x,t), I(x,t), R(x,t)$ are displayed as a function of x and t, with every fifth value of x from by=5.

```
#
# Display numerical solution
  for(it in 1:nout){
    cat(sprintf("\n      t      x        S(x,t)
                   I(x,t)       R(x,t)\n"));
    iv=seq(from=1,to=nx,by=5);
    for(i in iv){
      cat(sprintf(
        "%6.2f%6.1f%12.3e%12.3e%12.3e\n",
        tout[it],x[i],S[i,it],I[i,it],R[i,it]));
    }
  }
```

- The number of calls to pde1a is displayed at the end of the solution.

```
#
# Calls to ODE routine
  cat(sprintf("\n\n ncall = %5d\n\n",ncall));
```

- $S(x,t), I(x,t), R(x,t)$ are plotted as a function of x with t as a parameter.

```
#
# Plot PDE solutions
#
# S
  par(mfrow=c(1,1));
  matplot(x=x,y=S,type="l",xlab="x",
    ylab="S(x,t)",xlim=c(xl,xu),lty=1,
    main="",lwd=2,col="black");
```

```
    #
    # I
      par(mfrow=c(1,1));
      matplot(x=x,y=I,type="l",xlab="x",
        ylab="I(x,t)",xlim=c(xl,xu),lty=1,
        main="",lwd=2,col="black");
    #
    # R
      par(mfrow=c(1,1));
      matplot(x=x,y=R,type="l",xlab="x",
        ylab="R(x,t)",xlim=c(xl,xu),lty=1,
        main="",lwd=2,col="black");
```

This completes the main program. The ODE/MOL routine pde1a called by lsodes is considered next.

(3.2.2) ODE/MOL routine

pde1a called by lsodes is listed next.

```
  pde1a=function(t,u,parms){
#
# Function pde1a computes the t derivative
# vectors of S(x,t),I(x,t),R(x,t)
#
# One vector to three vectors
  S=rep(0,nx);I=rep(0,nx);R=rep(0,nx);
  for(i in 1:nx){
    S[i]=u[i];
    I[i]=u[i+nx];
    R[i]=u[i+2*nx];
  }
#
# S*I
  SI=rep(0,nx);
```

```
  for(i in 1:nx){SI[i]=S[i]*I[i];}
#
# Sx,Ix,Rx
  Sx=dss004(xl,xu,nx,S);
  Ix=dss004(xl,xu,nx,I);
  Rx=dss004(xl,xu,nx,R);
#
# BCs
  Sx[1]=0;Sx[nx]=0;
  Ix[1]=0;Ix[nx]=0;
  Rx[1]=0;Rx[nx]=0;
#
# Sxx,Ixx,Rxx
  Sxx=dss004(xl,xu,nx,Sx);
  Ixx=dss004(xl,xu,nx,Ix);
  Rxx=dss004(xl,xu,nx,Rx);
#
# SIx,SIxx
  SIx=dss004(xl,xu,nx,SI);
 SIxx=dss004(xl,xu,nx,SIx);
#
# PDEs
  St=rep(0,nx);It=rep(0,nx);Rt=rep(0,nx);
  for(i in 1:nx){
    St[i]=D_si*SIxx[i]+D_s*Sxx[i]+r_p1*S[i]-
          r_si*SI[i];
    It[i]=D_si*SIxx[i]+D_i*Ixx[i]+r_p2*I[i]+
          r_si*SI[i]-r_i*I[i];
    Rt[i]=D_r*Rxx[i]+r_p3*R[i]+r_i*I[i];
  }
#
# Three vectors to one vector
  ut=rep(0,3*nx);
  for(i in 1:nx){
```

```
    ut[i]      =St[i];
    ut[i+nx]   =It[i];
    ut[i+2*nx]=Rt[i];
  }
#
# Increment calls to pde1a
  ncall <<- ncall+1;
#
# Return derivative vector
  return(list(c(ut)));
  }
```

Listing 3.2: ODE/MOL routine for eqs. (3.2), (3.3), (3.4)

We can note the following details about Listing 3.2.

- The function is defined.

```
    pde1a=function(t,u,parms){
#
# Function pde1a computes the t derivative
# vectors of S(x,t),I(x,t),R(x,t)
```

  t is the current value of t in eqs. (3.2). u the 153-vector of ODE/MOL dependent variables. **parm** is an argument to pass parameters to **pde1a** (unused, but required in the argument list). The arguments must be listed in the order stated to properly interface with **lsodes** called in the main program of Listing 3.1. The derivative vector of the LHS of eqs. (3.2) is calculated next and returned to **lsodes**.

- u is placed in three vectors, S,I,R, to facilitate the programming of eqs. (3.2).

```
#
# One vector to three vectors
    S=rep(0,nx);I=rep(0,nx);R=rep(0,nx);
```

```
for(i in 1:nx){
  S[i]=u[i];
  I[i]=u[i+nx];
  R[i]=u[i+2*nx];
}
```

- The product of the two dependent variables of the terms $\pm r_{si} SI$ of eqs. (3.2a,b) is placed in SI.

```
#
# S*I
  SI=rep(0,nx);
  for(i in 1:nx){SI[i]=S[i]*I[i];}
```

- The derivatives $\dfrac{\partial S}{\partial x}, \dfrac{\partial I}{\partial x}, \dfrac{\partial R}{\partial x}$ are computed by dss004.

```
#
# Sx,Ix,Rx
  Sx=dss004(xl,xu,nx,S);
  Ix=dss004(xl,xu,nx,I);
  Rx=dss004(xl,xu,nx,R);
```

- BCs (3.4) are implemented (the subscripts 1,nx correspond to $x = x_l, x_u$).

```
#
# BCs
  Sx[1]=0;Sx[nx]=0;
  Ix[1]=0;Ix[nx]=0;
  Rx[1]=0;Rx[nx]=0;
```

- The derivatives $\dfrac{\partial^2 S}{\partial x^2}, \dfrac{\partial^2 I}{\partial x^2}, \dfrac{\partial^2 I}{\partial x^2}$ are computed by differentiating the first derivatives (stagewise or successive differentiation).

```
#
# Sxx,Ixx,Rxx
```

```
Sxx=dss004(xl,xu,nx,Sx);
Ixx=dss004(xl,xu,nx,Ix);
Rxx=dss004(xl,xu,nx,Rx);
```

- The cross second derivative is programmed as

$$\frac{\partial^2 SI}{\partial x^2} = \frac{\partial \left(\dfrac{\partial SI}{\partial x} \right)}{\partial x}$$

```
#
# SIx,SIxx
SIx=dss004(xl,xu,nx,SI)  ;
SIxx=dss004(xl,xu,nx,SIx);
```

- Eqs. (3.2) are programmed.

```
#
# PDEs
St=rep(0,nx);It=rep(0,nx);Rt=rep(0,nx);
for(i in 1:nx){
   St[i]=D_si*SIxx[i]+D_s*Sxx[i]+r_p1*S[i]-
        r_si*SI[i];
   It[i]=D_si*SIxx[i]+D_i*Ixx[i]+r_p2*I[i]+
        r_si*SI[i]-r_i*I[i];
   Rt[i]=D_r*Rxx[i]+r_p3*R[i]+r_i*I[i];
}
```

The four second derivatives in x with diffusivities D_s, D_i, D_r, D_{si} are clear.

- The derivatives $\dfrac{\partial S}{\partial t}, \dfrac{\partial I}{\partial t}, \dfrac{\partial R}{\partial t}$, (LHSs of eqs. (3.2)) are placed in ut.

```
#
# Three vectors to one vector
ut=rep(0,3*nx);
```

```
for(i in 1:nx){
  ut[i]      =St[i];
  ut[i+nx]   =It[i];
  ut[i+2*nx]=Rt[i];
}
```

- The counter for the calls to pde1a is incremented and returned to the main program of Listing 3.1 with <<-.

```
#
# Increment calls to pde1a
  ncall <<- ncall+1;
```

- ut is returned to lsodes as a list (required by lsodes). c is the R vector utility.

```
#
# Return derivative vector
  return(list(c(ut)));
}
```

The final } concludes pde1a.

The output from the main program and subordinate routine of Listings 3.1, 3.2 is considered next.

(3.2.3) Model output

For ncase=1, the model is the same as eq. (2.1), (2.2), (2.3) (since the cross diffusion term is deleted through $D_{si} = 0$). Consequently, the solutions are the same as in Table 2.1, Figs. (2.1a,b,c) and are therefore not repeated here.

For ncase=2, the model has cross diffusion only (the linear diffusion is dropped through $D_s = D_i = D_r = 0$). Abbreviated numerical output is in Table 3.1.

[1] 6

[1] 154

t	x	S(x,t)	I(x,t)	R(x,t)
0.00	-1.0	1.000e+00	3.720e-44	0.000e+00
0.00	-0.8	1.000e+00	1.604e-28	0.000e+00
0.00	-0.6	1.000e+00	2.320e-16	0.000e+00
0.00	-0.4	1.000e+00	1.125e-07	0.000e+00
0.00	-0.2	1.000e+00	1.832e-02	0.000e+00
0.00	0.0	1.000e+00	1.000e+00	0.000e+00
0.00	0.2	1.000e+00	1.832e-02	0.000e+00
0.00	0.4	1.000e+00	1.125e-07	0.000e+00
0.00	0.6	1.000e+00	2.320e-16	0.000e+00
0.00	0.8	1.000e+00	1.604e-28	0.000e+00
0.00	1.0	1.000e+00	3.720e-44	0.000e+00

.   .
.   .
.   .

Output for t=0.02,..., 0.08 removed

.   .
.   .
.   .

t	x	S(x,t)	I(x,t)	R(x,t)
0.10	-1.0	9.997e-01	-2.771e-03	-4.262e-04
0.10	-0.8	1.003e+00	8.159e-04	1.330e-04
0.10	-0.6	1.010e+00	1.051e-02	2.738e-03
0.10	-0.4	1.027e+00	5.283e-02	2.594e-02
0.10	-0.2	9.672e-01	1.266e-01	1.312e-01
0.10	0.0	3.511e-01	3.903e-01	5.697e-01
0.10	0.2	9.672e-01	1.266e-01	1.312e-01
0.10	0.4	1.027e+00	5.283e-02	2.594e-02
0.10	0.6	1.010e+00	1.051e-02	2.738e-03
0.10	0.8	1.003e+00	8.159e-04	1.330e-04
0.10	1.0	9.997e-01	-2.771e-03	-4.262e-04

```
ncall =    264
```

Table 3.1: Abbreviated output for eqs. (3.2), (3.3), (3.4),
ncase=2

We can note the following details about this output.

- The dimensions of the solution matrix out are *nout* $\times$ $3nx+1 = 6 \times 3(51)+1 = 154$. The offset $+1$ results from the value of t as the first element in each of the *nout* $= 6$ solution vectors. These same values of t are in tout,
- ICs (3.3) $(t = 0)$ are verified for $f_1(x)$, $f_2(x)$, $f_3(x)$.
- The output is for $x = -1, -0.8, ...1$ as programmed in Listing 3.1 (51 values at each value of t with every fifth value in x).
- The output is for $t = 0, 0.02, ..., 0.1$ as programmed in Listing 3.1.
- $S(x, t)$, $R(x, t)$ depart from their initial values as a consequence of the input from $I(x, t)$.
- The computational effort is modest, ncall = 264, indicating lsodes efficiently computes a solution to the 153 MOL/ODEs.

The graphical output is in Figs. 3.1a,b,c.

Fig. 3.1a indicates the cross diffusion (D_si*SIxx) gives an initial increase above $S(x, t = 0) = 1$ of about 3% (at $t = 0.02$). The location of this increase in x is resolved with the following steps:

- The number of output points is increased by changing by=5 to by=1 in the numerical display of the solution (51 output values of x are displayed).
- The format for x is changed from %6.1f to %8.3f (and the label for x is moved two spaces to the right).

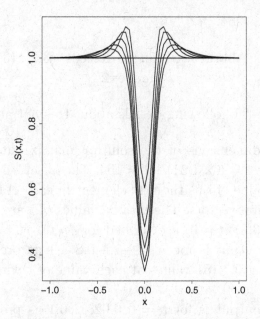

Figure 3.1a: Numerical solution $S(x,t)$ from eq. (3.2a), `ncase=2`

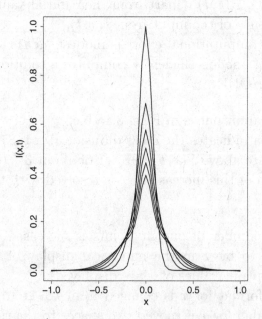

Figure 3.1b: Numerical solution $I(x,t)$ from eq. (3.2b), `ncase=2`

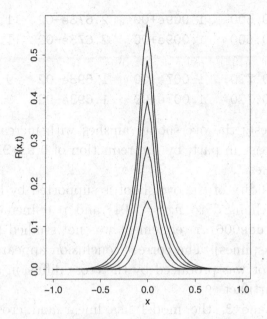

Figure 3.1c: Numerical solution $R(x,t)$ from eq. (3.2c), `ncase=2`

The output that results includes

```
    t       x       S(x,t)          I(x,t)          R(x,t)
  0.02   -0.280   1.033e+00       8.913e-02       1.361e-02
  0.02    0.280   1.033e+00       8.913e-02       1.361e-02
```

Thus, at $t = 0.02$, $x = \pm0.28$, $S(x, t = 0) = 1$ is exceeded by 0.033.

This overshoot decreases with increasing t and a shift in x toward the boundaries. For example,

```
    t       x       S(x,t)          I(x,t)          R(x,t)
  0.04   -0.400   1.020e+00       5.304e-02       1.470e-02
  0.04    0.400   1.020e+00       5.304e-02       1.470e-02

  0.06   -0.520   1.013e+00       3.231e-02       1.218e-02
  0.06    0.520   1.013e+00       3.231e-02       1.218e-02
```

```
0..08   -0.600   1.009e+00   2.673e-02   1.322e-02
0.08    0.600    1.009e+00   2.673e-02   1.322e-02

0.10   -0.720    1.007e+00   1.693e-02   9.477e-03
0.10    0.720    1.007e+00   1.693e-02   9.477e-03
```

which suggests the overshoot vanishes with increasing t. This is due, at least in part, by the reduction of D_si*SIxx through smaller values I.

The validity of the overshoot is supported by h refinement ($nx = 51$ changed to $nx = 101$) and p refinement (dss004 changed to dss006). r refinement was not studied (e.g., changing FDs to splines). The correct conclusion appears to be that the overshoot was produced by the cross diffusion and is not a numerical artifact.

For ncase=3, the model has linear and cross diffusion. Abbreviated numerical output is in Table 3.2.

[1] 6

[1] 154

```
   t      x      S(x,t)      I(x,t)      R(x,t)
 0.00   -1.0   1.000e+00   3.720e-44   0.000e+00
 0.00   -0.8   1.000e+00   1.604e-28   0.000e+00
 0.00   -0.6   1.000e+00   2.320e-16   0.000e+00
 0.00   -0.4   1.000e+00   1.125e-07   0.000e+00
 0.00   -0.2   1.000e+00   1.832e-02   0.000e+00
 0.00    0.0   1.000e+00   1.000e+00   0.000e+00
 0.00    0.2   1.000e+00   1.832e-02   0.000e+00
 0.00    0.4   1.000e+00   1.125e-07   0.000e+00
 0.00    0.6   1.000e+00   2.320e-16   0.000e+00
 0.00    0.8   1.000e+00   1.604e-28   0.000e+00
 0.00    1.0   1.000e+00   3.720e-44   0.000e+00
```

```
        Output for t=0.02,..., 0.08 removed
```

t	x	S(x,t)	I(x,t)	R(x,t)
0.10	-1.0	1.004e+00	3.578e-03	1.248e-03
0.10	-0.8	1.006e+00	9.838e-03	4.748e-03
0.10	-0.6	1.002e+00	3.478e-02	2.415e-02
0.10	-0.4	9.452e-01	8.754e-02	8.370e-02
0.10	-0.2	8.146e-01	1.601e-01	1.860e-01
0.10	0.0	7.357e-01	2.007e-01	2.458e-01
0.10	0.2	8.146e-01	1.601e-01	1.860e-01
0.10	0.4	9.452e-01	8.754e-02	8.370e-02
0.10	0.6	1.002e+00	3.478e-02	2.415e-02
0.10	0.8	1.006e+00	9.838e-03	4.748e-03
0.10	1.0	1.004e+00	3.578e-03	1.248e-03

```
ncall =   272
```

Table 3.2: Abbreviated output for eqs. (3.2), (3.3), (3.4),
ncase=3

We can note the following details about this output.

- The dimensions of the solution matrix out are again $nout \times 3nx + 1 = 6 \times 3(51) + 1 = 154$.
- ICs (3.3) ($t = 0$) are verified for $f_1(x)$, $f_2(x)$, $f_3(x)$.
- The output is for $x = -1, -0.8, ...1$ as programmed in Listing 3.1 (51 values at each value of t with every fifth value in x).
- The output is for $t = 0, 0.02, ..., 0.1$ as programmed in Listing 3.1.

- $S(x,t)$, $R(x,t)$ depart from their initial values as a consequence of the input from $I(x,t)$.
- The effect of cross diffusion on $S(x,t)$ is diminished (`ncase=3` rather than `ncase=2`). This is reflected in the following comparison.

```
Table 3.1 (ncase=2)
  0.10    0.0    3.511e-01    3.903e-01    5.697e-01

Table 3.2 (ncase=3)
  0.10    0.0    7.357e-01    2.007e-01    2.458e-01
```

In other words, the linear diffusion diminishes the effect of the cross diffusion on $S(x = 0, t)$ (but the $S(x,t)$ is more disperse in x).

- The computational effort is modest, `ncall = 272`.

The graphical output is in Figs. 3.2a,b,c.

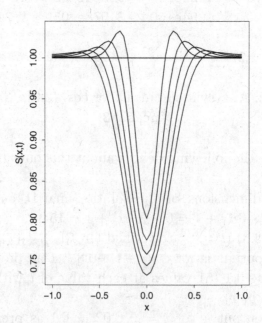

Figure 3.2a: Numerical solution $S(x,t)$ from eq. (3.2a), `ncase=3`

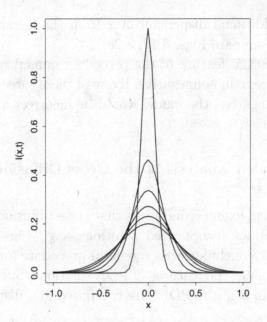

Figure 3.2b: Numerical solution $I(x,t)$ from eq. (3.2b), `ncase=3`

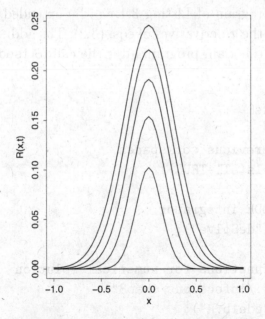

Figure 3.2c: Numerical solution $R(x,t)$ from eq. (3.2c), `ncase=3`

The additional dispersion in x from the linear diffusion is clear (e.g., compare Figs. 3.1c, 3.2c).

An essential feature of the preceding numerical solution is that S,I,R remain nonnegative. If any of these three populations should be negative, the model would be incorrect and therefore require revision.

(3.3) Detailed Analysis of the Cross Diffusion PDEs

The preceding example indicates that cross diffusion PDE models can produce complicated solutions, e.g., Figs. 3.1a, 3.2a. This chapter concludes with a general procedure for elucidating what determines the features of PDE solutions. Specifically, the derivatives in x in the PDEs are computed and displayed.

(3.3.1) Main program

The main program of Listing 3.1 can be extended to compute and display the x derivatives of eqs. (3.2). The additional coding is added to the main program after the call to lsodes.

```
#
# SIRC model
#
# Delete previous workspaces
  rm(list=ls(all=TRUE))
#
# Access ODE integrator
  library("deSolve");
#
# Access functions for numerical solution
  setwd("f:/infectious/chap3");
  source("pde1b.R");
  source("dss004.R");
```

```
#
# Parameters
  f1=function(x) 1;
  f2=function(x) exp(-100*x^2);
  f3=function(x) 0;
  r_p1=0.02;r_p2=0.02;r_p3=0.02;
  r_si=10;r_i=10;
#
# Select case
  ncase=1;
  if(ncase==1){D_s=0.25;D_i=0.25;D_r=0.25;D_si=0;    }
  if(ncase==2){D_s=0;   D_i=0;   D_r=0;   D_si=0.25;}
  if(ncase==3){D_s=0.25;D_i=0.25;D_r=0.25;D_si=0.25;}
#
# Spatial grid (in x)
  nx=51;
  xl=-1;xu=1;
  x=seq(from=xl,to=xu,by=(xu-xl)/(nx-1));
#
# Independent variable for ODE integration
  t0=0;tf=0.1;nout=6;
  tout=seq(from=t0,to=tf,by=(tf-t0)/(nout-1));
#
# Initial condition (t=0)
  u0=rep(0,3*nx);
  for(i in 1:nx){
    u0[i]      =f1(x[i]);
    u0[i+nx]   =f2(x[i]);
    u0[i+2*nx]=f3(x[i]);
  }
  ncall=0;
#
# ODE integration
  out=lsodes(y=u0,times=tout,func=pde1b,
```

```
      sparsetype="sparseint",rtol=1e-6,
      atol=1e-6,maxord=5);
  nrow(out)
  ncol(out)
#
# Display PDE solutions
#
# S,I,R
  S=matrix(0,nrow=nx,ncol=nout);
  I=matrix(0,nrow=nx,ncol=nout);
  R=matrix(0,nrow=nx,ncol=nout);
  for(it in 1:nout){
    for(i in 1:nx){
      S[i,it]=out[it,i+1];
      I[i,it]=out[it,i+1+nx];
      R[i,it]=out[it,i+1+2*nx];
    }
  }
#
# Arrays for x derivatives
    SI=matrix(0,nrow=nx,ncol=nout);
    Sx=matrix(0,nrow=nx,ncol=nout);
    Ix=matrix(0,nrow=nx,ncol=nout);
    Rx=matrix(0,nrow=nx,ncol=nout);
   SIx=matrix(0,nrow=nx,ncol=nout);
   Sxx=matrix(0,nrow=nx,ncol=nout);
   Ixx=matrix(0,nrow=nx,ncol=nout);
   Rxx=matrix(0,nrow=nx,ncol=nout);
  SIxx=matrix(0,nrow=nx,ncol=nout);
#
# S,I,R,SI x derivatives
  for(it in 1:nout){
    SI[,it]=S[,it]*I[,it];
    Sx[,it]=dss004(xl,xu,nx,S[,it]);
```

```
   Ix[,it]=dss004(xl,xu,nx,I[,it]);
   Rx[,it]=dss004(xl,xu,nx,R[,it]);
  SIx[,it]=dss004(xl,xu,nx,SI[,it]);
  }
#
# BCs
  Sx[1]=0;Sx[nx]=0;
  Ix[1]=0;Ix[nx]=0;
  Rx[1]=0;Rx[nx]=0;
#
# Sx,Ix,Rx,SIx x derivatives
  for(it in 1:nout){
   Sxx[,it]=dss004(xl,xu,nx,Sx[,it]);
   Ixx[,it]=dss004(xl,xu,nx,Ix[,it]);
   Rxx[,it]=dss004(xl,xu,nx,Rx[,it]);
  SIxx[,it]=dss004(xl,xu,nx,SIx[,it]);
#
# Display S,I,R,SI x, xx derivatives
    iv=seq(from=1,to=nx,by=5);
    for(i in iv){
    cat(sprintf("\n       t      x\n"));
    cat(sprintf("            S            I
                         R         SI\n"));
    cat(sprintf("            Sx           Ix
                         Rx        SIx\n"));
    cat(sprintf("            Sxx          Ixx
                         Rxx       SIxx\n"));
      cat(sprintf("%6.2f %5.1f\n",
          tout[it],x[i]));
      cat(sprintf("%12.3e %10.3e %10.3e %10.3e\n",
          S[i,it], I[i,it], R[i,it], SI[i,it]));
      cat(sprintf("%12.3e %10.3e %10.3e %10.3e\n",
          Sx[i,it], Ix[i,it], Rx[i,it], SIx[i,it]));
      cat(sprintf("%12.3e %10.3e %10.3e %10.3e\n",
```

```
         Sxx[i,it],Ixx[i,it],Rxx[i,it],SIxx[i,it]));
   }
 }
#
# Plot S,I,R,SI x, xx derivatives (12 plots)
#
# S
  par(mfrow=c(1,1));
  matplot(x=x,y=S,type="l",xlab="x",ylab="S(x,t)",
    xlim=c(xl,xu),lty=1,main="",lwd=2,col="black");
#
# I
  par(mfrow=c(1,1));
  matplot(x=x,y=I,type="l",xlab="x",ylab="I(x,t)",
    xlim=c(xl,xu),lty=1,main="",lwd=2,col="black");
#
# R
  par(mfrow=c(1,1));
  matplot(x=x,y=R,type="l",xlab="x",ylab="R(x,t)",
    xlim=c(xl,xu),lty=1,main="",lwd=2,col="black");
#
# SI
  par(mfrow=c(1,1));
  matplot(x=x,y=SI,type="l",xlab="x",ylab="SI(x,t)",
    xlim=c(xl,xu),lty=1,main="",lwd=2,col="black");
#
# Sx
  par(mfrow=c(1,1));
  matplot(x=x,y=Sx,type="l",xlab="x",ylab="Sx(x,t)",
    xlim=c(xl,xu),lty=1,main="",lwd=2,col="black");
#
# Ix
  par(mfrow=c(1,1));
  matplot(x=x,y=Ix,type="l",xlab="x",ylab="Ix(x,t)",
```

```
    xlim=c(xl,xu),lty=1,main="",lwd=2,col="black");
#
# Rx
  par(mfrow=c(1,1));
  matplot(x=x,y=Rx,type="l",xlab="x",ylab="Rx(x,t)",
    xlim=c(xl,xu),lty=1,main="",lwd=2,col="black");
#
# SIx
  par(mfrow=c(1,1));
  matplot(
    x=x,y=SIx,type="l",xlab="x",ylab="SIx(x,t)",
    xlim=c(xl,xu),lty=1,main="",lwd=2,col="black");
#
# Sxx
  par(mfrow=c(1,1));
  matplot(
    x=x,y=Sxx,type="l",xlab="x",ylab="Sxx(x,t)",
    xlim=c(xl,xu),lty=1,main="",lwd=2,col="black");
#
# Ixx
  par(mfrow=c(1,1));
  matplot(
    x=x,y=Ixx,type="l",xlab="x",ylab="Ixx(x,t)",
    xlim=c(xl,xu),lty=1,main="",lwd=2,col="black");
#
# Rxx
  par(mfrow=c(1,1));
  matplot(
    x=x,y=Rxx,type="l",xlab="x",ylab="Rxx(x,t)",
    xlim=c(xl,xu),lty=1,main="",lwd=2,col="black");
#
# SIxx
  par(mfrow=c(1,1));
  matplot(
```

```
    x=x,y=SIxx,type="l",xlab="x",ylab="SIxx(x,t)",
    xlim=c(xl,xu),lty=1,main="",lwd=2,col="black");
#
# Calls to ODE routine
  cat(sprintf("\n\n ncall = %5d\n\n",ncall));
```

Listing 3.3: Extended output from the main program for eqs.
(3.2), (3.3), (3.4)

We can note the following details about Listing 3.3.

- The code before the call to `lsodes` is the same as in Listing 3.1 except for the change in the name of the ODE/MOL routine from `pde1a` to `pde1b` (these two routines are the same, but given different names to distinguish the two cases of basic and extended output).
- `S,I,R` are placed in arrays for display as in Listing 3.1.

```
    #
    # Display PDE solutions
    #
    # S,I,R
      S=matrix(0,nrow=nx,ncol=nout);
      I=matrix(0,nrow=nx,ncol=nout);
      R=matrix(0,nrow=nx,ncol=nout);
      for(it in 1:nout){
        for(i in 1:nx){
          S[i,it]=out[it,i+1];
          I[i,it]=out[it,i+1+nx];
          R[i,it]=out[it,i+1+2*nx];
        }
      }
```

- Arrays for SI to $\dfrac{\partial^2 SI}{\partial x^2}$ (SIxx) are defined.

```
#
# Arrays for x derivatives
   SI=matrix(0,nrow=nx,ncol=nout);
   Sx=matrix(0,nrow=nx,ncol=nout);
   Ix=matrix(0,nrow=nx,ncol=nout);
   Rx=matrix(0,nrow=nx,ncol=nout);
  SIx=matrix(0,nrow=nx,ncol=nout);
  Sxx=matrix(0,nrow=nx,ncol=nout);
  Ixx=matrix(0,nrow=nx,ncol=nout);
  Rxx=matrix(0,nrow=nx,ncol=nout);
 SIxx=matrix(0,nrow=nx,ncol=nout);
```

- SI and the first derivatives in x are computed, concluding
  with $\dfrac{\partial SI}{\partial x} = SIx$.

```
#
# S,I,R,SI x derivatives
  for(it in 1:nout){
    SI[,it]=S[,it]*I[,it];
    Sx[,it]=dss004(xl,xu,nx,S[,it]);
    Ix[,it]=dss004(xl,xu,nx,I[,it]);
    Rx[,it]=dss004(xl,xu,nx,R[,it]);
    SIx[,it]=dss004(xl,xu,nx,SI[,it]);
  }
```

dss004 requires a 1D vector of values to be differentiated as the fourth input argument. This is accomplished
by using [,it] as the subscripting for the 2D matrices
S,I,R,SI, that is, all x referenced with , for particular
t referenced with it.

Similarly, dss004 returns a 1D vector of first derivatives which is specified with [,it] for the 2D matrices
Si,Sx,Ix,Rx,SIx.

- S,I,R homogeneous Neumann Bcs are defined.

```
#
# BCs
  Sx[1]=0;Sx[nx]=0;
  Ix[1]=0;Ix[nx]=0;
  Rx[1]=0;Rx[nx]=0;
```

- The second derivatives in x are computed, concluding with $\dfrac{\partial^2 SI}{\partial x^2} = \text{SIxx}$.

```
#
# Sx,Ix,Rx,SIx x derivatives
  for(it in 1:nout){
    Sxx[,it]=dss004(xl,xu,nx,Sx[,it]);
    Ixx[,it]=dss004(xl,xu,nx,Ix[,it]);
    Rxx[,it]=dss004(xl,xu,nx,Rx[,it]);
    SIxx[,it]=dss004(xl,xu,nx,SIx[,it]);
```

Again, [,it] is used to reference 2D matrices in applying differentiation in x a second time.

- S,I,R and the derivatives in x are displayed numerically with every fifth value of x from by=5.

```
#
# Display S,I,R,SI x, xx derivatives
    iv=seq(from=1,to=nx,by=5);
    for(i in iv){
    cat(sprintf("\n      t      x\n"));
    cat(sprintf("              S              I
                        R            SI\n"));
    cat(sprintf("             Sx             Ix
                        Rx           SIx\n"));
    cat(sprintf("            Sxx            Ixx
                        Rxx          SIxx\n"));
      cat(sprintf("%6.2f %5.1f\n",
          tout[it],x[i]));
```

```
      cat(sprintf(
        "%12.3e %10.3e %10.3e %10.3e\n",
        S[i,it],  I[i,it],  R[i,it],  SI[i,it]));
      cat(sprintf(
        "%12.3e %10.3e %10.3e %10.3e\n",
        Sx[i,it], Ix[i,it], Rx[i,it], SIx[i,it]));
      cat(sprintf(
        "%12.3e %10.3e %10.3e %10.3e\n",
        Sxx[i,it],Ixx[i,it],Rxx[i,it],SIxx[i,it]));
    }
  }
```

- $S(x,t)$ to $\dfrac{\partial^2 SI}{\partial x^2}$ are plotted against x with t as a parameter.

```
#
# Plot S,I,R,SI x, xx derivatives (12 plots)
#
# S
  par(mfrow=c(1,1));
  matplot(
    x=x,y=S,type="l",xlab="x",ylab="S(x,t)",
    xlim=c(xl,xu),lty=1,main="",lwd=2,
    col="black");
```

```
#
# SIxx
  par(mfrow=c(1,1));
  matplot(
    x=x,y=SIxx,type="l",xlab="x",ylab="SIxx(x,t)",
    xlim=c(xl,xu),lty=1,main="",lwd=2,
    col="black");
```

- The number of calls to **pde1b** is displayed at the end of the solution.

```
#
# Calls to ODE routine
  cat(sprintf("\n\n ncall = %5d\n\n",ncall));
```

(3.3.2) ODE/MOL routine

As noted previously, **pde1b** is the same as **pde1a** of Listing 3.2, except for the change of name, so it is not listed here.

(3.3.3) Model output

The extensive numerical and graphical output from the preceding coding is presented next in abbreviated form for **ncase=3** in Listing 3.1.

[1] 6

[1] 154

t	x			
	S	I	R	SI
	Sx	Ix	Rx	SIx
	Sxx	Ixx	Rxx	SIxx
0.00	-1.0			
	1.000e+00	3.720e-44	0.000e+00	3.720e-44
	0.000e+00	0.000e+00	0.000e+00	-1.411e-30
	0.000e+00	1.043e-24	0.000e+00	1.043e-24

t	x			
	S	I	R	SI
	Sx	Ix	Rx	SIx
	Sxx	Ixx	Rxx	SIxx
0.00	-0.8			

```
1.000e+00   1.604e-28   0.000e+00   1.604e-28
0.000e+00  -6.245e-23   0.000e+00  -6.245e-23
0.000e+00   6.493e-18   0.000e+00   6.493e-18
              .                         .
              .                         .
              .                         .

       Output for x = -0.6,...,0.6 removed
              .                         .
              .                         .
              .                         .


   t    x
        S           I           R           SI
        Sx          Ix          Rx          SIx
        Sxx         Ixx         Rxx         SIxx
0.00    0.8
1.000e+00   1.604e-28   0.000e+00   1.604e-28
0.000e+00   6.245e-23   0.000e+00   6.245e-23
0.000e+00   6.493e-18   0.000e+00   6.493e-18


   t    x
        S           I           R           SI
        Sx          Ix          Rx          SIx
        Sxx         Ixx         Rxx         SIxx
0.00    1.0
1.000e+00   3.720e-44   0.000e+00   3.720e-44
0.000e+00   0.000e+00   0.000e+00   1.411e-30
0.000e+00   1.043e-24   0.000e+00   1.043e-24
              .                         .
              .                         .
              .                         .

       Output for t = 0.02,...,0.08 removed
              .                         .
              .                         .
              .                         .
```

```
                S           I           R           SI
               Sx          Ix          Rx          SIx
              Sxx         Ixx         Rxx         SIxx
    0.10   -1.0
         1.004e+00   3.578e-03   1.248e-03   3.594e-03
        -1.632e-05   8.648e-05   6.133e-05   8.746e-05
         1.209e-01   2.785e-01   1.368e-01   2.801e-01


       t     x
                S           I           R           SI
               Sx          Ix          Rx          SIx
              Sxx         Ixx         Rxx         SIxx
    0.10   -0.8
         1.006e+00   9.838e-03   4.748e-03   9.898e-03
         1.297e-02   6.862e-02   4.215e-02   6.917e-02
        -7.290e-02   4.580e-01   3.571e-01   4.619e-01


                      .            .
                      .            .
                      .            .

          Output for x = -0.6,...,0.6 removed

                      .            .
                      .            .
                      .            .


       t     x
                S           I           R           SI
               Sx          Ix          Rx          SIx
              Sxx         Ixx         Rxx         SIxx
    0.10    0.8
         1.006e+00   9.838e-03   4.748e-03   9.898e-03
        -1.297e-02  -6.862e-02  -4.215e-02  -6.917e-02
        -7.290e-02   4.580e-01   3.571e-01   4.619e-01


       t     x
                S           I           R           SI
```

	Sx	Ix	Rx	SIx
	Sxx	Ixx	Rxx	SIxx
0.10	1.0			
	1.004e+00	3.578e-03	1.248e-03	3.594e-03
	1.630e-05	-8.649e-05	-6.133e-05	-8.748e-05
	1.209e-01	2.785e-01	1.368e-01	2.801e-01

ncall =   272

Table 3.3: Abbreviated output for eqs. (3.2), (3.3), (3.4),
ncase=3

An understanding of the solution is facilitated by the graphical output. For example, Figs. 3.3,a,b,c are the three plots pertaining to SI in eqs. (3.2a,b).

These plots demonstrate that each of the RHS terms of a PDE system can be computed from the numerical solutions. Further, if all of the RHS terms are computed and summed, they give the LHS derivatives in t which provides a direct indication of

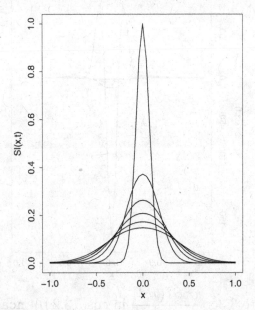

Figure 3.3a: $SI(x, t)$ in eqs. (3.2,b), ncase=3

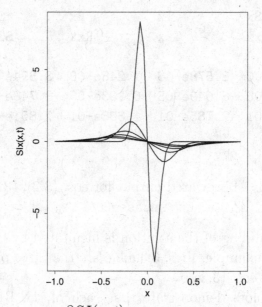

Figure 3.3b: $\dfrac{\partial SI(x,t)}{\partial x}$ in eqs. (3.2,b), ncase=3

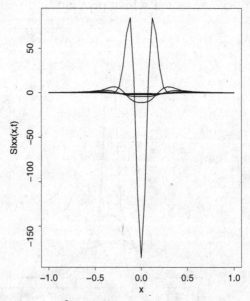

Figure 3.3c: $\dfrac{\partial^2 SI(x,t)}{\partial x^2}$ in eqs. (3.2,b), ncase=3

how the solutions evolve through integration of the MOL/ODEs. The calculation of the LHS of eqs. (3.2) is illustrated with the following extension of the main program of Listing 3.3.

- The code before the calculation of $\frac{\partial^2 SI}{\partial x^2} = $ SIxx is the same as in Listing 3.3 except for the change in the name of the ODE/MOL routine from pde1b to pde1c (these two routines are the same, but given different names to distinguish the two cases of extended and t derivative output).

- Arrays for the t derivatives $\frac{\partial S}{\partial t}, \frac{\partial I}{\partial t}, \frac{\partial R}{\partial t}$ are declared,

```
#
# t derivatives
  St=matrix(0,nrow=nx,ncol=nout);
  It=matrix(0,nrow=nx,ncol=nout);
  Rt=matrix(0,nrow=nx,ncol=nout);
```

- The RHS terms of eqs. (3.2) are summed to give the LHS t derivatives.

```
#
# PDEs
  for(it in 1:nout){
    for(i in 1:nx){
      St[i,it]=D_si*SIxx[i,it]+D_s*Sxx[i,it]+
               r_p1*S[i,it]-r_si*SI[i,it];
      It[i,it]=D_si*SIxx[i,it]+D_i*Ixx[i,it]+
               r_p2*I[i,it]+r_si*SI[i,it]-
               r_i*I[i,it];
      Rt[i,it]=D_r*Rxx[i,it]+r_p3*R[i,it]+
               r_i*I[i,it];
    }
  }
```

This code is taken from `pde1c` with the addition of a second subscript `it` to include the variation in t (the outer `for`).

- The t derivatives are plotted.

```
#
# Plot St,It,Rt
#
# St
  par(mfrow=c(1,1));
  matplot(
    x=x,y=St,type="l",xlab="x",ylab="St(x,t)",
    xlim=c(xl,xu),lty=1,main="",lwd=2,
    col="black");
#
# It
  par(mfrow=c(1,1));
  matplot(
    x=x,y=It,type="l",xlab="x",ylab="It(x,t)",
    xlim=c(xl,xu),lty=1,main="",lwd=2,
    col="black");
#
# Rt
  par(mfrow=c(1,1));
  matplot(
    x=x,y=Rt,type="l",xlab="x",ylab="Rt(x,t)",
    xlim=c(xl,xu),lty=1,main="",lwd=2,
    col="black");
```

Listing 3.4: Calculation of t derivatives for eqs. (3.2), (3.3), (3.4)

The numerical output is limited to

```
[1]  6
```

```
[1]  154
```

```
ncall =    272
```

The graphical output is in Figs. 3.4a,b,c.

Figs. 3.4a,b,c appear to indicate that the solutions are approaching an equilibrium (steady state) solution with $\dfrac{\partial S(x, t \to \infty)}{\partial t} = \dfrac{\partial I(x, t \to \infty)}{\partial t} = \dfrac{\partial R(x, t \to \infty)}{\partial t} = 0$. In other words, the solution for $S(x, t), I(x, t), R(x, t)$ appears to be stable (as also indicated in Figs. 3.1a,b,c) and the infecteds decay with t as the recovereds increase.

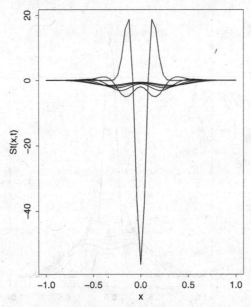

Figure 3.4a: $\dfrac{\partial S(x, t)}{\partial t}$ in eqs. (3.2,b), ncase=3

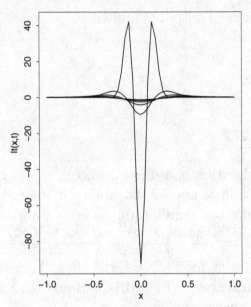

Figure 3.4b: $\dfrac{\partial I(x,t)}{\partial t}$ in eqs. (3.2,b), ncase=3

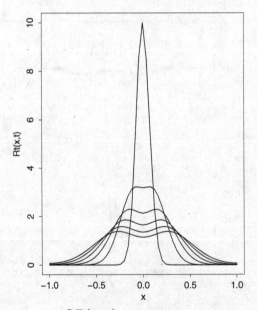

Figure 3.4c: $\dfrac{\partial R(x,t)}{\partial t}$ in eqs. (3.2,b), ncase=3

Fig. (3.4a) provides an explanation of the 3% overshoot in $S(x, t = 0.02)$ discussed previously. Specifically, $\dfrac{\partial S(x, t)}{\partial t}$ is positive at approximately where the overshoot occurs. This positive derivative decays with t, as does the overshoot in Fig. 3.1a.

The source of the positive derivative $\dfrac{\partial S(x, t)}{\partial t}$ can be ascertained by considering the relative magnitudes of all of the RHS terms of eq. (3.2a). SI and the derivatives in x were computed and displayed previously, so the only additional term to be examined is $r_{p1}S$. This is left as an exercise for the reader, and in particular, to look at the relative contributions of the RHS terms of eq. (3.2a).

This detailed insight into the PDE solutions can demonstrate the contributions of the individual terms which can be used for refinement of the models such as the addition, deletion or revision of the terms. Also, the addition of PDEs is straightforward. This detailed analysis is essential in the development of PDE models.

Two additional points can be added at this point.

(1) The expanded form of $\dfrac{\partial^2 SI}{\partial x^2}$ in eq. (3.1c)

$$D_{si}\left(S\frac{\partial I}{\partial x} + I\frac{\partial S}{\partial x}\right)$$

has an interpretation of the corresponding diffusion. $D_{si}S\dfrac{\partial I}{\partial x}$ represents chemotaxis[4] in eq. (3.1a) and $D_{si}I\dfrac{\partial S}{\partial x}$ represents nonlinear diffusion (with the diffusivity $D_{si}I$). Thus, if these

---

[4]Chemotaxis has the feature of a diffusivity as a function of the PDE dependent variable, e.g., $D_{si}S$ for eq. (3.2a), and a gradient of another dependent variable, e.g., $\dfrac{\partial I}{\partial x}$.

terms are used one at a time, chemotaxis and nonlinear diffusion in eq. (3.2a) can be studied separately.

Conversely, $D_{si}S\dfrac{\partial I}{\partial x}$ is nonlinear diffusion in eq. (3.2b) and $D_{si}I\dfrac{\partial S}{\partial x}$ is chemotaxis.

(2) The spatial interval $-1 \leq x \leq 1$ is nondimensionalized to ± 1 at the boundaries $x = x_l, x_u$. If dimensional boundaries are of interest, the diffusivities which define the spatial scale of the model can be adjusted accordingly. For example, if the boundaries are ± 100 km and the diffusivity units are km^2/yr, the diffusivities are multiplied by 100^2 and the Gaussian IC is changed to $I(x, t = 0) = e^{-0.01x^2}$ to obtain the same solution as for ± 1.

(3.4) Summary and Conclusions

The examples, in this chapter demonstrate

- The addition of PDEs to a model, e.g., a $R(x, t)$ balance added to the SI model of Chapter 1 to give a SIR model.
- The formulation of a SIRC model, including the special case of a constant total population (eq. (2.4h)).
- Numerical and graphical output for the solutions as a function of x and parameterized in t (solutions as a function of t at a particular x are illustrated in Chapter 2).
- The use of cross diffusion to represent the spatial distribution of SI interactions.
- The calculation of the RHS and LHS terms in the PDEs from the solutions.

The MOL analysis of these variants is straightforward and can be readily applied to other models as demonstrated in the next chapter with the use of different coordinate systems.

One possible complication of the various models considered previously and subsequently is the requirement to assign physically valid numerical values to the parameters, e.g., D_s, D_i, D_r, D_{si} in eqs. (3.2a,b). This is the *parameterization* requirement and the model may be *over-parameterized* in the sense that it contains parameters that might be considered physically meaningful, but are unavailable and/or unattainable numerically. In other words, in formulating a model, consideration should be given to whether the model parameters can be given estimated values that are physically realistic. The parameterization requirement is discussed in later chapters.

References

[1] Berres, S., and R. Ruiz-Baier (2011), A fully adaptive numerical approximation for a two-dimensional epidemic model with nonlinear cross-diffusion, *Nonlinear Analysis: Real World Applications*, **12**, pp 28882903

[2] Cai, Y., and W. Wang (2015), Stability and Hopf bifurcation of the stationary solutions to an epidemic model with cross-diffusion, *Computers and Mathematics with Applications*, **70**, no. 8, pp 1906-1920

[3] Ling, Z., L. Zhang and Z. Lin (2014), Turing pattern formation in a predatorprey system with cross diffusion, *Applied Mathmatical Modelling*, **38**, no. 2122, pp 5022-5032

[4] Ruiz-Baier, R., and C. Tian (2013), Mathematical analysis and numerical simulation of pattern formation under cross-diffusion, *Nonlinear Analysis: Real World Applications*, **14**, pp 601-612

[5] Tian,C., Z. Lin, and M. Pedersen (2010), Instability induced by cross-diffusion in reaction-diffusion systems, *Nonlinear Analysis: Real World Applications*, **11**, pp 1036-1045

[6] Zemskov, E.P., K. Kassner and M. J. B. Hauser (2008), Wavy fronts and speed bifurcation in excitable systems with cross diffusion, *Physical Review* **E 77**, pp 036219(1-6)

[7] Zenga, X., and Z. Liu (2010), Nonconstant positive steady states for a ratio-dependent predator-prey system with cross-diffusion, *Nonlinear Analysis: Real World Applications*, **11**, pp 372-390

Chapter 4

Alternative Coordinate Systems

(4.1) Introduction

In the preceding chapters, the PDE models were expressed in 1D Cartesian coordinates with spatial variable x. However, this geometric specification may not fit the physical system since the infectious disease evolution may occur over two dimensions, e.g., over a geographical area. Extension of the geometry to 2D via a second coordinate, that is, x, y has two possible problems.

- The number of grid points equals **nx*ny** which increases rapidly with **nx** and **ny** so that the number of MOL/ODEs is large (the so-called *curse of dimensionality*).
- Cartesian coordinates may not represent the physical system very well, particularly at the boundaries.

One approach to circumvent these difficulties is to use a coordinate system that more closely corresponds to the physical system. This alternative is considered in this chapter.

(4.2) Model in Radial Coordinates

To start, the PDE models considered previously can be expressed in coordinate-free format. For example, the SIR model of eqs. (3.2a,b,c) can be written as

$$\frac{\partial S}{\partial t} = D_s \nabla^2 S + D_{si} \nabla^2 SI + r_{p1} S - r_{si} SI \qquad (4.1a)$$

$$\frac{\partial I}{\partial t} = D_i \nabla^2 I + D_{si} \nabla^2 SI + r_{p2} I + r_{si} SI - r_i I \qquad (4.1b)$$

$$\frac{\partial R}{\partial t} = D_r \nabla^2 R + r_{p3} I + r_i I \qquad (4.1c)$$

The Laplacian in Cartesian coordinates is

$$\nabla^2 = \frac{\partial^2}{\partial x^2} + \frac{\partial^2}{\partial y^2} + \frac{\partial^2}{\partial z^2} \qquad (4.1d)$$

With only x considered, the second derivative $\dfrac{\partial^2}{\partial x^2}$ is used in eqs. (3.2a,b,c).

In cylindrical coordinates (r, θ, z), the Laplacian is

$$\nabla^2 = \frac{\partial^2}{\partial r^2} + \frac{1}{r} \frac{\partial}{\partial r} + \frac{1}{r^2} \frac{\partial^2}{\partial \theta^2} + \frac{\partial^2}{\partial z^2} \qquad (4.1e)$$

If an epidemic is considered to move radially from $r = 0$, with variations in θ, z neglected, the PDEs for S, I, R are

$$\frac{\partial S}{\partial t} = D_s \left(\frac{\partial^2 S}{\partial r^2} + \frac{1}{r} \frac{\partial S}{\partial r} \right) + D_{si} \left(\frac{\partial^2 SI}{\partial r^2} + \frac{1}{r} \frac{\partial SI}{\partial r} \right)$$

$$+ r_{p1} S - r_{si} SI \qquad (4.2a)$$

$$\frac{\partial I}{\partial t} = D_i \left(\frac{\partial^2 I}{\partial r^2} + \frac{1}{r} \frac{\partial I}{\partial r} \right) + D_{si} \left(\frac{\partial^2 SI}{\partial r^2} + \frac{1}{r} \frac{\partial SI}{\partial r} \right)$$

$$+ r_{p2} I + r_{si} SI - r_i I \qquad (4.2b)$$

$$\frac{\partial R}{\partial t} = D_r \left(\frac{\partial^2 R}{\partial r^2} + \frac{1}{r} \frac{\partial R}{\partial r} \right)$$

$$+ r_{p3}I + r_i I \tag{4.2c}$$

Eqs. (4.2) are first order in t and each requires one IC.

$$S(r, t = 0) = f_1(r); \quad I(r, t = 0) = f_2(r); \quad R(r, t = 0) = f_3(r)$$
$$\tag{4.3a,b,c}$$

Eqs. (4.2) are second order in r and each requires two BCs.

$$\frac{\partial S(r = 0, t)}{\partial r} = \frac{\partial S(r = r_0, t)}{\partial r} = 0 \tag{4.4a,b}$$

$$\frac{\partial I(r = 0, t)}{\partial r} = \frac{\partial I(r = r_0, t)}{\partial r} = 0 \tag{4.4c,d}$$

$$\frac{\partial R(r = 0, t)}{\partial r} = \frac{\partial R(r = r_0, t)}{\partial r} = 0 \tag{4.4e,f}$$

The *radial coordinate* form of eqs. (4.2) has the advantage of an outer boundary at $r = r_0$ that is circular, which better corresponds to the physical situation than a SIR model in 2D Cartesian coordinates (as well as the advantage of 1D rather than 2D).

The SIR model of eqs. (4.2), (4.3), (4.4) is next implemented with a main program and ODE/MOL routine, in analogy with the routines of Listings 3.1, 3.2.

(4.2.1) Main program

```
#
# SIRC model
#
# Delete previous workspaces
```

```
  rm(list=ls(all=TRUE))
#
# Access ODE integrator
  library("deSolve");
#
# Access functions for numerical solution
  setwd("f:/infectious/chap4");
  source("pde1a.R");
  source("dss044.R");
#
# Parameters
  f1=function(r) 1;
  f2=function(r) exp(-100*r^2);
  f3=function(r) 0;
  r_p1=0.02;r_p2=0.02;r_p3=0.02;
  r_si=10;r_i=10;
#
# Select case
  ncase=1;
  if(ncase==1){D_s=0.25;D_i=0.25;
                D_r=0.25;D_si=0    ;}
  if(ncase==2){D_s=0;    D_i=0;
                D_r=0;    D_si=0.25;}
  if(ncase==3){D_s=0.25; D_i=0.25;
                D_r=0.25;D_si=0.25;}
#
# Spatial grid (in r)
  nr=51;
  rl=0;ru=1;
  r=seq(from=rl,to=ru,by=(ru-rl)/(nr-1));
#
# Independent variable for ODE integration
  t0=0;tf=0.1;nout=6;
  tout=seq(from=t0,to=tf,by=(tf-t0)/(nout-1));
```

```
#
# Initial condition (t=0)
  u0=rep(0,3*nr);
  for(i in 1:nr){
    u0[i]      =f1(r[i]);
    u0[i+nr]   =f2(r[i]);
    u0[i+2*nr]=f3(r[i]);
  }
  ncall=0;
#
# ODE integration
  out=lsodes(y=u0,times=tout,func=pde1a,
      sparsetype="sparseint",rtol=1e-6,
      atol=1e-6,maxord=5);
  nrow(out)
  ncol(out)
#
# Arrays for plotting numerical solution
  S=matrix(0,nrow=nr,ncol=nout);
  I=matrix(0,nrow=nr,ncol=nout);
  R=matrix(0,nrow=nr,ncol=nout);
  for(it in 1:nout){
    for(i in 1:nr){
      S[i,it]=out[it,i+1];
      I[i,it]=out[it,i+1+nr];
      R[i,it]=out[it,i+1+2*nr];
    }
  }
#
# Display numerical solution
  for(it in 1:nout){
    cat(sprintf("\n     t      r      S(r,t)
                I(r,t)      R(r,t)\n"));
    iv=seq(from=1,to=nr,by=5);
```

```
    for(i in iv){
      cat(sprintf(
        "%6.2f%6.1f%12.3e%12.3e%12.3e\n",
         tout[it],r[i],S[i,it],I[i,it],R[i,it]));
    }
  }
#
# Calls to ODE routine
  cat(sprintf("\n\n  ncall = %5d\n\n",ncall));
#
# Plot PDE solutions
#
# S
  par(mfrow=c(1,1));
  matplot(x=r,y=S,type="l",xlab="r",ylab="S(r,t)",
    xlim=c(rl,ru),lty=1,main="",lwd=2,col="black");
#
# I
  par(mfrow=c(1,1));
  matplot(x=r,y=I,type="l",xlab="r",ylab="I(r,t)",
    xlim=c(rl,ru),lty=1,main="",lwd=2,col="black");
#
# R
  par(mfrow=c(1,1));
  matplot(x=r,y=R,type="l",xlab="r",ylab="R(r,t)",
    xlim=c(rl,ru),lty=1,main="",lwd=2,col="black");
```

Listing 4.1: Main program for eqs. (4.2a,b,c)

We can note the following details about Listing 4.1.

- Previous workspaces are deleted.

```
#
# SIRC model
#
```

```
# Delete previous workspaces
  rm(list=ls(all=TRUE))
```

- The R ODE integrator library `deSolve` is accessed. Then the directory with the files for the solution of eqs. (4.2a,b,c) is designated. Note that `setwd` (set working directory) uses / rather than the usual \.

```
#
# Access ODE integrator
  library("deSolve");
#
# Access functions for numerical solution
  setwd("f:/infectious/chap4");
  source("pde1a.R");
  source("dss044.R");
```

Direct differentiation with `dss044` is used as discussed in Chapter 1 and next when the ODE/MOL `pde1a` routine is discussed.

- A subset of the model parameters is defined numerically (the same values as in Listing 3.1).

```
#
# Parameters
  f1=function(r) 1;
  f2=function(r) exp(-100*r^2);
  f3=function(r) 0;
  r_p1=0.02;r_p2=0.02;r_p3=0.02;
  r_si=10;r_i=10;
```

The IC functions `f1,f2,f3` are also defined (further discussion is given after Listing 3.1)

- The four diffusivities of eqs. (4.2) are defined for three cases.

```
#
```

```
# Select case
  ncase=1;
  if(ncase==1){D_s=0.25;D_i=0.25;
              D_r=0.25;D_si=0    ;}
  if(ncase==2){D_s=0;    D_i=0;
              D_r=0;    D_si=0.25;}
  if(ncase==3){D_s=0.25;  D_i=0.25;
              D_r=0.25;D_si=0.25;}
```

For `ncase=1`, only linear (Fickian) diffusion is used with the diffusivities D_s, D_i, D_r.

For `ncase=2`, only cross diffusion is used with the diffusivity D_{si}.

For `ncase=3`, linear and cross diffusion are used with the diffusivities D_s, D_i, D_r, D_{si}.

The units are 1/yr (r is normalized to the interval $0 \leq r \leq 1$).

- A normalized spatial grid of 51 points is defined for $r_l = 0 \leq r \leq r_u = 1$, so that r=0,1/50=0.02,...,1.

```
#
# Spatial grid (in r)
  nr=51;
  rl=0;ru=1;
  r=seq(from=rl,to=ru,by=(ru-rl)/(nr-1));
```

- An interval in t of 6 points is defined for $0 \leq t \leq 0.1$ yr so that `tout=0,0.02,...,0.1`.

```
#
# Independent variable for ODE integration
  t0=0;tf=0.1;nout=6;
  tout=seq(from=t0,to=tf,by=(tf-t0)/(nout-1));
```

- ICs (4.3) are defined.

```
#
```

```
# Initial condition (t=0)
  u0=rep(0,3*nr);
  for(i in 1:nr){
    u0[i]      =f1(r[i]);
    u0[i+nr]   =f2(r[i]);
    u0[i+2*nr]=f3(r[i]);
  }
  ncall=0;
```

u0 therefore has $(3)(51) = 153$ elements. The counter for the calls to the ODE/MOL routine pde1a is also initialized.

- The system of 153 MOL/ODEs is integrated by the library integrator lsodes (available in deSolve). As expected, the inputs to lsodes are the ODE function, pde1a, the IC vector u0, and the vector of output values of t, tout. The length of u0 (153) informs lsodes how many ODEs are to be integrated. func,y,times are reserved names.

```
#
# ODE integration
  out=lsodes(y=u0,times=tout,func=pde1a,
      sparsetype="sparseint",rtol=1e-6,
      atol=1e-6,maxord=5);
  nrow(out)
  ncol(out)
```

The numerical solution to the ODEs is returned in matrix out. In this case, out has the dimensions $nout \times (3nr + 1) = 6 \times 3(51) + 1 = 153 + 1 = 154$, which are confirmed by the output from nrow(out),ncol(out) (included in the numerical output considered subsequently).

The offset $153 + 1$ is required since the first element of each column has the output t (also in tout), and the

$2, ..., 3nr + 1 = 2, ..., 154$ column elements have the 153 ODE solutions.

- The solutions of the 153 ODEs returned in out by lsodes are placed in arrays S,I,R.

```
#
# Arrays for plotting numerical solution
  S=matrix(0,nrow=nr,ncol=nout);
  I=matrix(0,nrow=nr,ncol=nout);
  R=matrix(0,nrow=nr,ncol=nout);
  for(it in 1:nout){
    for(i in 1:nr){
      S[i,it]=out[it,i+1];
      I[i,it]=out[it,i+1+nr];
      R[i,it]=out[it,i+1+2*nr];
    }
  }
```

- $S(r,t), I(r,t), R(r,t)$ are displayed as a function of r and t, with every fifth value of r from by=5.

```
#
# Display numerical solution
  for(it in 1:nout){
    cat(sprintf("\n      t      r         S(r,t)
                  I(r,t)         R(r,t)\n"));
    iv=seq(from=1,to=nr,by=5);
    for(i in iv){
      cat(sprintf(
        "%6.2f%6.1f%12.3e%12.3e%12.3e\n",
          tout[it],r[i],S[i,it],I[i,it],R[i,it]));
    }
  }
```

- The number of calls to `pde1a` is displayed at the end of the solution.

```
#
# Calls to ODE routine
  cat(sprintf("\n\n  ncall = %5d\n\n",ncall));
```

- $S(r,t)$, $I(r,t)$, $R(r,t)$ are plotted as a function of r with t as a parameter.

```
#
# Plot PDE solutions
#
# S
  par(mfrow=c(1,1));
  matplot(
    x=r,y=S,type="l",xlab="r",ylab="S(r,t)",
    xlim=c(rl,ru),lty=1,main="",lwd=2,
    col="black");
#
# I
  par(mfrow=c(1,1));
  matplot(
    x=r,y=I,type="l",xlab="r",ylab="I(r,t)",
    xlim=c(rl,ru),lty=1,main="",lwd=2,
    col="black");
#
# R
  par(mfrow=c(1,1));
  matplot(
    x=r,y=R,type="l",xlab="r",ylab="R(r,t)",
    xlim=c(rl,ru),lty=1,main="",lwd=2,
    col="black");
```

This completes the main program. The ODE/MOL routine `pde1a` called by `lsodes` is considered next.

(4.2.2) ODE/MOL routine

```
  pde1a=function(t,u,parms){
#
# Function pde1a computes the t derivative
# vectors of S(r,t),I(r,t),R(r,t)
#
# One vector to three vectors
  S=rep(0,nr);I=rep(0,nr);R=rep(0,nr);
  for(i in 1:nr){
    S[i]=u[i];
    I[i]=u[i+nr];
    R[i]=u[i+2*nr];
  }
#
# S*I
  SI=rep(0,nr);
  for(i in 1:nr){SI[i]=S[i]*I[i];}
#
# Sr,Ir,R,Sir
    Sr=rep(0,nr);  Ir=rep(0,nr);
    Rr=rep(0,nr);SIr=rep(0,nr);
#
# BCs
    Sr[1]=0;Sr[nr] =0;
    Ir[1]=0;Ir[nr] =0;
    Rr[1]=0;Rr[nr] =0;
   SIr[1]=0;SIr[nr]=0;
#
# Srr,Irr,Rrr,SIrr
    nl=2;nu=2;
    Srr=dss044(rl,ru,nr,S,Sr,nl=2,nu=2);
    Irr=dss044(rl,ru,nr,I,Ir,nl=2,nu=2);
    Rrr=dss044(rl,ru,nr,R,Rr,nl=2,nu=2);
```

```
  SIrr=dss044(rl,ru,nr,SI,SIr,nl=2,nu=2);
#
# PDEs
  St=rep(0,nr);It=rep(0,nr);Rt=rep(0,nr);
#
# r=0
  for(i in 1:nr){
    if(i==1){
      St[i]=2*D_si*SIrr[i]+2*D_s*Srr[i]+
            r_p1*S[i]-r_si*SI[i];
      It[i]=2*D_si*SIrr[i]+2*D_i*Irr[i]+
            r_p2*I[i]+r_si*SI[i]-r_i*I[i];
      Rt[i]=2*D_r*Rrr[i]+r_p3*R[i]+
            r_i*I[i];
    }
#
# r > 0
    if(i>1){
    ri=1/r[i];
    St[i]=D_si*(SIrr[i]+ri*SIr[i])+
          D_s*( Srr[i]+ri* Sr[i])+
          r_p1*S[i]-r_si*SI[i];
    It[i]=D_si*(SIrr[i]+ri*SIr[i])+
          D_i*( Irr[i]+ri* Ir[i])+
          r_p2*I[i]+r_si*SI[i]-r_i*I[i];
    Rt[i]= D_r*( Rrr[i]+ri* Rr[i])+
          r_p3*R[i]+r_i*I[i];
    }
#
# Next i
    }
#
# Three vectors to one vector
  ut=rep(0,3*nr);
```

```
for(i in 1:nr){
  ut[i]     =St[i];
  ut[i+nr]  =It[i];
  ut[i+2*nr]=Rt[i];
  }
#
# Increment calls to pde1a
  ncall <<- ncall+1;
#
# Return derivative vector
  return(list(c(ut)));
  }
```

Listing 4.2: ODE/MOL routine for eqs. (4.2), (4.3), (4.4)

We can note the following details about Listing 4.2.

- The function is defined.

```
pde1a=function(t,u,parms){
#
# Function pde1a computes the t derivative
# vectors of S(r,t),I(r,t),R(r,t)
```

t is the current value of t in eqs. (4.2). u the 153-vector of ODE/MOL dependent variables. **parm** is an argument to pass parameters to **pde1a** (unused, but required in the argument list). The arguments must be listed in the order stated to properly interface with **lsodes** called in the main program of Listing 4.1. The derivative vector of the LHS of eqs. (4.2) is calculated next and returned to **lsodes**.

- u is placed in three vectors, **S,I,R**, to facilitate the programming of eqs. (4.2).

```
#
# One vector to three vectors
```

```
S=rep(0,nr);I=rep(0,nr);R=rep(0,nr);
for(i in 1:nr){
  S[i]=u[i];
  I[i]=u[i+nr];
  R[i]=u[i+2*nr];
}
```

- The product of the two dependent variables of the terms $\pm r_{si} SI$ of eqs. (4.2a,b) is placed in SI.

```
#
# S*I
SI=rep(0,nr);
for(i in 1:nr){SI[i]=S[i]*I[i];}
```

- Arrays for the first derivative in r are allocated.

```
#
# Sr,Ir,Rr,SIr
  Sr=rep(0,nr);  Ir=rep(0,nr);
  Rr=rep(0,nr);SIr=rep(0,nr);
```

- BCs 4.4 are implemented. 1,nr correspond to $r = 0, 1$.

```
#
# BCs
  Sr[1]=0;Sr[nr] =0;
  Ir[1]=0;Ir[nr] =0;
  Rr[1]=0;Rr[nr] =0;
SIr[1]=0;SIr[nr]=0;
```

Also, homogeneous Neumann BCs for the derivative of SI are defined.

- The second derivatives in r are computed by direct differentiation of S, I, R.

```
#
# Srr,Irr,Rrr,SIrr
```

```
nl=2;nu=2;
 Srr=dss044(rl,ru,nr,S,Sr,nl=2,nu=2);
 Irr=dss044(rl,ru,nr,I,Ir,nl=2,nu=2);
 Rrr=dss044(rl,ru,nr,R,Rr,nl=2,nu=2);
 SIrr=dss044(rl,ru,nr,SI,SIr,nl=2,nu=2);
```

Stagewise differentiation (dss004) as in Listing 3.2 failed in the sense that negative values for S, I, R developed in the neightborhood of $r = 0$, so direct differentiation (dss044) was used[1].

- The derivatives in t (the LHSs of eqs. (4.2)) are computed, first for $r = 0$ (i=1).

```
#
# PDEs
 St=rep(0,nr);It=rep(0,nr);Rt=rep(0,nr);
#
# r=0
 for(i in 1:nr){
  if(i==1){
   St[i]=2*D_si*SIrr[i]+2*D_s*Srr[i]+
       r_p1*S[i]-r_si*SI[i];
   It[i]=2*D_si*SIrr[i]+2*D_i*Irr[i]+
       r_p2*I[i]+r_si*SI[i]-r_i*I[i];
   Rt[i]=2*D_r*Rrr[i]+r_p3*R[i]+
       r_i*I[i];
  }
```

---

[1]Experience has indicated that stagewise differentiation is not as robust as direct differentiation. In fact, this was a principal reason for developing the direct differentiation routines dss042 (second order) to dss050 (tenth order) with Dirichlet BCs (nl=nu=1) and Neumann BCs (nl=nu=2). The guidance and suggestions of Professor Gilbert Stengle in the development of these routines is gratefully acknowledged.

This programming requires some additional explanation.

- The derivative terms in eqs. (4.2), $\dfrac{1}{r}\dfrac{\partial SI}{\partial r}$, $\dfrac{1}{r}\dfrac{\partial S}{\partial r}$, $\dfrac{1}{r}\dfrac{\partial I}{\partial r}$, $\dfrac{1}{r}\dfrac{\partial R}{\partial r}$ are indeterminant $(0/0)$ at $r = 0$ since the first derivatives are also zero from BCs (4.4a,c,e).
- The indeterminant terms are resolved by *l'Hospital's rule*, e.g.,

$$\lim_{r\to 0}\frac{1}{r}\frac{\partial SI}{\partial r} = \frac{\partial^2 SI}{\partial r^2}$$

so that

$$\frac{\partial^2 SI}{\partial r^2} + \frac{1}{r}\frac{\partial SI}{\partial r} = 2\frac{\partial^2 SI}{\partial r^2}$$

which is programmed as 2*D_si*SIrr[i].

- The multiplication of the second derivatives by 2 for the other first derivative radial groups is programmed in the same way.

```
2*D_s*Srr[i]
```

```
2*D_i*Sii[i]
```

```
2*D_r*Rrr[i]
```

- For $r > 0$, the programming is

```
#
# r > 0
    if(i>1){
    ri=1/r[i];
    St[i]=D_si*(SIrr[i]+ri*SIr[i])+
          D_s*( Srr[i]+ri* Sr[i])+
```

```
                    r_p1*S[i]-r_si*SI[i];
        It[i]=D_si*(SIrr[i]+ri*SIr[i])+
              D_i*( Irr[i]+ri* Ir[i])+
              r_p2*I[i]+r_si*SI[i]-r_i*I[i];
        Rt[i]= D_r*( Rrr[i]+ri* Rr[i])+
              r_p3*R[i]+r_i*I[i];
        }
```

- The derivatives $\dfrac{\partial S}{\partial t}, \dfrac{\partial I}{\partial t}, \dfrac{\partial R}{\partial t}$, (LHSs of eqs. (4.2)) are placed in ut.

```
#
# Three vectors to one vector
  ut=rep(0,3*nr);
  for(i in 1:nr){
    ut[i]      =St[i];
    ut[i+nr]   =It[i];
    ut[i+2*nr]=Rt[i];
  }
```

- The counter for the calls to pde1a is incremented and returned to the main program of Listing 4.1 with <<-.

```
#
# Increment calls to pde1a
  ncall <<- ncall+1;
```

-

- ut is returned to lsodes as a list (required by lsodes). c is the R vector utility.

```
#
# Return derivative vector
  return(list(c(ut)));
  }
```

The final } concludes pde1a.

The output from the main program and subordinate routine of Listings 4.1, 4.2 is considered next.

(4.2.3) Model output

Abbreviated output for `ncase=1` in Listing 4.1 follows.

[1] 6

[1] 154

t	r	S(r,t)	I(r,t)	R(r,t)
0.00	0.0	1.000e+00	1.000e+00	0.000e+00
0.00	0.1	1.000e+00	3.679e-01	0.000e+00
0.00	0.2	1.000e+00	1.832e-02	0.000e+00
0.00	0.3	1.000e+00	1.234e-04	0.000e+00
0.00	0.4	1.000e+00	1.125e-07	0.000e+00
0.00	0.5	1.000e+00	1.389e-11	0.000e+00
0.00	0.6	1.000e+00	2.320e-16	0.000e+00
0.00	0.7	1.000e+00	5.243e-22	0.000e+00
0.00	0.8	1.000e+00	1.604e-28	0.000e+00
0.00	0.9	1.000e+00	6.640e-36	0.000e+00
0.00	1.0	1.000e+00	3.720e-44	0.000e+00

. .
. .
. .

Output for t=0.02,..., 0.08 removed

. .
. .
. .

t	r	S(r,t)	I(r,t)	R(r,t)
0.10	0.0	7.610e-01	2.557e-01	2.795e-01
0.10	0.1	7.793e-01	2.359e-01	2.566e-01
0.10	0.2	8.279e-01	1.833e-01	1.970e-01
0.10	0.3	8.876e-01	1.195e-01	1.262e-01

```
0.10    0.4    9.393e-01    6.493e-02    6.746e-02
0.10    0.5    9.735e-01    2.931e-02    3.005e-02
0.10    0.6    9.912e-01    1.098e-02    1.114e-02
0.10    0.7    9.986e-01    3.412e-03    3.441e-03
0.10    0.8    1.001e+00    8.808e-04    8.849e-04
0.10    0.9    1.002e+00    1.938e-04    1.943e-04
0.10    1.0    1.002e+00    6.739e-05    6.752e-05


ncall =    276
```

Table 4.1: Abbreviated output for eqs. (4.2), (4.3), (4.4),
ncase=1

We can note the following details about this output.

- The dimensions of the solution matrix out are $nout \times 3nr + 1 = 6 \times 3(51) + 1 = 154$. The offset $+1$ results from the value of t as the first element in each of the $nout = 6$ solution vectors. These same values of t are in tout,

   [1] 6

   [1] 154

- ICs (4.3) ($t = 0$) are verified for $f_1(r)$, $f_2(r)$, $f_3(r)$.
- The output is for $r = 0, 0.02, ...1$ as programmed in Listing 4.1 (51 values at each value of t with every fifth value in r).
- The output is for $t = 0, 0.02, ..., 0.1$ as programmed in Listing 4.1.
- $S(r, t)$, $R(r, t)$ depart from their initial values as a consequence of the input from $I(r, t)$.
- The computational effort is modest, ncall = 276, indicating lsodes efficiently computes a solution to the 153 MOL/ODEs.

The graphical output is in Figs. 4.1a,b,c.

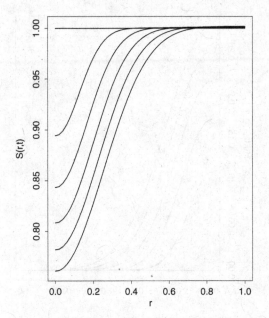

Figure 4.1a: Numerical solution $S(r,t)$ from eq. (4.2a), `ncase=1`

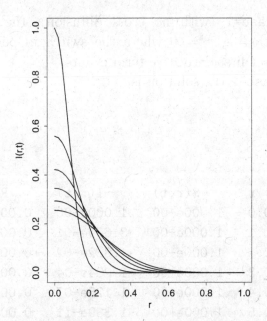

Figure 4.1b: Numerical solution $I(r,t)$ from eq. (4.2b), `ncase=1`

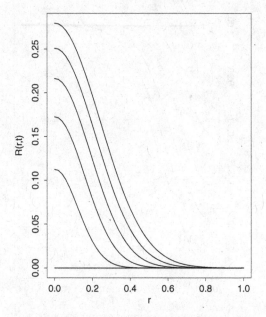

Figure 4.1c: Numerical solution $R(r,t)$ from eq. (4.2c), ncase=1

For ncase=1 (with no cross diffusion), the solution is smooth, including $r = 0$ where the switch in pde1a for the indeterminant first derivative term occurs.

For ncase=2 the solution is

[1] 6

[1] 154

t	r	S(r,t)	I(r,t)	R(r,t)
0.00	0.0	1.000e+00	1.000e+00	0.000e+00
0.00	0.1	1.000e+00	3.679e-01	0.000e+00
0.00	0.2	1.000e+00	1.832e-02	0.000e+00
0.00	0.3	1.000e+00	1.234e-04	0.000e+00
0.00	0.4	1.000e+00	1.125e-07	0.000e+00
0.00	0.5	1.000e+00	1.389e-11	0.000e+00
0.00	0.6	1.000e+00	2.320e-16	0.000e+00

```
0.00    0.7    1.000e+00    5.243e-22    0.000e+00
0.00    0.8    1.000e+00    1.604e-28    0.000e+00
0.00    0.9    1.000e+00    6.640e-36    0.000e+00
0.00    1.0    1.000e+00    3.720e-44    0.000e+00
         .                        .
         .                        .
         .                        .
```

Output for t=0.02,..., 0.08 removed

```
         .                        .
         .                        .
         .                        .

   t     r      S(r,t)       I(r,t)       R(r,t)
0.10    0.0    3.509e-01    3.858e-01    5.631e-01
0.10    0.1    6.525e-01    2.079e-01    2.922e-01
0.10    0.2    9.671e-01    1.252e-01    1.301e-01
0.10    0.3    1.022e+00    8.721e-02    6.177e-02
0.10    0.4    1.027e+00    5.230e-02    2.569e-02
0.10    0.5    1.019e+00    2.589e-02    9.100e-03
0.10    0.6    1.010e+00    1.042e-02    2.718e-03
0.10    0.7    1.005e+00    3.409e-03    6.835e-04
0.10    0.8    1.003e+00    9.127e-04    1.448e-04
0.10    0.9    1.002e+00    2.063e-04    2.634e-05
0.10    1.0    1.002e+00    7.303e-05    7.779e-06


ncall =    310
```

Table 4.2: Abbreviated output for eqs. (4.2), (4.3), (4.4),
ncase=2

The graphical output is in Figs. 4.2a,b,c.

The previous points for ncase=1 also apply to this solution (with no linear diffusion), but the solutions are markedly different (between ncase=1 and ncase=2). For example, $S(r,t)$ has an initial overshoot of the IC that decays with t. This is indicated

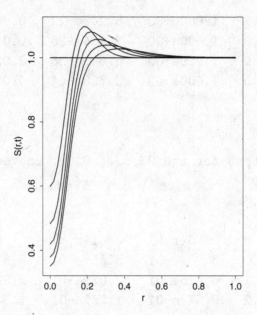

Figure 4.2a: Numerical solution $S(r, t)$ from eq. (4.2a), `ncase=2`

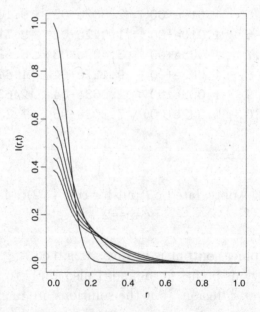

Figure 4.2b: Numerical solution $I(r, t)$ from eq. (4.2b), `ncase=2`

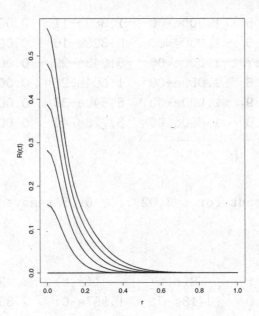

Figure 4.2c: Numerical solution $R(r,t)$ from eq. (4.2c), `ncase=2`

by $S(r = 0.2, t = 0.02) = 1.095e + 00$ and can be observed in Fig. 4.2a.

t	r	S(r,t)	I(r,t)	R(r,t)
0.02	0.2	1.095e+00	1.333e-01	1.751e-02

For `ncase=3` the solution is

```
[1] 6
```

```
[1] 154
```

t	r	S(r,t)	I(r,t)	R(r,t)
0.00	0.0	1.000e+00	1.000e+00	0.000e+00
0.00	0.1	1.000e+00	3.679e-01	0.000e+00
0.00	0.2	1.000e+00	1.832e-02	0.000e+00
0.00	0.3	1.000e+00	1.234e-04	0.000e+00
0.00	0.4	1.000e+00	1.125e-07	0.000e+00

```
0.00    0.5    1.000e+00    1.389e-11    0.000e+00
0.00    0.6    1.000e+00    2.320e-16    0.000e+00
0.00    0.7    1.000e+00    5.243e-22    0.000e+00
0.00    0.8    1.000e+00    1.604e-28    0.000e+00
0.00    0.9    1.000e+00    6.640e-36    0.000e+00
0.00    1.0    1.000e+00    3.720e-44    0.000e+00
         .                                 .
         .                                 .
         .                                 .
      Output for t=0.02,..., 0.08 removed
         .                                 .
         .                                 .
         .                                 .

   t       r       S(r,t)        I(r,t)        R(r,t)
0.10    0.0    7.413e-01    1.957e-01    2.395e-01
0.10    0.1    7.619e-01    1.852e-01    2.239e-01
0.10    0.2    8.173e-01    1.570e-01    1.824e-01
0.10    0.3    8.861e-01    1.212e-01    1.303e-01
0.10    0.4    9.457e-01    8.621e-02    8.250e-02
0.10    0.5    9.838e-01    5.670e-02    4.673e-02
0.10    0.6    1.001e+00    3.432e-02    2.386e-02
0.10    0.7    1.006e+00    1.902e-02    1.105e-02
0.10    0.8    1.006e+00    9.727e-03    4.700e-03
0.10    0.9    1.005e+00    4.980e-03    1.976e-03
0.10    1.0    1.004e+00    3.554e-03    1.243e-03


ncall =    302
```

Table 4.3: Abbreviated output for eqs. (4.2), (4.3), (4.4), ncase=3

The graphical output is in Figs. 4.3a,b,c.

The linear diffusion (ncase=1) gives a dispersion to the cross diffusion (ncase=2). The overshoot in $S(r,t)$ for ncase=3

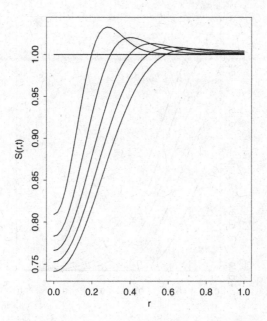

Figure 4.3a: Numerical solution $S(r,t)$ from eq. (4.2a), `ncase=3`

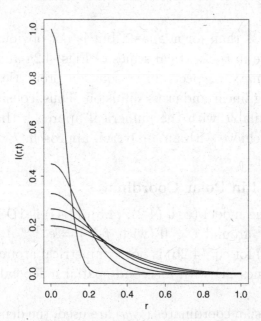

Figure 4.3b: Numerical solution $I(r,t)$ from eq. (4.2b), `ncase=3`

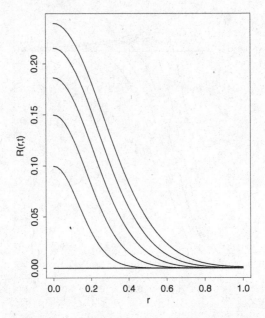

Figure 4.3c: Numerical solution $R(r, t)$ from eq. (4.2c), `ncase=3`

is actually less than for `ncase=2`, but is not obvious because of the difference in the vertical scales of Figs. 4.2a and 4.3a.

   In summary, a spectrum of solution properties is possible by combining linear and cross diffusion. Thus, considerable flexibility is available with the numerical approach that would be difficult to achieve with an analytical approach.

(4.3) Model in Polar Coordinates

The preceding model (eqs. (4.2), (4.3), (4.4)) is 1D in r because of symmetry around $r = 0$ (with $f_2(r) = e^{-100r^2}$). However, if the IC (4.3b) for eq. (4.2b) is not symmetrical around $r = 0$, the model becomes 2D with a second spatial independent variable required.

   If Cartesian coordinates (x, y) are used, the definition of the BCs is not straightforward for the representation of a physical system (e.g., dispersion from a source of infecteds). If *polar* coordinates (r, θ) are used, the addition of the terms $\dfrac{1}{r^2}\dfrac{\partial^2 S}{\partial \theta^2}, \dfrac{1}{r^2}\dfrac{\partial^2 I}{\partial \theta^2},$ $\dfrac{1}{r^2}\dfrac{\partial^2 R}{\partial \theta^2}$ to eqs. (4.2) would be required (see eq. (4.1e)), as well as two BCs in θ.

If approximations of the spatial derivatives in θ are developed and then included in the approximation of eqs. (4.2) on a (r, θ) grid, the resulting system of ODEs could then be integrated numerically. This extension from 1D to 2D MOL is not considered further here.

(4.4) 3D Plotting

In this concluding section, plotting of the solution of eqs. (4.2) to (4.4) in 3D perspective is presented. A main program is listed next.

(4.4.1) Main program

```
#
# SIRC model
#
# Delete previous workspaces
  rm(list=ls(all=TRUE))
#
# Access ODE integrator
  library("deSolve");
#
# Access functions for numerical solution
  setwd("f:/infectious/chap4");
  source("pde1b.R");
  source("dss044.R");
#
# Parameters
```

```
  f1=function(r) 1;
  f2=function(r) exp(-100*r^2);
  f3=function(r) 0;
  r_p1=0.02;r_p2=0.02;r_p3=0.02;
  r_si=10;r_i=10;
#
# Select case
  ncase=1;
  if(ncase==1){D_s=0.25;D_i=0.25;
               D_r=0.25;D_si=0    ;}
  if(ncase==2){D_s=0;    D_i=0;
               D_r=0;    D_si=0.25;}
  if(ncase==3){D_s=0.25; D_i=0.25;
               D_r=0.25;D_si=0.25;}
#
# Spatial grid (in r)
  nr=51;
  rl=0;ru=1;
  r=seq(from=rl,to=ru,by=(ru-rl)/(nr-1));
#
# Independent variable for ODE integration
  t0=0;tf=0.1;nout=31;
  tout=seq(from=t0,to=tf,by=(tf-t0)/(nout-1));
#
# Initial condition (t=0)
  u0=rep(0,3*nr);
  for(i in 1:nr){
    u0[i]      =f1(r[i]);
    u0[i+nr]   =f2(r[i]);
    u0[i+2*nr]=f3(r[i]);
  }
  ncall=0;
#
# ODE integration
```

```
out=lsodes(y=u0,times=tout,func=pde1b,
    sparsetype="sparseint",rtol=1e-6,
    atol=1e-6,maxord=5);
nrow(out)
ncol(out)
#
# Arrays for plotting numerical solution
  S=matrix(0,nrow=nr,ncol=nout);
  I=matrix(0,nrow=nr,ncol=nout);
  R=matrix(0,nrow=nr,ncol=nout);
  for(it in 1:nout){
    for(i in 1:nr){
      S[i,it]=out[it,i+1];
      I[i,it]=out[it,i+1+nr];
      R[i,it]=out[it,i+1+2*nr];
    }
  }
#
# Display numerical solution
  for(it in 1:nout){
    if((it-1)*(it-16)*(it-nout)==0){
    cat(sprintf("\n      t      r        S(r,t)
                I(r,t)        R(r,t)\n"));
    iv=seq(from=1,to=nr,by=5);
    for(i in iv){
      cat(sprintf(
        "%6.2f%6.1f%12.3e%12.3e%12.3e\n",
        tout[it],r[i],S[i,it],I[i,it],R[i,it]));
    }
  }
}
#
# Calls to ODE routine
  cat(sprintf("\n\n ncall = %5d\n\n",ncall));
```

```
#
# Plot PDE solutions
#
# S(r,t)
  persp(
    r,tout,S,theta=25,phi=45,xlim=c(rl,ru),
    ylim=c(t0,tf),xlab="r",ylab="t",
    zlab="S(r,t)");
#
# I(r,t)
  persp(
    r,tout,I,theta=55,phi=45,xlim=c(rl,ru),
    ylim=c(t0,tf),xlab="r",ylab="t",
    zlab="I(r,t)");
#
# R(r,t)
  persp(
    r,tout,R,theta=55,phi=45,xlim=c(rl,ru),
    ylim=c(t0,tf),xlab="r",ylab="t",
    zlab="R(r,t)");
```

Listing 4.3: Main program for eqs. (4.2a,b,c) with 3D plotting

Listing 4.3 is similar to Listing 4.1, so the differences are explained (refer to the discussion of Listing 4.1 for additional details).

- Previous files are cleared and **deSolve** is accessed.

  ```
  #
  # SIRC model
  #
  # Delete previous workspaces
    rm(list=ls(all=TRUE))
  #
  # Access ODE integrator
  ```

```
library("deSolve");
#
# Access functions for numerical solution
setwd("f:/infectious/chap4");
source("pde1b.R");
source("dss044.R");
```

The ODE/MOL routine pde1b is the same as pde1a of Listing 4.2. The name change is used for a complete example application.

- The parameters and cases are defined as in Listing 4.1.

```
#
# Parameters
f1=function(r) 1;
f2=function(r) exp(-100*r^2);
f3=function(r) 0;
r_p1=0.02;r_p2=0.02;r_p3=0.02;
r_si=10;r_i=10;
#
# Select case
ncase=1;
if(ncase==1){D_s=0.25;D_i=0.25;
             D_r=0.25;D_si=0    ;}
if(ncase==2){D_s=0;    D_i=0;
             D_r=0;    D_si=0.25;}
if(ncase==3){D_s=0.25; D_i=0.25;
             D_r=0.25;D_si=0.25;}
```

- The spatial grid in r and time interval in t are defined.

```
#
# Spatial grid (in r)
nr=51;
rl=0;ru=1;
r=seq(from=rl,to=ru,by=(ru-rl)/(nr-1));
```

```
#
# Independent variable for ODE integration
  t0=0;tf=0.1;nout=31;
  tout=seq(from=t0,to=tf,by=(tf-t0)/(nout-1));
```

The time interval of Listing 4.1, t0=0;tf=0.1;nout=6;,
is changed to t0=0;tf=0.1;nout=31; so that additional
output in t is produced to give acceptable resolution of
the 3D plots (this will be clear when the plotted output
is discussed subsequently).

• The IC vector u0 is defined as in Listing 4.1.

```
#
# Initial condition (t=0)
  u0=rep(0,3*nr);
  for(i in 1:nr){
    u0[i]     =f1(r[i]);
    u0[i+nr]  =f2(r[i]);
    u0[i+2*nr]=f3(r[i]);
  }
  ncall=0;
```

• The system of $3(51) = 153$ MOL/ODEs is integrated by
lsodes. **pde1b** is the MOL/ODE routine.

```
#
# ODE integration
  out=lsodes(y=u0,times=tout,func=pde1b,
    sparsetype="sparseint",rtol=1e-6,
    atol=1e-6,maxord=5);
  nrow(out)
  ncol(out)
```

• $S(r, t), I(r, t), R(r, t)$ are placed in arrays for subsequent
numerical and graphical output. The subscripting of the
solution matrix out is explained with Listing 4.1.

```
#
# Arrays for plotting numerical solution
  S=matrix(0,nrow=nr,ncol=nout);
  I=matrix(0,nrow=nr,ncol=nout);
  R=matrix(0,nrow=nr,ncol=nout);
  for(it in 1:nout){
    for(i in 1:nr){
      S[i,it]=out[it,i+1];
      I[i,it]=out[it,i+1+nr];
      R[i,it]=out[it,i+1+2*nr];
    }
  }
```

- The numerical output is limited in t with if((it-1)*(it-16)*(it-nout)==0) (output at $t = 0, 0.05, 0.1$) and every fifth value in r (with by=5).

```
#
# Display numerical solution
  for(it in 1:nout){
    if((it-1)*(it-16)*(it-nout)==0){
    cat(sprintf("\n      t      r        S(r,t)
                I(r,t)        R(r,t)\n"));
    iv=seq(from=1,to=nr,by=5);
    for(i in iv){
      cat(sprintf(
        "%6.2f%6.1f%12.3e%12.3e%12.3e\n",
        tout[it],r[i],S[i,it],I[i,it],R[i,it]));
    }
    }
  }
```

- The number of calls to **pde1b** is displayed.

```
#
# Calls to ODE routine
```

```
cat(sprintf("\n\n ncall = %5d\n\n",ncall));
```

- $S(r,t)$ is plotted in 3D perspective with persp.

```
#
# Plot PDE solutions
#
# S(r,t)
  persp(
    r,tout,S,theta=25,phi=45,xlim=c(rl,ru),
    ylim=c(t0,tf),xlab="r",ylab="t",
    zlab="S(r,t)");
```

The arguments of persp are:

  - r: Radial grid (51 values).
  - tout: Output values of t (31 values).
  - S: Solution of eq. (4.2a), $S(r,t)$ (51 × 31 values).
  - theta=55: Angle (in degrees) in the $x-y$ plane with theta=0 for the x axis.
  - phi=45: Angle (in degrees) relative to the z axis with phi=0 corresponding to the z axis.
  - xlim=c(rl,ru): Limits of the x (r) axis.
  - ylim=c(t0,tf): Limits of the y (t) axis.
  - xlab="r",ylab="t": Labels of the r, t axes.
  - zlab="S(r,t)": Label for the z $(S(r,t))$ axis.

- $I(r,t)$ is plotted in 3D perspective.

```
#
# I(r,t)
  persp(
    r,tout,I,theta=55,phi=45,xlim=c(rl,ru),
    ylim=c(t0,tf),xlab="r",ylab="t",
    zlab="I(r,t)");
```

- $R(r,t)$ is plotted in 3D perspective.

```
#
# R(r,t)
  persp(
    r,tout,R,theta=55,phi=45,xlim=c(rl,ru),
    ylim=c(t0,tf),xlab="r",ylab="t",
    zlab="R(r,t)");
```

The angles theta,phi were determined by trial and error to give 3D plots with a clear perspective.

(4.4.2) ODE/MOL routine

The ODE/MOL routine, pde1b is the same as pde1a of Listing 4.2 except for the name change. The output from Listing 4.3 is considered next.

(4.4.3) Model output

[1] 31

[1] 154

t	r	S(r,t)	I(r,t)	R(r,t)
0.00	0.0	1.000e+00	1.000e+00	0.000e+00
0.00	0.1	1.000e+00	3.679e-01	0.000e+00
0.00	0.2	1.000e+00	1.832e-02	0.000e+00
0.00	0.3	1.000e+00	1.234e-04	0.000e+00
0.00	0.4	1.000e+00	1.125e-07	0.000e+00
0.00	0.5	1.000e+00	1.389e-11	0.000e+00
0.00	0.6	1.000e+00	2.320e-16	0.000e+00
0.00	0.7	1.000e+00	5.243e-22	0.000e+00
0.00	0.8	1.000e+00	1.604e-28	0.000e+00
0.00	0.9	1.000e+00	6.640e-36	0.000e+00
0.00	1.0	1.000e+00	3.720e-44	0.000e+00

t	r	S(r,t)	I(r,t)	R(r,t)
0.05	0.0	7.742e-01	2.933e-01	1.691e-01
0.05	0.1	8.121e-01	2.630e-01	1.491e-01
0.05	0.2	9.006e-01	1.922e-01	1.018e-01
0.05	0.3	9.785e-01	1.195e-01	5.510e-02
0.05	0.4	1.013e+00	6.412e-02	2.423e-02
0.05	0.5	1.015e+00	2.917e-02	8.778e-03
0.05	0.6	1.008e+00	1.105e-02	2.638e-03
0.05	0.7	1.004e+00	3.461e-03	6.608e-04
0.05	0.8	1.002e+00	8.986e-04	1.387e-04
0.05	0.9	1.001e+00	1.984e-04	2.495e-05
0.05	1.0	1.001e+00	6.919e-05	7.306e-06

t	r	S(r,t)	I(r,t)	R(r,t)
0.10	0.0	7.413e-01	1.957e-01	2.395e-01
0.10	0.1	7.619e-01	1.852e-01	2.239e-01
0.10	0.2	8.173e-01	1.570e-01	1.824e-01
0.10	0.3	8.861e-01	1.212e-01	1.303e-01
0.10	0.4	9.457e-01	8.621e-02	8.250e-02
0.10	0.5	9.838e-01	5.670e-02	4.673e-02
0.10	0.6	1.001e+00	3.432e-02	2.386e-02
0.10	0.7	1.006e+00	1.902e-02	1.105e-02
0.10	0.8	1.006e+00	9.727e-03	4.700e-03
0.10	0.9	1.005e+00	4.980e-03	1.976e-03
0.10	1.0	1.004e+00	3.554e-03	1.243e-03

```
ncall =    287
```

Table 4.4: Numerical output for eqs. (4.2), (4.3), (4.4), ncase=3

We can note the following details about this output.

- out has the dimensions $31 \times 153 + 1 = 154$ as explained with Listing 4.1.
- The ICs are confirmed (as in Listing 4.1).

- The solutions are for $t = 0, 0.05, 0.1$ and $r = 0, 0.1, ..., 1$ as explained previously.
- The solutions are the same at $t = 0.1$ as in Table 4.3.
- The computational effort is modest, with `ncall` = 287.

The graphical output is in Figs. 4.4a,b,c.

These figures display the evolution of the SIRC model with r and t. Note in particular $S(r, t = 0), I(r, t = 0), R(r, t = 0)$ and the approaching equilibrium solution for $S(r, t = 0.1), I(r, t = 0.1), R(r, t = 0.1)$.

They also demonstrate the symmetry BCs (4.4a,c,e). In other words, the solution for $r = -ru = -1 \leq r \leq r = rl = 0$ is the same as for $r = rl = 0 \leq r \leq r = ru = 1$. This symmetry can be displayed by extending the r axis to negative r, which could be accomplished by (1) computing a solution for $-1 \leq r \leq 1$ or (2) using the solution for $0 \leq r \leq 1$ over the interval $-1 \leq r \leq 0$. The second approach is demonstrated with the following changes to Listing 4.3.

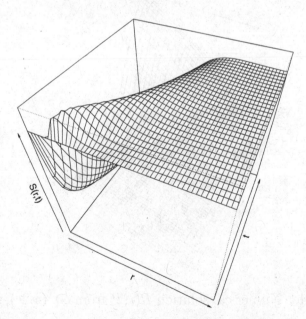

Figure 4.4a: Numerical solution $S(r, t)$ from eq. (4.2a), `ncase=3`

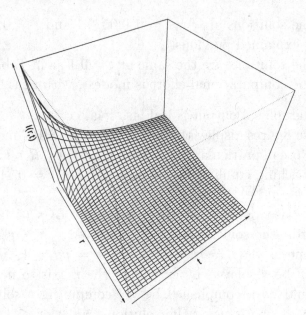

Figure 4.4b: Numerical solution $I(r, t)$ from eq. (4.2b), `ncase=3`

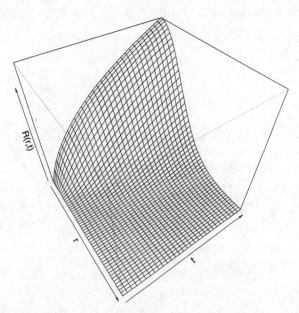

Figure 4.4c: Numerical solution $R(r, t)$ from eq. (4.2c), `ncase=3`

```
#
# SIRC model
#
# Delete previous workspaces
  rm(list=ls(all=TRUE))
#
# Access ODE integrator
  library("deSolve");
#
# Access functions for numerical solution
  setwd("f:/infectious/chap4");
  source("pde1c.R");
  source("dss044.R");
#
# Parameters
  f1=function(r) 1;
  f2=function(r) exp(-100*r^2);
  f3=function(r) 0;
  r_p1=0.02;r_p2=0.02;r_p3=0.02;
  r_si=10;r_i=10;
#
# Select case
  ncase=3;
  if(ncase==1){D_s=0.25;D_i=0.25;
               D_r=0.25;D_si=0   ;}
  if(ncase==2){D_s=0;    D_i=0;
               D_r=0;    D_si=0.25;}
  if(ncase==3){D_s=0.25; D_i=0.25;
               D_r=0.25;D_si=0.25;}
#
# Spatial grid (in r)
  nr=26;
  rl=0;ru=1;
  r=seq(from=rl,to=ru,by=(ru-rl)/(nr-1));
```

```
#
# Independent variable for ODE integration
  t0=0;tf=0.1;nout=31;
  tout=seq(from=t0,to=tf,by=(tf-t0)/(nout-1));
#
# Initial condition (t=0)
  u0=rep(0,3*nr);
  for(i in 1:nr){
    u0[i]     =f1(r[i]);
    u0[i+nr]  =f2(r[i]);
    u0[i+2*nr]=f3(r[i]);
  }
  ncall=0;
#
# ODE integration
  out=lsodes(y=u0,times=tout,func=pde1c,
      sparsetype="sparseint",rtol=1e-6,
      atol=1e-6,maxord=5);
  nrow(out)
  ncol(out)
#
# Arrays for plotting numerical solution
  S=matrix(0,nrow=nr,ncol=nout);
  I=matrix(0,nrow=nr,ncol=nout);
  R=matrix(0,nrow=nr,ncol=nout);
  for(it in 1:nout){
    for(i in 1:nr){
      S[i,it]=out[it,i+1];
      I[i,it]=out[it,i+1+nr];
      R[i,it]=out[it,i+1+2*nr];
    }
  }
#
# Display numerical solution
```

```
  for(it in 1:nout){
    if((it-1)*(it-16)*(it-nout)==0){
    cat(sprintf("\n        t       r        S(r,t)
                I(r,t)        R(r,t)\n"));
    iv=seq(from=1,to=nr,by=5);
    for(i in iv){
      cat(sprintf(
        "%6.2f%6.1f%12.3e%12.3e%12.3e\n",
         tout[it],r[i],S[i,it],I[i,it],R[i,it]));
      }
    }
  }
#
# Calls to ODE routine
  cat(sprintf("\n\n ncall = %5d\n\n",ncall));
#
# Plot PDE solutions, -r0 <= r <= r0
  Sr2=matrix(0,nrow=(2*nr-1),ncol=nout);
  Ir2=matrix(0,nrow=(2*nr-1),ncol=nout);
  Rr2=matrix(0,nrow=(2*nr-1),ncol=nout);
  r2=rep(0,(2*nr-1));
  for(it in 1:nout){
    for(i in 1:(2*nr-1)){
      if(i<=26){
        r2[i]=-r[nr-(i-1)];
        Sr2[i,it]=S[nr-(i-1),it];
        Ir2[i,it]=I[nr-(i-1),it];
        Rr2[i,it]=R[nr-(i-1),it]};
      if(i>26){
        r2[i]=r[i-(nr-1)];
        Sr2[i,it]=S[i-(nr-1),it];
        Ir2[i,it]=I[i-(nr-1),it];
        Rr2[i,it]=R[i-(nr-1),it]};
#     if((it-1)*(it-16)*(it-nout)==0){
```

```
#      cat(sprintf(
#        "\n %5d %5d %10.4f %10.4f %10.4f
#        %10.4f",
#        it,i,r2[i],Sr2[i,it],Ir2[i,it],
#        Rr2[i,it]));
#      }
    }
  }
#
# S(r,t)
  persp(
    r,tout,S,theta=25,phi=45,xlim=c(rl,ru),
    ylim=c(t0,tf),xlab="r",ylab="t",
    zlab="S(r,t)");
#
# I(r,t)
  persp(
    r,tout,I,theta=55,phi=45,xlim=c(rl,ru),
    ylim=c(t0,tf),xlab="r",ylab="t",
    zlab="I(r,t)");
#
# R(r,t)
  persp(
    r,tout,R,theta=55,phi=45,xlim=c(rl,ru),
    ylim=c(t0,tf),xlab="r",ylab="t",
    zlab="R(r,t)");
```

Listing 4.4: Main program for eqs. (4.2a,b,c) with 3D plotting, $-1 \leq r \leq 1$

Listing 4.4 is similar to Listing 4.3, so the differences are explained (refer to the discussion of Listings 4.1, 4.3 for additional details).

- The ODE/MOL routine is `pde1c` which is the same as `pde1a` of Listing 4.2 with only a name change.

```
#
# Access functions for numerical solution
  setwd("f:/infectious/chap4");
  source("pde1c.R");
  source("dss044.R");
```

- The spatial grid is for $0 \le r \le 1$ with 26 points (subsequently redefined for $-1 \le r \le 1$).

```
#
# Spatial grid (in r)
  nr=26;
  rl=0;ru=1;
  r=seq(from=rl,to=ru,by=(ru-rl)/(nr-1));
```

- `pde1c` is used in the ODE/MOL integration by `lsodes`.

```
#
# ODE integration
  out=lsodes(y=u0,times=tout,func=pde1c,
      sparsetype="sparseint",rtol=1e-6,
      atol=1e-6,maxord=5);
  nrow(out)
  ncol(out)
```

- Solution arrays for $-1 \le r \le 1$ are defined.

```
#
# Calls to ODE routine
  cat(sprintf("\n\n ncall = %5d\n\n",ncall));
#
# Plot PDE solutions, -r0 <= r <= r0
  Sr2=matrix(0,nrow=(2*nr-1),ncol=nout);
  Ir2=matrix(0,nrow=(2*nr-1),ncol=nout);
```

```
          Rr2=matrix(0,nrow=(2*nr-1),ncol=nout);
          r2=rep(0,(2*nr-1));
          for(it in 1:nout){
            for(i in 1:(2*nr-1)){
              if(i<=26){
                r2[i]=-r[nr-(i-1)];
                Sr2[i,it]=S[nr-(i-1),it];
                Ir2[i,it]=I[nr-(i-1),it];
                Rr2[i,it]=R[nr-(i-1),it]};
              if(i>26){
                r2[i]=r[i-(nr-1)];
                Sr2[i,it]=S[i-(nr-1),it];
                Ir2[i,it]=I[i-(nr-1),it];
                Rr2[i,it]=R[i-(nr-1),it]};
#             if((it-1)*(it-16)*(it-nout)==0){
#             cat(sprintf(
#             "\n %5d %5d %10.4f %10.4f %10.4f
#             %10.4f",
#             it,i,r2[i],Sr2[i,it],Ir2[i,it],
#             Rr2[i,it]));
#           }
          }
        }
```

Some additional explanation follows.

- Solution arrays Sr2,Ir2,Rr2 are defined for $-1 \leq r \leq 1$. These arrays have an r dimension of 51.

```
          #
          # Plot PDE solutions, -r0 <= r <= r0
          Sr2=matrix(0,nrow=(2*nr-1),ncol=nout);
          Ir2=matrix(0,nrow=(2*nr-1),ncol=nout);
          Rr2=matrix(0,nrow=(2*nr-1),ncol=nout);
          r2=rep(0,(2*nr-1));
```

r is also extended to $r2$ with 51 elements.
- Two **fors** step through t and r. For $r \leq 0$ (i<=26),

```
for(it in 1:nout){
  for(i in 1:(2*nr-1)){
    if(i<=26){
      r2[i]=-r[nr-(i-1)];
      Sr2[i,it]=S[nr-(i-1),it];
      Ir2[i,it]=I[nr-(i-1),it];
      Rr2[i,it]=R[nr-(i-1),it]};
```

which uses the solutions for $r > 0$ to reflect symmetry around $r = 0$.
- For $r > 0$, the previous solutions are used.

```
if(i>26){
  r2[i]=r[i-(nr-1)];
  Sr2[i,it]=S[i-(nr-1),it];
  Ir2[i,it]=I[i-(nr-1),it];
  Rr2[i,it]=R[i-(nr-1),it]};
```

- The resulting arrays and vector can be viewed at $t = 0, 0.05, 0.1$ (by deactivating the comments).

```
#      if((it-1)*(it-16)*(it-nout)==0){
#      cat(sprintf(
#      "\n %5d %5d %10.4f %10.4f %10.4f
#      %10.4f",
#      it,i,r2[i],Sr2[i,it],Ir2[i,it],
#      Rr2[i,it]));
#      }
     }
   }
```

The two } conclude the **fors**.

- The solutions are plotted with **persp**. Note the use of r2, Sr2, Ir2, Rr2 for $-1 \leq r \leq 1$.

```
#
# S(r,t)
  persp(r2,tout,Sr2,theta=60,phi=45,
         xlim=c(-ru,ru),ylim=c(t0,tf),xlab="r",
         ylab="t",zlab="S(r,t)");
#
# I(r,t)
  persp(r2,tout,Ir2,theta=55,phi=45,
         xlim=c(-ru,ru),ylim=c(t0,tf),xlab="r",
         ylab="t",zlab="I(r,t)");
#
# R(r,t)
  persp(r2,tout,Rr2,theta=55,phi=45,
         xlim=c(-ru,ru),ylim=c(t0,tf),xlab="r",
         ylab="t",zlab="R(r,t)");
```

The numerical output is the same as in Table 4.5.

[1] 31

[1] 79

t	r	S(r,t)	I(r,t)	R(r,t)
0.00	0.0	1.000e+00	1.000e+00	0.000e+00
0.00	0.2	1.000e+00	1.832e-02	0.000e+00
0.00	0.4	1.000e+00	1.125e-07	0.000e+00
0.00	0.6	1.000e+00	2.320e-16	0.000e+00
0.00	0.8	1.000e+00	1.604e-28	0.000e+00
0.00	1.0	1.000e+00	3.720e-44	0.000e+00

t	r	S(r,t)	I(r,t)	R(r,t)
0.05	0.0	7.777e-01	2.875e-01	1.658e-01
0.05	0.2	9.007e-01	1.901e-01	1.008e-01
0.05	0.4	1.012e+00	6.367e-02	2.411e-02

```
0.05    0.6    1.008e+00    1.100e-02    2.631e-03
0.05    0.8    1.002e+00    8.964e-04    1.382e-04
0.05    1.0    1.001e+00    6.939e-05    7.373e-06


   t      r       S(r,t)       I(r,t)       R(r,t)
0.10    0.0    7.456e-01    1.919e-01    2.346e-01
0.10    0.2    8.191e-01    1.548e-01    1.798e-01
0.10    0.4    9.459e-01    8.527e-02    8.169e-02
0.10    0.6    1.001e+00    3.402e-02    2.369e-02
0.10    0.8    1.006e+00    9.660e-03    4.674e-03
0.10    1.0    1.004e+00    3.534e-03    1.238e-03


ncall =    210
```

Table 4.5: Numerical output for eqs. (4.2), (4.3), (4.4),
ncase=3

We can note the following details about this output.

- out has the dimensions $31 \times 3(26) + 1 = 79$ since nr was reduced from 51 to 26.
- The ICs are confirmed (as in Listing 4.1).
- The solutions are for $t = 0, 0.05, 0.1$ and $r = 0$, $0.1, ..., 1$ as explained previously. They are slightly different than in Table 4.4 since the gridding in r is different.
- The computational effort is smaller than in Table 4.4 (ncall = 210 rather than 287) which is not unexpected since the MOL/ODEs are less stiff with a larger grid spacing of $(1 - 0)/(26 - 1)$ rather than $(1 - 0)/(51 - 1)$.

The resulting plots, Figs. 4.5a,b,c, indicate (1) the reduction in $S(r, t)$ from conversion of susceptibles to infecteds and then recovereds (Fig. 4.5a), (2) the initial infecteds at $r = 0$ which eventually decay with t (Fig. 4.5b), and

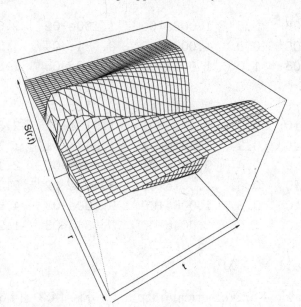

Figure 4.5a: Numerical solution $S(r, t)$ from eq. (4.2a), `ncase=3`, $-1 \leq r \leq 1$

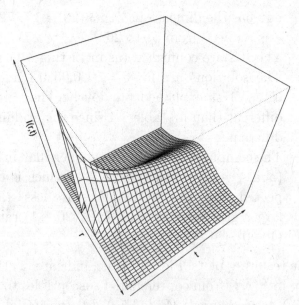

Figure 4.5b: Numerical solution $I(r, t)$ from eq. (4.2b), `ncase=3`, $-1 \leq r \leq 1$

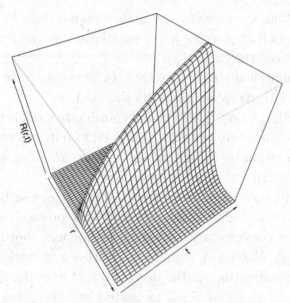

Figure 4.5c: Numerical solution $R(r, t)$ from eq. (4.2c), `ncase=3`, $-1 \leq r \leq 1$

(3) the increase in recovereds as the infecteds diminish (Fig. 4.5c).

In summary, this graphical output indicates (1) the symmetry of the solution around $r = 0$ and (2) the epidemic is stable with eventual recovery. The use of the spatial grid $-1 \leq r \leq 1$ can be viewed as the use of polar coordinates with $\theta = 0$ for $0 \leq r \leq 1$ and $\theta = \pi$ for $-1 \leq r \leq 0$.

(4.5) Summary and Conclusions

The following conclusions summarize the preceding discussion of cross diffusion PDEs defined on radial grids.

(1) The ease of programming the nonlinear cross diffusion product `SI` is demonstrated. Additionally, any of the coefficients in eqs. (4.2) can be programmed as a function of r and t. For example, the diffusivities D_{si}, D_s, D_i, D_r could vary with r,

which might represent the higher populations in an urban area (small r), and the lower populations in the surrounding rural areas (large r).

(2) The numerical solutions of eqs. (4.2) to (4.4) are displayed in 2D with `matplots` and 3D with `persp`.

(3) A 1D PDE model with a radial coordinate models the spread of infection from a central point. This contrasts with Cartesian coordinates which would require 2D that would not naturally fit the physical system.

(4) Consideration of physical systems with irregular boundaries would be a logical next step, but this probably could not be done conveniently within an orthogonal coordinate system, e.g., Cartesian, cylindrical. Rather a numerical method for approximating spatial derivatives on irregular geometries would be required, such as finite elements. This approach could still be used within the MOL framework (approximation of PDEs as systems of ODEs).

(5) Also, a numerical method for approximating spatial derivatives that does not require a coordinate system (a meshless or mesh-free method) could be used such as radial basis functions (RBFs) [1] Chapter 7. These extended methods are not considered here.

We can now consider applications of the cross diffusion equations in radial coordinates, eqs. (4.2).

Reference

[1] Griffiths, G.W. (2016), *Numerical Analysis Using R: Solutions to ODEs and PDEs*, Cambridge University Press, Cambridge, UK.

Chapter 5

Vector-Borne Diseases, Malaria

(5.1) Introduction

The application of the preceding ODE/PDE analysis to malaria is considered in this chapter. A distinguishing feature of malaria is that it is vector-borne and the vector is a mosquito. Therefore, the models that are considered include human and mosquito dynamics.

(5.2) ODE Malaria Model, Low Transmission

The model is from [2] stated as ODEs in t. The ODE model is then extended to PDEs to include spatial effects, that is, a spatiotemporal model.

The model is a 7×7 (seven equations in seven unknowns) ODE system.

$$\frac{dS_h}{dt} = \Lambda_h + \Psi_h N_h + \rho_h R_h - f_h(N_h) S_h \qquad (5.1a)$$

$$\frac{dE_h}{dt} = \lambda_h(t) S_h - \nu_h E_h - f_h(N_h) E_h \qquad (5.1b)$$

$$\frac{dI_h}{dt} = \nu_h E_h - \gamma_h I_h - f_h(N_h) I_h - \delta_h I_h \qquad (5.1c)$$

$$\frac{dR_h}{dt} = \gamma_h I_h - \rho_h R_h - f_h(N_h) R_h \qquad (5.1d)$$

$$\frac{dS_v}{dt} = \Psi_v N_v - \lambda_v(t)S_v - f_v(N_v)S_v \qquad (5.1e)$$

$$\frac{dE_v}{dt} = \lambda_v(t)S_v - \nu_v E_v - f_v(N_v)E_v \qquad (5.1f)$$

$$\frac{dI_v}{dt} = \nu_v E_v - f_v(N_v)I_v \qquad (5.1g)$$

The dependent (state) variables of equations (5.1) are listed in Table 5.1.

Variable	Description
$S_h(t)$	susceptible humans
$E_h(t)$	exposed humans
$I_h(t)$	infected humans
$R_h(t)$	recovered humans
$S_v(t)$	susceptible mosquitoes
$E_v(t)$	exposed mosquitoes
$I_v(t)$	infected mosquitoes

Table 5.1: Dependent (state) variables of eqs. (5.1)

Note that subscript h pertains to humans and subscript v pertains to mosquitoes.

A few of the RHS terms of eqs. (5.1) require additional explanation.

(1) N_h, N_v: The total number of humans and mosquitoes at a particular time t.

$$N_h = S_h + E_h + I_h + R_h; \quad N_v = S_v + E_v + I_v \qquad (5.2a,b)$$

(2) Functions of the dependent variables.

$$f_h(N_h) = \mu_{1h} + \mu_{2h} N_h \tag{5.2c}$$

$$f_v(N_v) = \mu_{1v} + \mu_{2v} N_v \tag{5.2d}$$

$$\lambda_h = \frac{\sigma_v N_v \sigma_h}{\sigma_v N_v + \sigma_h N_h} \beta_{hv} \frac{I_v}{N_v} \tag{5.2e}$$

$$\lambda_v = \frac{\sigma_v N_h \sigma_h}{\sigma_v N_v + \sigma_h N_h} \left(\beta_{vh} \frac{I_h}{N_h} + \bar{\beta}_{vh} \frac{R_h}{N_h} \right) \tag{5.2f}$$

The parameters (constants) in eqs. (5.1) and (5.2) are explained in detail in [2], Table 2.

Eqs. (5.1) are first order in t so that each requires one initial condition (IC).

$$S_h(t = 0) = S_{h0}; \quad E_h(t = 0) = E_{h0} \tag{5.3a,b}$$

$$I_h(t = 0) = I_{h0}; \quad R_h(t = 0) = R_{h0} \tag{5.3c,d}$$

$$S_v(t = 0) = S_{v0}; \quad E_v(t = 0) = E_{v0}; \quad I_v(t = 0) = I_{v0} \tag{5.3e,f,g}$$

Two sets of the constants S_{h0} to I_{v0} are defined numerically, corresponding to high transmission and low transmission ([2], Table 3) analyzed subsequently as two cases.

Parameter	Units	High transmission	Low transmission
Λ_h	humans days^{-1}	0.033	0.041
Ψ_h	days^{-1}	1.1×10^{-4}	5.5×10^{-5}
Ψ_v	days^{-1}	0.13	0.13
σ_v	days^{-1}	0.50	0.33
σ_h	days^{-1}	19	4.3
β_{hv}	1	0.022	0.022
β_{vh}	1	0.48	0.24
$\bar{\beta}_{vh}$	1	0.048	0.024
ν_h	days^{-1}	0.10	0.10
ν_v	days^{-1}	0.091	0.083
γ_h	days^{-1}	0.0035	0.0035
δ_h	days^{-1}	9.0×10^{-5}	1.8×10^{-5}
ρ_h	days^{-1}	5.5×10^{-4}	2.7×10^{-3}
μ_{1h}	days^{-1}	1.6×10^{-5}	8.8×10^{-6}
μ_{2h}	humans^{-1} days^{-1}	3.0×10^{-7}	2.0×10^{-7}
μ_{1v}	days^{-1}	0.033	0.033
μ_{2v}	mosquitoes^{-1} days^{-1}	2.0×10^{-5}	4.0×10^{-5}

Table 5.2: Parameters in eqs. (5.1), (5.2)

As an additional feature of the ODE model, a *reproductive number (reproduction ratio)*, R_o, is defined in [2]

$$R_o = \sqrt{K_{vh} K_{hv}} \tag{5.4a}$$

with

$$K_{hv} = \left(\frac{\nu_v}{\nu_v + \mu_{1v} + \mu_{2v} N_v^e} \right) \left(\frac{\sigma_v \sigma_h N_h^e}{\sigma_v N_v^e + \sigma_h N_h^e} \right)$$

$$(\beta_{hv}) \left(\frac{1}{\mu_{1v} + \mu_{2v} N_v^e} \right). \tag{5.4b}$$

$$K_{vh} = \left(\frac{\nu_h}{\nu_h + \mu_{1h} + \mu_{2h} N_h^e} \right) \left(\frac{\sigma_v \sigma_h N_v^e}{\sigma_v N_v^e + \sigma_h N_h^e} \right)$$

$$\left(\frac{1}{\gamma_h + \delta_h + \mu_{1h} + \mu_{2h} N_h^e} \right) \left[\beta_{vh} + \bar{\beta}_{vh} \left(\frac{\gamma_h}{\rho_h + \mu_{1h} + \mu_{2h} N_h^e} \right) \right]$$

$$(5.4c)$$

Eqs. (5.4) are implemented in a R routine that follows. R_o is an indicator of the increase of human infections from a base case. For $R_o > 1$, infections will increase, while for $R_o < 1$ they will decrease. For the low and high transmission cases that are discussed subsequently, R_o is calculated according to eqs. (5.4) and is greater than one.

Also, a parameter sensitivity, Υ_p^{Ro} is defined as

$$\Upsilon_p^{Ro} = \frac{\partial Ro}{\partial p} \times \frac{p}{Ro} \qquad (5.5a)$$

Two parameters are of particular interest, one with the largest sensitivity, σ_v, and one with the smallest sensitivity, ν_h ([2], Table 4)

$$\Upsilon_{\sigma_v}^{Ro} = \frac{\sigma_h N_h^e}{\sigma_v N_v^e + \sigma_h N_h^e} \qquad (5.5b)$$

$$\Upsilon_{\sigma_v}^{Ro} = \frac{(19)(514.4)}{(0.50)(4850) + (19)(514.4)} = 0.8012$$

$$\Upsilon_{\nu_h}^{Ro} = 0.00086 \qquad (5.5c)$$

(5.2.1) Main program

A main program for eqs. (5.1), (5.2) and (5.3) for the low transmission case follows.

```
#
# SEIRV ODE malaria model
```

```
#
# Delete previous workspaces
  rm(list=ls(all=TRUE))
#
# Access ODE integrator
  library("deSolve");
#
# Access functions for numerical solution
  setwd("f:/infectious/chap5/sevenODE");
  source("ode1a.R");
#
# Parameters
  Lambda_h=0.041;
  Psi_h=5.5e-05;
  Psi_v=0.13;
  sigma_v=0.33;
  sigma_h=4.3;
  beta_hv=0.022;
  beta_vh=0.24;
  beta_vhb=0.024;
  nu_h=0.10;
  nu_v=0.083;
  gamma_h=0.0035;
  delta_h=1.8e-05;
  rho_h=2.7e-03;
  mu_1h=8.8e-06;
  mu_2h=2.0e-07;
  mu_1v=0.033;
  mu_2v=4.0e-05;
#
# Independent variable for ODE integration
  t0=0;tf=10000;
  tout=seq(from=t0,to=tf,by=250);
# print(tout);
```

```
#
# Initial condition (t=0)
  ncase=1;
  u0=rep(0,7);
  if(ncase==1){
    u0[1]=600;
    u0[2]=20;
    u0[3]=3;
    u0[4]=0;
    u0[5]=2400;
    u0[6]=30;
    u0[7]=5;
  }
  if(ncase==2){
    u0[1]=481.6;
    u0[2]=1.7;
    u0[3]=45.6;
    u0[4]=56.4;
    u0[5]=2330.6;
    u0[6]=57.6;
    u0[7]=36.8;
  }
  ncall=0;
#
# ODE integration
  out=lsodes(y=u0,times=tout,func=ode1a,
      sparsetype="sparseint",rtol=1e-6,
      atol=1e-6,maxord=5);
  nrow(out)
  ncol(out)
#
# Arrays for plotting numerical solution
  nout=41;
  Sh=rep(0,nout);
```

```
Eh=rep(0,nout);
Ih=rep(0,nout);
Rh=rep(0,nout);
Sv=rep(0,nout);
Ev=rep(0,nout);
Iv=rep(0,nout);
Nh=rep(0,nout);
Nv=rep(0,nout);
for(it in 1:nout){
  Sh[it]=out[it,2];
  Eh[it]=out[it,3];
  Ih[it]=out[it,4];
  Rh[it]=out[it,5];
  Sv[it]=out[it,6];
  Ev[it]=out[it,7];
  Iv[it]=out[it,8];
  Nh[it]=Sh[it]+Eh[it]+Ih[it]+Rh[it];
  Nv[it]=Sv[it]+Ev[it]+Iv[it];
}
#
# Display numerical solution
  for(it in 1:nout){
  if((it-1)*(it-21)*(it-nout)==0){
  cat(sprintf("\n"));
  cat(sprintf("\n        t        Sh(t)        Eh(t)"));
  cat(sprintf("\n                 Ih(t)        Rh(t)"));
  cat(sprintf("\n                 Sv(t)        Ev(t)"));
  cat(sprintf("\n                 Iv(t)              "));
  cat(sprintf("\n                 Nh(t)        Nv(t)"));
  cat(sprintf("\n %6.0f %10.1f %10.1f",
              tout[it],Sh[it],Eh[it]));
  cat(sprintf(
     "\n          %10.1f %10.1f",Ih[it],Rh[it]));
  cat(sprintf(
```

```
      "\n          %10.1f %10.1f",Sv[it],Ev[it]));
  cat(sprintf(
      "\n          %10.1f          ",Iv[it]));
  cat(sprintf(
      "\n          %10.1f %10.1f",Nh[it],Nv[it]));
  }
  }
#
# Calls to ODE routine
  cat(sprintf("\n\n ncall = %5d\n\n",ncall));
#
# Plot ODE solutions
#
# Sh
  par(mfrow=c(1,1));
  plot(tout,Sh,type="l",xlab="t",ylab="Sh(t)",
    lty=1,main="",lwd=2,col="black");
#
# Eh
  par(mfrow=c(1,1));
  plot(tout,Eh,type="l",xlab="t",ylab="Eh(t)",
    lty=1,main="",lwd=2,col="black");
#
# Ih
  par(mfrow=c(1,1));
  plot(tout,Ih,type="l",xlab="t",ylab="Ih(t)",
    lty=1,main="",lwd=2,col="black");
#
# Rh
  par(mfrow=c(1,1));
  plot(tout,Rh,type="l",xlab="t",ylab="Rh(t)",
    lty=1,main="",lwd=2,col="black");
#
# Eh,Ih,Rh
```

```
plot(
  tout,Eh,type="l",xlab="t",ylab="Eh(t),
  Ih(t),Rh(t)",ylim=c(0,60),lty=1,main="",
  lwd=2,col="black");
points(tout,Eh, pch="1",lwd=2);
 lines(tout,Ih,type="l",lwd=2);
points(tout,Ih, pch="2",lwd=2);
 lines(tout,Rh,type="l",lwd=2);
points(tout,Rh, pch="3",lwd=2);
#
# Sv
 par(mfrow=c(1,1));
 plot(tout,Sv,type="l",xlab="t",ylab="Sv(t)",
   lty=1,main="",lwd=2,col="black");
#
# Ev
 par(mfrow=c(1,1));
 plot(tout,Ev,type="l",xlab="t",ylab="Ev(t)",
   lty=1,main="",lwd=2,col="black");
#
# Iv
 par(mfrow=c(1,1));
 plot(tout,Iv,type="l",xlab="t",ylab="Iv(t)",
   lty=1,main="",lwd=2,col="black");
#
# Ev,Iv
 par(mfrow=c(1,1));
 plot(
   tout,Ev,type="l",xlab="t",
   ylab="Ev(t),Iv(t)",ylim=c(0,60),
   lty=1,main="",lwd=2,col="black");
points(tout,Ev, pch="1",lwd=2);
 lines(tout,Iv,type="l",lwd=2);
points(tout,Iv, pch="2",lwd=2);
```

Listing 5.1: Main program for eqs. (5.1), (5.2), (5.3), low transmission

We can note the following details about Listing 5.1.

- Previous workspaces are deleted.

```
#
# SEIRV ODE malaria model
#
# Delete previous workspaces
  rm(list=ls(all=TRUE))
```

- The R ODE integrator library deSolve is accessed. Then the directory with the files for the solution of eqs. (5.1), (5.2), (5.3) is designated. Note that setwd (set working directory) uses / rather than the usual \.

```
#
# Access ODE integrator
  library("deSolve");
#
# Access functions for numerical solution
  setwd("f:/infectious/chap5/sevenODE");
  source("ode1a.R");
```

The ODE routine, ode1a.R, is discussed next.

- The parameters for the low transmission case of Table 5.2 are defined numerically.

```
#
# Parameters
  Lambda_h=0.041;
  Psi_h=5.5e-05;
  Psi_v=0.13;
  sigma_v=0.33;
  sigma_h=4.3;
```

```
beta_hv=0.022;
beta_vh=0.24;
beta_vhb=0.024;
nu_h=0.10;
nu_v=0.083;
gamma_h=0.0035;
delta_h=1.8e-05;
rho_h=2.7e-03;
mu_1h=8.8e-06;
mu_2h=2.0e-07;
mu_1v=0.033;
mu_2v=4.0e-05;
```

- A time interval is defined as $0 \leq t \leq 10000$ with $41 = 10000/250 + 1$ output points so that tout = $0, 250, \ldots, 10000$.

```
#
# Independent variable for ODE integration
  t0=0;tf=10000;
  tout=seq(from=t0,to=tf,by=250);
# print(tout);
```

The #print(tout) can be activated (decommented) to confirm the values of tout.

- ICs (5.3) are defined for two cases. For ncase=1, the ICs from [2] are used. For ncase=2, the equilibrium (steady state) solution from ncase=1 is used as ICs so that the solution does not change with t (it remains at the equilibrium point).

```
#
# Initial condition (t=0)
  ncase=2;
  u0=rep(0,7);
  if(ncase==1){
```

```
  u0[1]=600;
  u0[2]=20;
  u0[3]=3;
  u0[4]=0;
  u0[5]=2400;
  u0[6]=30;
  u0[7]=5;
}
if(ncase==2){
  u0[1]=481.6;
  u0[2]=1.7;
  u0[3]=45.6;
  u0[4]=56.4;
  u0[5]=2330.6;
  u0[6]=57.6;
  u0[7]=36.8;
}
ncall=0;
```

The number of calls to ode1a is also initialized.

- t is defined on the interval $0 \leq t \leq 10000$ days with $10000/250 + 1 = 41$ output points so that tout has the values $0, 250, \ldots, 10000$.

```
#
# Independent variable for ODE integration
  t0=0;tf=10000;
  tout=seq(from=t0,to=tf,by=250);
# print(tout);
```

-

- The system of 7 ODEs is integrated by the library integrator lsodes (available in deSolve). As expected, the inputs to lsodes are the ODE function, ode1a, the IC vector u0, and the vector of output values of t, tout. The length of u0

(7) informs `lsodes` how many ODEs are to be integrated. `func,y,times` are reserved names.

```
#
# ODE integration
  out=lsodes(y=u0,times=tout,func=ode1a,
     sparsetype="sparseint",rtol=1e-6,
     atol=1e-6,maxord=5);
  nrow(out)
  ncol(out)
```

- The seven ODE dependent variables returned by `lsodes` in out and N_h, N_v are placed in vectors for plotting.

```
#
# Arrays for plotting numerical solution
  nout=41;
  Sh=rep(0,nout);
  Eh=rep(0,nout);
  Ih=rep(0,nout);
  Rh=rep(0,nout);
  Sv=rep(0,nout);
  Ev=rep(0,nout);
  Iv=rep(0,nout);
  Nh=rep(0,nout);
  Nv=rep(0,nout);
  for(it in 1:nout){
    Sh[it]=out[it,2];
    Eh[it]=out[it,3];
    Ih[it]=out[it,4];
    Rh[it]=out[it,5];
    Sv[it]=out[it,6];
    Ev[it]=out[it,7];
    Iv[it]=out[it,8];
    Nh[it]=Sh[it]+Eh[it]+Ih[it]+Rh[it];
```

```
    Nv[it]=Sv[it]+Ev[it]+Iv[it];
    }
```

- The ODE solutions, N_h, N_v are displayed at $t = 0, 5000, 10000$.

```
#
# Display numerical solution
  for(it in 1:nout){
  if((it-1)*(it-21)*(it-nout)==0){
  cat(sprintf("\n"));
  cat(sprintf("\n          t         Sh(t)        Eh(t)"));
  cat(sprintf("\n                    Ih(t)        Rh(t)"));
  cat(sprintf("\n                    Sv(t)        Ev(t)"));
  cat(sprintf("\n                    Iv(t)               "));
  cat(sprintf("\n                    Nh(t)        Nv(t)"));
  cat(sprintf("\n %6.0f %10.1f %10.1f",
             tout[it],Sh[it],Eh[it]));
  cat(sprintf(
     "\n          %10.1f %10.1f",Ih[it],Rh[it]));
  cat(sprintf(
     "\n          %10.1f %10.1f",Sv[it],Ev[it]));
  cat(sprintf(
     "\n          %10.1f        ",Iv[it]));
  cat(sprintf(
     "\n          %10.1f %10.1f",Nh[it],Nv[it]));
  }
  }
```

- The number of calls to ode_1a is displayed as a measure of the computational effort for the complete solution.

```
#
# Calls to ODE routine
  cat(sprintf("\n\n ncall = %5d\n\n",ncall));
```

- Plots for the human variables are produced with plot.

```
#
# Plot ODE solutions
#
# Sh
  par(mfrow=c(1,1));
  plot(tout,Sh,type="l",xlab="t",ylab="Sh(t)",
    lty=1,main="",lwd=2,col="black");
#
# Eh
  par(mfrow=c(1,1));
  plot(tout,Eh,type="l",xlab="t",ylab="Eh(t)",
    lty=1,main="",lwd=2,col="black");
#
# Ih
  par(mfrow=c(1,1));
  plot(tout,Ih,type="l",xlab="t",ylab="Ih(t)",
    lty=1,main="",lwd=2,col="black");
#
# Rh
  par(mfrow=c(1,1));
  plot(tout,Rh,type="l",xlab="t",ylab="Rh(t)",
    lty=1,main="",lwd=2,col="black");
```

- E_h, I_h, R_h are then superimposed on a composite plot (discussed subsequently), with the markers $1, 2, 3$, respectively.

```
#
# Eh,Ih,Rh
  plot(
    tout,Eh,type="l",xlab="t",ylab="Eh(t),
    Ih(t),Rh(t)",ylim=c(0,60),lty=1,main="",
    lwd=2,col="black");
  points(tout,Eh, pch="1",lwd=2);
```

```
  lines(tout,Ih,type="l",lwd=2);
  points(tout,Ih,  pch="2",lwd=2);
  lines(tout,Rh,type="l",lwd=2);
  points(tout,Rh,  pch="3",lwd=2);
```

- Plots for the vector variables are produced with plot.

```
  #
  # Sv
  par(mfrow=c(1,1));
  plot(tout,Sv,type="l",xlab="t",ylab="Sv(t)",
    lty=1,main="",lwd=2,col="black");
  #
  # Ev
  par(mfrow=c(1,1));
  plot(tout,Ev,type="l",xlab="t",ylab="Ev(t)",
    lty=1,main="",lwd=2,col="black");
  #
  # Iv
  par(mfrow=c(1,1));
  plot(tout,Iv,type="l",xlab="t",ylab="Iv(t)",
    lty=1,main="",lwd=2,col="black");
```

- E_v, I_v are then superimposed on a composite plot (discussed subsequently), with the markers $1, 2$, respectively.

```
  #
  # Ev,Iv
  par(mfrow=c(1,1));
  plot(
    tout,Ev,type="l",xlab="t",
    ylab="Ev(t),Iv(t)",ylim=c(0,60),
    lty=1,main="",lwd=2,col="black");
  points(tout,Ev,  pch="1",lwd=2);
  lines(tout,Iv,type="l",lwd=2);
  points(tout,Iv,  pch="2",lwd=2);
```

ODE routine ode1a is discussed next.

(5.2.2) ODE/MOL routine

Routine ode1a for eqs. (5.1), (5.2), (5.3) follows.

```
  ode1a=function(t,u,parms){
#
# Function ode1a computes the t derivative
# vectors of Sh(t),Eh(t),Ih(t),Rh(t),
# Sv(t),Ev(t),Iv(t)
#
# One vector to seven scalars
  Sh=u[1];
  Eh=u[2];
  Ih=u[3];
  Rh=u[4];
  Sv=u[5];
  Ev=u[6];
  Iv=u[7];
#
# Algebra
  Nh=Sh+Eh+Ih+Rh;
  Nv=Sv+Ev+Iv;
  fhNh=mu_1h+mu_2h*Nh;
  fvNv=mu_1v+mu_2v*Nv;
  lambda_h=(sigma_v*Nv*sigma_h)/
          (sigma_v*Nv+sigma_h*Nh)*
           beta_hv*(Iv/Nv);
  lambda_v=(sigma_v*Nh*sigma_h)/
          (sigma_v*Nv+sigma_h*Nh)*
          (beta_vh*(Ih/Nh)+beta_vhb*(Rh/Nh));
#
# ODEs
  Sht=Lambda_h+Psi_h*Nh+rho_h*Rh-lambda_h*Sh-
```

```
      fhNh*Sh;
  Eht=lambda_h*Sh-nu_h*Eh-fhNh*Eh;
  Iht=nu_h*Eh-gamma_h*Ih-fhNh*Ih-delta_h*Ih;
  Rht=gamma_h*Ih-rho_h*Rh-fhNh*Rh;
  Svt=Psi_v*Nv-lambda_v*Sv-fvNv*Sv;
  Evt=lambda_v*Sv-nu_v*Ev-fvNv*Ev;
  Ivt=nu_v*Ev-fvNv*Iv;
#
# Seven scalars to one vector
  ut=rep(0,7);
    ut[1]=Sht;
    ut[2]=Eht;
    ut[3]=Iht;
    ut[4]=Rht;
    ut[5]=Svt;
    ut[6]=Evt;
    ut[7]=Ivt;
#
# Increment calls to ode1a
  ncall <<- ncall+1;
#
# Return derivative vector
  return(list(c(ut)));
  }
```

Listing 5.2: ODE routine **ode1a** for eqs. (5.1), (5.2), (5.3), low transmission

We can note the following details about Listing 5.2.

- The function is defined.

```
  ode1a=function(t,u,parms){
#
# Function ode1a computes the t derivative
# vectors of Sh(t),Eh(t),Ih(t),Rh(t),
```

```
# Sv(t),Ev(t),Iv(t)
```

t is the current value of t in eqs. (5.1). u the 7-vector of ODE dependent variables. parm is an argument to pass parameters to ode1a (unused, but required in the argument list). The arguments must be listed in the order stated to properly interface with lsodes called in the main program of Listing 5.1. The derivative vector of the LHS of eqs. (5.1) is calculated next and returned to lsodes.

- u is placed in seven scalars to facilitate the programming of eqs. (5.1), (5.2).

```
#
# One vector to seven scalars
  Sh=u[1];
  Eh=u[2];
  Ih=u[3];
  Rh=u[4];
  Sv=u[5];
  Ev=u[6];
  Iv=u[7];
```

- The algebra of eqs. (5.2) is programmed.

```
#
# Algebra
  Nh=Sh+Eh+Ih+Rh;
  Nv=Sv+Ev+Iv;
  fhNh=mu_1h+mu_2h*Nh;
  fvNv=mu_1v+mu_2v*Nv;
  lambda_h=(sigma_v*Nv*sigma_h)/
          (sigma_v*Nv+sigma_h*Nh)*
          beta_hv*(Iv/Nv);
  lambda_v=(sigma_v*Nh*sigma_h)/
          (sigma_v*Nv+sigma_h*Nh)*
          (beta_vh*(Ih/Nh)+beta_vhb*(Rh/Nh));
```

- ODEs (5.1) are programmed. For example, $\dfrac{dS_h}{dt} = \text{Sht}$ for eq. (5.1a).

```
#
# ODEs
  Sht=Lambda_h+Psi_h*Nh+rho_h*Rh-lambda_h*Sh-
      fhNh*Sh;
  Eht=lambda_h*Sh-nu_h*Eh-fhNh*Eh;
  Iht=nu_h*Eh-gamma_h*Ih-fhNh*Ih-delta_h*Ih;
  Rht=gamma_h*Ih-rho_h*Rh-fhNh*Rh;
  Svt=Psi_v*Nv-lambda_v*Sv-fvNv*Sv;
  Evt=lambda_v*Sv-nu_v*Ev-fvNv*Ev;
  Ivt=nu_v*Ev-fvNv*Iv;
```

- The t derivatives of the seven ODEs are placed in a vector ut to return to lsodes for the next step along the solution.

```
#
# Seven scalars to one vector
  ut=rep(0,7);
    ut[1]=Sht;
    ut[2]=Eht;
    ut[3]=Iht;
    ut[4]=Rht;
    ut[5]=Svt;
    ut[6]=Evt;
    ut[7]=Ivt;
```

- The number of calls to ode1a is incremented and returned to the main program of Listing 5.1 via <<-.

```
#
# Increment calls to ode1a
  ncall <<- ncall+1;
```

- The derivative vector ut is returned to lsodes as a list (required by lsodes). c is the vector operator in R.

```
#
# Return derivative vector
  return(list(c(ut)));
  }
```

The final } concludes ode1a.

The numerical and graphical output is discussed next.

(5.2.3) Model output

The numerical output from the main program of Listing 5.1 and ODE routine of Listing 5.2 follows.

[1] 41

[1] 8

t	Sh(t)	Eh(t)
	Ih(t)	Rh(t)
	Sv(t)	Ev(t)
	Iv(t)	
	Nh(t)	Nv(t)
0	600.0	20.0
	3.0	0.0
	2400.0	30.0
	5.0	
	623.0	2435.0

t	Sh(t)	Eh(t)
	Ih(t)	Rh(t)
	Sv(t)	Ev(t)
	Iv(t)	

	Nh(t)	Nv(t)
5000	498.6	1.6
	43.2	52.7
	2336.9	53.8
	34.3	
	596.1	2425.0

t	Sh(t)	Eh(t)
	Ih(t)	Rh(t)
	Sv(t)	Ev(t)
	Iv(t)	
	Nh(t)	Nv(t)
10000	481.6	1.7
	45.6	56.4
	2330.6	57.6
	36.8	
	585.3	2425.0

```
ncall =    247
```

Table 5.3: Numerical output, ncase=1

We can note the following details about this output.

- The dimensions of the solution matrix out are $nout = 41 \times 7 + 1 = 8$. The offset +1 results from the value of t as the first element in each of the $nout = 41$ solution vectors. These same values of t are in tout,

```
[1] 41
```

```
[1] 8
```

- ICs (5.3) ($t = 0$) are verified (set in Listing 5.1).
- The output is for $t = 0, 5000, 10000$ as explained previously for Listing 5.1.

- The output for $t = 10000$ is close to an equilibrium (steady state) solution for which the LHS derivatives of eqs. (5.1) are close to zero. This property is used for the ICs of ncase=2 that follows.

Nine plots are produced by the main program of Listing 5.1. Four are indicated next.

The approach to an equilibrium solution is clear, e.g., Figs. 5.1-1, 5.1-6. Figs. 5.1-1,5,6,9 correspond to the solution in Fig. 2 of [2].

The solutions for ncase=2 are next. The ICs defined in Listing 5.1 are

```
if(ncase==2){
   u0[1]=481.6;
   u0[2]=1.7;
   u0[3]=45.6;
   u0[4]=56.4;
```

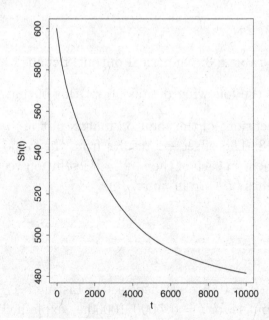

Figure 5.1-1: Numerical solution $S_h(t)$ from eq. (5.1a), ncase=1

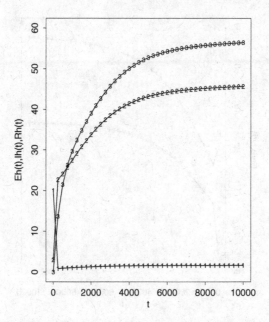

Figure 5.1-5: Numerical solutions $E_h(t), I_h(t), R_h(t)$ from eqs. (5.1b,c,d), `ncase=1`

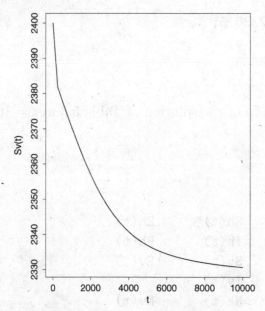

Figure 5.1-6: Numerical solution $S_v(t)$ from eq. (5.1e), `ncase=1`

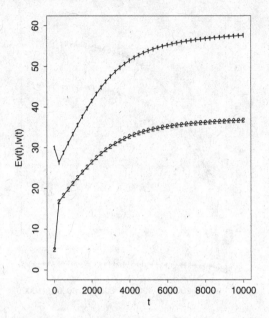

Figure 5.1-9: Numerical solutions $E_v(t)$, $I_v(t)$ from eqs. (5.1f,g), ncase=1

```
   u0[5]=2330.6;
   u0[6]=57.6;
   u0[7]=36.8;
}
```

which follow from the solution of Table 5.3 at $t = 10000$.

```
[1] 41
```

```
[1] 8
```

t	Sh(t)	Eh(t)
	Ih(t)	Rh(t)
	Sv(t)	Ev(t)
	Iv(t)	
	Nh(t)	Nv(t)
0	481.6	1.7

	45.6	56.4
	2330.6	57.6
	36.8	
	585.3	2425.0

t	Sh(t)	Eh(t)
	Ih(t)	Rh(t)
	Sv(t)	Ev(t)
	Iv(t)	
	Nh(t)	Nv(t)
5000	476.1	1.7
	46.2	57.2
	2329.1	58.6
	37.4	
	581.1	2425.0

t	Sh(t)	Eh(t)
	Ih(t)	Rh(t)
	Sv(t)	Ev(t)
	Iv(t)	
	Nh(t)	Nv(t)
10000	473.9	1.7
	46.4	57.4
	2328.5	58.9
	37.6	
	579.4	2425.0

```
ncall =    135
```

Table 5.4: Numerical output, ncase=2

We can note the following details about this output.

- The dimensions of the solution matrix out are again *nout* = $41 \times 7 + 1 = 8$.

[1] 41

[1] 8

- ICs (5.3) ($t = 0$) are verified (set in Listing 5.1 for `ncase=2`).
- The output is again for $t = 0, 5000, 10000$ as explained previously for Listing 5.1.
- The output remains close to the equilibrium solution set as the IC. For example,

  - $S_h(t = 0) = 481.6$
  - $S_h(t = 5000) = 476.1$
  - $S_h(t = 10000) = 473.9$

  This equilibrium solution could also be verified by displaying the t derivatives (LHSs of eqs. (5.1)). The derivatives are small, but not zero. They would be closer to zero if $t_f > 10000$ (set in the main program of Listing 5.1). This verification is left as an exercise for the reader.

- The computational effort is small, `ncall = 135`, since the changes in the solutions are small.

Again, nine plots are produced by the main program of Listing 5.1. Four are indicated next.

The vertical scales of Figs. 5.2-1,6 indicate a small change in $S_h(t), S_v(t)$. This is confirmed by the vertical scales of Fig. 5.2-5,9.

The reproduction number R_o from eqs. (5.4) is computed with the following routine.

```
#
# SEIRV ODE model
#
# Ro calculation, low transmission
#
# Delete previous workspaces
```

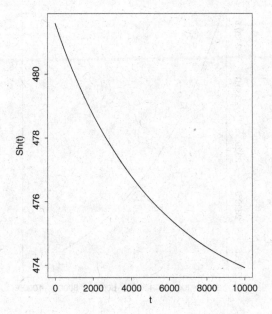

Figure 5.2-1: Numerical solution $S_h(t)$ from eq. (5.1a), `ncase=2`

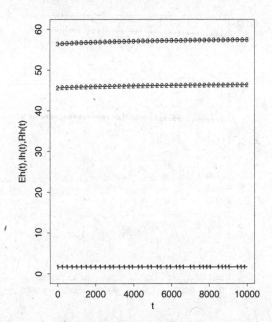

Figure 5.2-5: Numerical solutions $E_h(t), I_h(t), R_h(t)$ from eqs. (5.1b,c,d), `ncase=2`

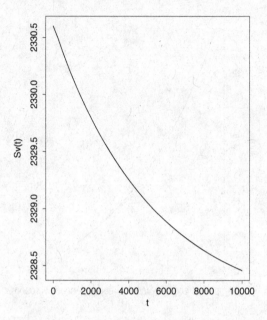

Figure 5.2-6: Numerical solution $S_v(t)$ from eq. (5.1e), `ncase=2`

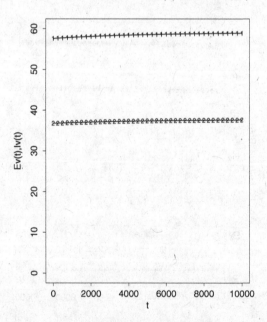

Figure 5.2-9: Numerical solutions $E_v(t)$, $I_v(t)$ from eqs. (5.1f,g), `ncase=2`

```
  rm(list=ls(all=TRUE))
#
# Parameters
  Lambda_h=0.041;
  Psi_h=5.5e-05;
  Psi_v=0.13;
  sigma_v=0.33;
  sigma_h=4.3;
  beta_hv=0.022;
  beta_vh=0.24;
  beta_vhb=0.024;
  nu_h=0.10;
  nu_v=0.083;
  gamma_h=0.0035;
  delta_h=1.8e-05;
  rho_h=2.7e-03;
  mu_1h=8.8e-06;
  mu_2h=2.0e-07;
  mu_1v=0.033;
  mu_2v=4.0e-05;
#
# Equilibrium (t=tf=10000) solution
# (ode1a_main.R, ode1a.R, ncase=2)
  Nh=579.4
  Nv=2425.0
#
# K_hv
  fact1=nu_v/(nu_v+mu_1v+mu_2v*Nv);
  fact2=(sigma_v*sigma_h*Nh)/(sigma_v*Nv+
         sigma_h*Nh);
  fact3=beta_hv;
  fact4=1/(mu_1v+mu_2v*Nv);
  K_hv=fact1*fact2*fact3*fact4;
#
```

```
# K_vh
  fact1=nu_h/(nu_h+mu_1h+mu_2h*Nv);
  fact2=(sigma_v*sigma_h*Nv)/(sigma_v*Nv+
        sigma_h*Nh);
  fact3=1/(gamma_h+delta_h+mu_1h+mu_2h*Nh);
  fact4=beta_vh+beta_vhb*(gamma_h/(rho_h+mu_1h+
        mu_2h*Nh));
  K_vh=fact1*fact2*fact3*fact4;
#
# Ro
  Ro_s=K_vh*K_hv;
  Ro  =Ro_s^{1/2};
#
# Output
  cat(sprintf("\n K_hv = %10.4f
               \n K_vh = %10.4f
               \n Ro_s = %10.4f
               \n   Ro = %10.4f",
              K_hv,K_vh,Ro_s,Ro));
```

Listing 5.3: Routine for the calculation of R_o, eqs. (5.4), low transmission

We can note the following details about Listing 5.3.

- Previous workspaces are cleared.

```
  #
  # SEIRV ODE model
  #
  # Ro calculation, low transmission
  #
  # Delete previous workspaces
    rm(list=ls(all=TRUE))
```

- The parameters for the low transmission case (Table 5.2) are specified.

```
#
# Parameters
  Lambda_h=0.041;
  Psi_h=5.5e-05;
  Psi_v=0.13;
  sigma_v=0.33;
  sigma_h=4.3;
  beta_hv=0.022;
  beta_vh=0.24;
  beta_vhb=0.024;
  nu_h=0.10;
  nu_v=0.083;
  gamma_h=0.0035;
  delta_h=1.8e-05;
  rho_h=2.7e-03;
  mu_1h=8.8e-06;
  mu_2h=2.0e-07;
  mu_1v=0.033;
  mu_2v=4.0e-05;
```

- The equilibrium values of N_h, N_v from Table 5.4 are specified.

```
#
# Equilibrium (t=tf=10000) solution
# (ode1a_main.R, ode1a.R, ncase=2)
  Nh=579.4
  Nv=2425.0
```

- K_{hv} from eq. (5.4b) is computed.

```
#
# K_hv
```

```
fact1=nu_v/(nu_v+mu_1v+mu_2v*Nv);
fact2=(sigma_v*sigma_h*Nh)/(sigma_v*Nv+
      sigma_h*Nh);
fact3=beta_hv;
fact4=1/(mu_1v+mu_2v*Nv);
K_hv=fact1*fact2*fact3*fact4;
```

- K_{vh} from eq. (5.4c) is computed.

```
#
# K_vh
fact1=nu_h/(nu_h+mu_1h+mu_2h*Nv);
fact2=(sigma_v*sigma_h*Nv)/(sigma_v*Nv+
      sigma_h*Nh);
fact3=1/(gamma_h+delta_h+mu_1h+mu_2h*Nh);
fact4=beta_vh+beta_vhb*(gamma_h/(rho_h+mu_1h+
      mu_2h*Nh));
K_vh=fact1*fact2*fact3*fact4;
```

- R_o from eq. (5.4a) is computed.

```
#
# Ro
Ro_s=K_vh*K_hv;
Ro  =Ro_s^{1/2};
```

- The various computed constants are displayed.

```
#
# Output
cat(sprintf("\n K_hv = %10.4f
             \n K_vh = %10.4f
             \n Ro_s = %10.4f
             \n   Ro = %10.4f",
            K_hv,K_vh,Ro_s,Ro));
```

Execution of the preceding routine gives the following output.

```
K_hv =      0.0165

K_vh =     77.0299

Ro_s =      1.2688

  Ro =      1.1264
```

In partcular, R_o is slightly greater than one (corresponding to the low transmission case of Table 5.2 which also has a long response time, $t_f = 10000$).

(5.3) ODE Malaria Model, High Transmission

An analogous development of Listings 5.1, 5.2 and 5.3 for high transmission with the parameters of Table 5.2 follows, starting with the main program.

(5.3.1) Main program

```
#
# SEIRV ODE malaria model
#
# Delete previous workspaces
  rm(list=ls(all=TRUE))
#
# Access ODE integrator
  library("deSolve");
#
# Access functions for numerical solution
  setwd("f:/infectious/chap5/sevenODE");
  source("ode1b.R");
#
# Parameters
  Lambda_h=0.033;
```

```
    Psi_h=1.1e-04;
    Psi_v=0.13;
    sigma_v=0.50;
    sigma_h=19;
    beta_hv=0.022;
    beta_vh=0.48;
    beta_vhb=0.048;
    nu_h=0.10;
    nu_v=0.091;
    gamma_h=0.0035;
    delta_h=9.0e-05;
    rho_h=5.5e-04;
    mu_1h=1.6e-05;
    mu_2h=3.0e-07;
    mu_1v=0.033;
    mu_2v=2.0e-05;
#
# Independent variable for ODE integration
    t0=0;tf=1200;
    tout=seq(from=t0,to=tf,by=30);
# print(tout);
#
# Initial condition (t=0)
    ncase=1;
    u0=rep(0,7);
    if(ncase==1){
      u0[1]=500;
      u0[2]=10;
      u0[3]=30;
      u0[4]=0;
      u0[5]=4000;
      u0[6]=100;
      u0[7]=50;
    }
```

```
  if(ncase==2){
    u0[1]=34.1;
    u0[2]=3;
    u0[3]=83.2;
    u0[4]=401.4;
    u0[5]=3590.2;
    u0[6]=740.9;
    u0[7]=518.9;
  }
  ncall=0;
#
# ODE integration
  out=lsodes(y=u0,times=tout,func=ode1b,
      sparsetype="sparseint",rtol=1e-6,
      atol=1e-6,maxord=5);
  nrow(out)
  ncol(out)
#
# Arrays for plotting numerical solution
  nout=41;
  Sh=rep(0,nout);
  Eh=rep(0,nout);
  Ih=rep(0,nout);
  Rh=rep(0,nout);
  Sv=rep(0,nout);
  Ev=rep(0,nout);
  Iv=rep(0,nout);
  Nh=rep(0,nout);
  Nv=rep(0,nout);
  for(it in 1:nout){
    Sh[it]=out[it,2];
    Eh[it]=out[it,3];
    Ih[it]=out[it,4];
    Rh[it]=out[it,5];
```

```
    Sv[it]=out[it,6];
    Ev[it]=out[it,7];
    Iv[it]=out[it,8];
    Nh[it]=Sh[it]+Eh[it]+Ih[it]+Rh[it];
    Nv[it]=Sv[it]+Ev[it]+Iv[it];
  }
#
# Display numerical solution
  for(it in 1:nout){
  if((it-1)*(it-21)*(it-nout)==0){
  cat(sprintf("\n"));
  cat(sprintf("\n           t          Sh(t)        Eh(t)"));
  cat(sprintf("\n                       Ih(t)        Rh(t)"));
  cat(sprintf("\n                       Sv(t)        Ev(t)"));
  cat(sprintf("\n                       Iv(t)             "));
  cat(sprintf("\n                       Nh(t)        Nv(t)"));
  cat(sprintf("\n %6.0f %10.1f %10.1f",
              tout[it],Sh[it],Eh[it]));
  cat(sprintf(
     "\n           %10.1f %10.1f",Ih[it],Rh[it]));
  cat(sprintf(
     "\n           %10.1f %10.1f",Sv[it],Ev[it]));
  cat(sprintf(
     "\n           %10.1f          ",Iv[it]));
  cat(sprintf(
     "\n           %10.1f %10.1f",Nh[it],Nv[it]));
  }
  }
#
# Calls to ODE routine
  cat(sprintf("\n\n ncall = %5d\n\n",ncall));
#
# Plot ODE solutions
#
```

```
# Sh
  par(mfrow=c(1,1));
  plot(tout,Sh,type="l",xlab="t",ylab="Sh(t)",
    lty=1,main="",lwd=2,col="black");
#
# Eh
  par(mfrow=c(1,1));
  plot(tout,Eh,type="l",xlab="t",ylab="Eh(t)",
    lty=1,main="",lwd=2,col="black");
#
# Ih
  par(mfrow=c(1,1));
  plot(tout,Ih,type="l",xlab="t",ylab="Ih(t)",
    lty=1,main="",lwd=2,col="black");
#
# Rh
  par(mfrow=c(1,1));
  plot(tout,Rh,type="l",xlab="t",ylab="Rh(t)",
    lty=1,main="",lwd=2,col="black");
#
# Eh,Ih,Rh
  plot(
    tout,Eh,type="l",xlab="t",ylab="Eh(t),
    Ih(t),Rh(t)",ylim=c(0,60),lty=1,main="",
    lwd=2,col="black");
  points(tout,Eh, pch="1",lwd=2);
   lines(tout,Ih,type="l",lwd=2);
  points(tout,Ih, pch="2",lwd=2);
   lines(tout,Rh,type="l",lwd=2);
  points(tout,Rh, pch="3",lwd=2);
#
# Sv
  par(mfrow=c(1,1));
  plot(tout,Sv,type="l",xlab="t",ylab="Sv(t)",
```

```
      lty=1,main="",lwd=2,col="black");
#
# Ev
  par(mfrow=c(1,1));
  plot(tout,Ev,type="l",xlab="t",ylab="Ev(t)",
    lty=1,main="",lwd=2,col="black");
#
# Iv
  par(mfrow=c(1,1));
  plot(tout,Iv,type="l",xlab="t",ylab="Iv(t)",
    lty=1,main="",lwd=2,col="black");
#
# Ev,Iv
  par(mfrow=c(1,1));
  plot(tout,Ev,type="l",xlab="t",ylab="Ev(t),Iv(t)",
    ylim=c(0,60),lty=1,main="",lwd=2,col="black");
  points(tout,Ev, pch="1",lwd=2);
   lines(tout,Iv,type="l",lwd=2);
  points(tout,Iv, pch="2",lwd=2);
```

Listing 5.4: Main program for eqs. (5.1), (5.2), (5.3), high transmission

Listing 5.4 is similar to Listing 5.1 so only the differences are considered here.

- The ODE routine is changed from **ode1a** to **ode1b**. The two routines are the same and the name change was made to give a self-contained set of R routines for the high transmission case.

```
#
# SEIRV ODE malaria model
#
# Delete previous workspaces
  rm(list=ls(all=TRUE))
```

```
#
# Access ODE integrator
  library("deSolve");
#
# Access functions for numerical solution
  setwd("f:/infectious/chap5/sevenODE");
  source("ode1b.R");
```

- The parameters for the high transmission case (from Table 5.2) are used.

```
#
# Parameters
  Lambda_h=0.033;
  Psi_h=1.1e-04;
  Psi_v=0.13;
  sigma_v=0.50;
  sigma_h=19;
  beta_hv=0.022;
  beta_vh=0.48;
  beta_vhb=0.048;
  nu_h=0.10;
  nu_v=0.091;
  gamma_h=0.0035;
  delta_h=9.0e-05;
  rho_h=5.5e-04;
  mu_1h=1.6e-05;
  mu_2h=3.0e-07;
  mu_1v=0.033;
  mu_2v=2.0e-05;
```

- The interval in t is $0 \leq t \leq 1200$. The reduction tf=10000 to tf=1200 reflects the faster response for the high transmission case. tout=0,30,...,1200 for 41 output points.

```
#
```

```
# Independent variable for ODE integration
  t0=0;tf=1200;
  tout=seq(from=t0,to=tf,by=30);
# print(tout);
```

- For ncase=2, the equilibrium solution for ncase=1 is used as the ICs.

```
if(ncase==2){
  u0[1]=34.1;
  u0[2]=3;
  u0[3]=83.2;
  u0[4]=401.4;
  u0[5]=3590.2;
  u0[6]=740.9;
  u0[7]=518.9;
}
```

- ode1b is used in the ODE integration.

```
#
# ODE integration
  out=lsodes(y=u0,times=tout,func=ode1b,
      sparsetype="sparseint",rtol=1e-6,
      atol=1e-6,maxord=5);
  nrow(out)
  ncol(out)
```

(5.3.2) ODE/MOL routine

ODE routine ode1b follows.

```
ode1b=function(t,u,parms){
#
# Function ode1b computes the t derivative
# vectors of Sh(t),Eh(t),Ih(t),Rh(t),
# Sv(t),Ev(t),Iv(t)
```

```
#
# One vector to seven scalars
  Sh=u[1];
  Eh=u[2];
  Ih=u[3];
  Rh=u[4];
  Sv=u[5];
  Ev=u[6];
  Iv=u[7];
#
# Algebra
  Nh=Sh+Eh+Ih+Rh;
  Nv=Sv+Ev+Iv;
  fhNh=mu_1h+mu_2h*Nh;
  fvNv=mu_1v+mu_2v*Nv;
  lambda_h=(sigma_v*Nv*sigma_h)/
          (sigma_v*Nv+sigma_h*Nh)*
           beta_hv*(Iv/Nv);
  lambda_v=(sigma_v*Nh*sigma_h)/
          (sigma_v*Nv+sigma_h*Nh)*
          (beta_vh*(Ih/Nh)+beta_vhb*(Rh/Nh));
#
# ODEs
  Sht=Lambda_h+Psi_h*Nh+rho_h*Rh-lambda_h*Sh-
      fhNh*Sh;
  Eht=lambda_h*Sh-nu_h*Eh-fhNh*Eh;
  Iht=nu_h*Eh-gamma_h*Ih-fhNh*Ih-delta_h*Ih;
  Rht=gamma_h*Ih-rho_h*Rh-fhNh*Rh;
  Svt=Psi_v*Nv-lambda_v*Sv-fvNv*Sv;
  Evt=lambda_v*Sv-nu_v*Ev-fvNv*Ev;
  Ivt=nu_v*Ev-fvNv*Iv;
#
# Seven scalars to one vector
  ut=rep(0,7);
```

```
    ut[1]=Sht;
    ut[2]=Eht;
    ut[3]=Iht;
    ut[4]=Rht;
    ut[5]=Svt;
    ut[6]=Evt;
    ut[7]=Ivt;
#
# Increment calls to ode1b
  ncall <<- ncall+1;
#
# Return derivative vector
  return(list(c(ut)));
  }
```

Listing 5.5: ODE routine **ode1b** for eqs. (5.1), (5.2), (5.3), high transmission

Listing 5.5 is the same as Listing 5.2 except for the name change from **ode1a** to **ode1b**. The latter is included here for completness of the high transmission case.

(5.3.3) Model output

The output from Listings (5.4), (5.5) follows.

```
  ncase=1


[1] 41


[1] 8



          t         Sh(t)        Eh(t)
                    Ih(t)        Rh(t)
                    Sv(t)        Ev(t)
```

	Iv(t)	
	Nh(t)	Nv(t)
0	500.0	10.0
	30.0	0.0
	4000.0	100.0
	50.0	
	540.0	4150.0

	Sh(t)	Eh(t)
t	Ih(t)	Rh(t)
	Sv(t)	Ev(t)
	Iv(t)	
	Nh(t)	Nv(t)
600	22.7	2.5
	139.3	362.6
	3236.4	946.3
	667.3	
	527.2	4850.0

	Sh(t)	Eh(t)
t	Ih(t)	Rh(t)
	Sv(t)	Ev(t)
	Iv(t)	
	Nh(t)	Nv(t)
1200	34.1	3.0
	83.2	401.4
	3590.2	740.9
	518.9	
	521.7	4850.0

ncall = 272

ncase=2

[1] 41

[1] 8

t	Sh(t)	Eh(t)
	Ih(t)	Rh(t)
	Sv(t)	Ev(t)
	Iv(t)	
	Nh(t)	Nv(t)
0	34.1	3.0
	83.2	401.4
	3590.2	740.9
	518.9	
	521.7	4850.0

t	Sh(t)	Eh(t)
	Ih(t)	Rh(t)
	Sv(t)	Ev(t)
	Iv(t)	
	Nh(t)	Nv(t)
600	34.8	3.0
	80.9	399.1
	3604.5	732.6
	512.9	
	517.8	4850.0

t	Sh(t)	Eh(t)
	Ih(t)	Rh(t)
	Sv(t)	Ev(t)
	Iv(t)	
	Nh(t)	Nv(t)
1200	34.4	3.0
	80.5	396.5
	3604.9	732.4

```
512.7
514.4        4850.0
```

```
ncall =    99
```

Table 5.5: Numerical output, ncase=1,2

The graphical output for ncase=1 (Figs. 5.3-1,5,6,9) and ncase=2 (Figs. 5.4-1,5,6,9) follows.

The approach to an equilibrium solution is clear, e.g., Figs. 5.3-1, 5.3-6. Figs. 5.3-1,5,6,9 correspond to the solution in Fig. 3 of [2].

Figs. 5.3 and 5.4 indicate that the solutions approach an equilibrium well before $t_f = 1200$, in contrast to Figs. 5.1, 5.2 in which the solutions are still evolving at $t_f = 10000$. The vertical scales of Figs. 5.4-1,6 indicate a small change in $S_h(t), S_v(t)$. This is confirmed by the vertical scales of Fig. 5.4-5,9.

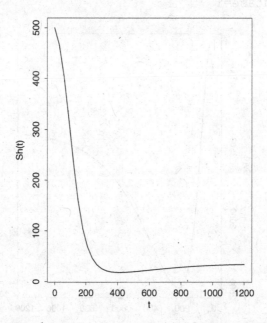

Figure 5.3-1: Numerical solution $S_h(t)$ from eq. (5.1a), ncase=1

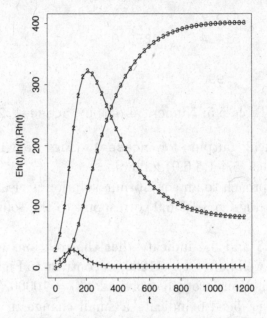

Figure 5.3-5: Numerical solutions $E_h(t), I_h(t), R_h(t)$ from eqs. (5.1b,c,d), `ncase=1`

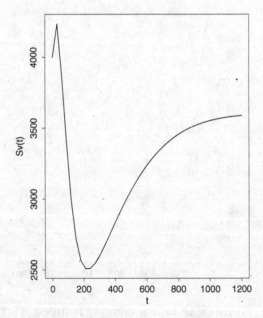

Figure 5.3-6: Numerical solution $S_v(t)$ from eq. (5.1e), `ncase=1`

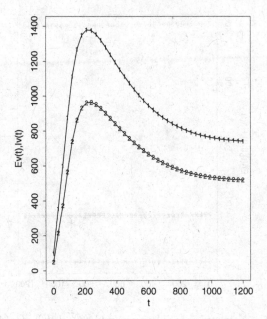

Figure 5.3-9: Numerical solutions $E_v(t), I_v(t)$ from eqs. (5.1f,g), ncase=1

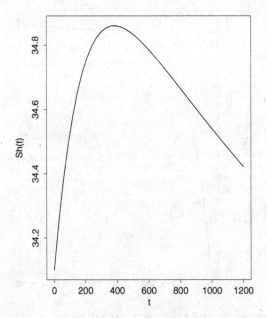

Figure 5.4-1: Numerical solution $S_h(t)$ from eq. (5.1a), ncase=2

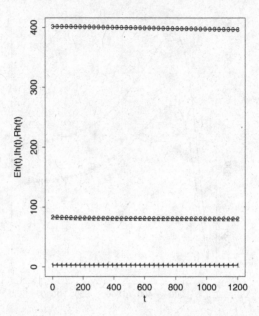

Figure 5.4-5: Numerical solutions $E_h(t), I_h(t), R_h(t)$ from eqs. (5.1b,c,d), ncase=2

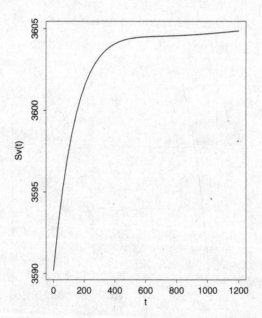

Figure 5.4-6: Numerical solution $S_v(t)$ from eq. (5.1e), ncase=2

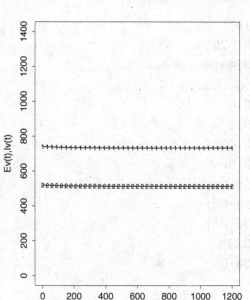

Figure 5.4-9: Numerical solutions $E_v(t)$, $I_v(t)$ from eqs. (5.1f,g), ncase=2

The preceding R_o analysis is repeated in the following routine for the high transmission case of Table 5.2.

```
#
# SEIRV ODE model
#
# Ro calculation, high transmission
#
# Delete previous workspaces
  rm(list=ls(all=TRUE))
#
# Parameters
  Lambda_h=0.033;
  Psi_h=1.1e-04;
  Psi_v=0.13;
  sigma_v=0.50;
```

```
    sigma_h=19;
    beta_hv=0.022;
    beta_vh=0.48;
    beta_vhb=0.048;
    nu_h=0.10;
    nu_v=0.091;
    gamma_h=0.0035;
    delta_h=9.0e-05;
    rho_h=5.5e-04;
    mu_1h=1.6e-05;
    mu_2h=3.0e-07;
    mu_1v=0.033;
    mu_2v=2.0e-05;
#
# Equilibrium (t=tf=1200) solution
# (ode1a_main.R, ode1a.R, ncase=1)
    Nh=514.4;
    Nv=4850.0;
#
# K_hv
    fact1=nu_v/(nu_v+mu_1v+mu_2v*Nv);
    fact2=(sigma_v*sigma_h*Nh)/(sigma_v*Nv+
        sigma_h*Nh);
    fact3=beta_hv;
    fact4=1/(mu_1v+mu_2v*Nv);
    K_hv=fact1*fact2*fact3*fact4;
#
# K_vh
    fact1=nu_h/(nu_h+mu_1h+mu_2h*Nv);
    fact2=(sigma_v*sigma_h*Nv)/(sigma_v*Nv+
        sigma_h*Nh);
    fact3=1/(gamma_h+delta_h+mu_1h+mu_2h*Nh);
    fact4=beta_vh+beta_vhb*(gamma_h/(rho_h+mu_1h+
        mu_2h*Nh));
```

```
  K_vh=fact1*fact2*fact3*fact4;
#
# Ro
  Ro_s=K_vh*K_hv;
  Ro  =Ro_s^{1/2};
#
# Output
  cat(sprintf("\n K_hv = %10.4f
             \n K_vh = %10.4f
             \n Ro_s = %10.4f
             \n   Ro = %10.4f",
           K_hv,K_vh,Ro_s,Ro));
```

Listing 5.6: Routine for the calculation of R_o, eqs. (5.4), high transmission

The routine in Listing 5.6 is a straightforward variant of the routine in Listing 5.3. The output is

```
K_hv =      0.0279

K_vh =    706.0216

Ro_s =     19.7088

  Ro =      4.4395
```

$R_o = 4.4395$ reflects a higher and faster transmission with $t_f = 1200$ than the previous Ro = 1.1264 for the low transmission case.

This completes the discussion of the ODE malaria model, eqs. (5.1) to (5.5). It is now extended to a PDE model by adding derivatives in r (radial coordinate) to eqs. (5.1)

(5.4) PDE Malaria Model, Linear Diffusion

Eqs. (5.1) can be extended to a 7×7 PDE system by adding partial derivatives in r to reflect linear (Fickian) diffusion (cross diffusion will be considered subsequently).

$$\frac{\partial S_h}{\partial t} = \Lambda_h + \Psi_h N_h + \rho_h R_h - f_h(N_h)S_h + D_{Sh}\left(\frac{\partial^2 S_h}{\partial r^2} + \frac{1}{r}\frac{\partial S_h}{\partial r}\right)$$
$$(5.6a)$$

$$\frac{\partial E_h}{\partial t} = \lambda_h(t)S_h - \nu_h E_h - f_h(N_h)E_h + D_{Eh}\left(\frac{\partial^2 E_h}{\partial r^2} + \frac{1}{r}\frac{\partial E_h}{\partial r}\right)$$
$$(5.6b)$$

$$\frac{\partial I_h}{\partial t} = \nu_h E_h - \gamma_h I_h - f_h(N_h)I_h - \delta_h I_h + D_{Ih}\left(\frac{\partial^2 I_h}{\partial r^2} + \frac{1}{r}\frac{\partial I_h}{\partial r}\right)$$
$$(5.6c)$$

$$\frac{\partial R_h}{\partial t} = \gamma_h I_h - \rho_h R_h - f_h(N_h)R_h + D_{Rh}\left(\frac{\partial^2 R_h}{\partial r^2} + \frac{1}{r}\frac{\partial R_h}{\partial r}\right) \quad (5.6d)$$

$$\frac{\partial S_v}{\partial t} = \Psi_v N_v - \lambda_v(t)S_v - f_v(N_v)S_v + D_{Sv}\left(\frac{\partial^2 S_v}{\partial r^2} + \frac{1}{r}\frac{\partial S_v}{\partial r}\right)$$
$$(5.6e)$$

$$\frac{\partial E_v}{\partial t} = \lambda_v(t)S_v - \nu_v E_v - f_v(N_v)E_v + D_{Ev}\left(\frac{\partial^2 E_v}{\partial r^2} + \frac{1}{r}\frac{\partial E_v}{\partial r}\right)$$
$$(5.6f)$$

$$\frac{\partial I_v}{\partial t} = \nu_v E_v - f_v(N_v)I_v + D_{Iv}\left(\frac{\partial^2 I_v}{\partial r^2} + \frac{1}{r}\frac{\partial I_v}{\partial r}\right) \quad (5.6g)$$

where $D_{Sh}, ..., D_{Iv}$ are diffusivities (dispersion coefficients). Eqs. (5.2) define functions that are used in eqs. (5.6)

Eqs. (5.6) are first order in t and second order in r so that each requires one IC and two BCs.

$$S_h(r, t = 0) = S_{h0}(r); \quad E_h(r, t = 0) = E_{h0}(r) \qquad (5.7\text{a,b})$$

$$I_h(r, t = 0) = I_{h0}(r); \quad R_h(r, t = 0) = R_{h0}(r) \qquad (5.7\text{c,d})$$

$$S_v(r, t = 0) = S_{v0}(r); \quad E_v(r, t = 0) = E_{v0}(r); \quad I_v(r, t = 0) = I_{v0}(r)$$
$$(5.7\text{e,f,g})$$

$$\frac{\partial S_h(r = r_l, t)}{\partial r} = \frac{\partial S_h(r = r_u, t)}{\partial r} = 0 \qquad (5.8\text{a})$$

$$\frac{\partial E_h(r = r_l, t)}{\partial r} = \frac{\partial E_h(r = r_u, t)}{\partial r} = 0 \qquad (5.8\text{b})$$

$$\frac{\partial I_h(r = r_l, t)}{\partial r} = \frac{\partial I_h(r = r_u, t)}{\partial r} = 0 \qquad (5.8\text{c})$$

$$\frac{\partial R_h(r = r_l, t)}{\partial r} = \frac{\partial R_h(r = r_u, t)}{\partial r} = 0 \qquad (5.8\text{d})$$

$$\frac{\partial S_v(r = r_l, t)}{\partial r} = \frac{\partial S_v(r = r_u, t)}{\partial r} = 0 \qquad (5.8\text{e})$$

$$\frac{\partial E_v(r = r_l, t)}{\partial r} = \frac{\partial R_v(r = r_u, t)}{\partial r} = 0 \qquad (5.8\text{f})$$

$$\frac{\partial I_v(r = r_l, t)}{\partial r} = \frac{\partial I_v(r = r_u, t)}{\partial r} = 0 \qquad (5.8\text{g})$$

Eqs. (5.6), (5.7), (5.8) (along with eqs. (5.2)) constitute the PDE malaria model.

(5.4.1) Main program

A main program for (5.6), (5.7), (5.8) follows.

```
#
# SEIRV PDE malaria model
#
# Delete previous workspaces
  rm(list=ls(all=TRUE))
#
# Access ODE integrator
  library("deSolve");
#
# Access functions for numerical solution
  setwd("f:/infectious/chap5/sevenPDE");
  source("pde1a.R");
  source("dss044.R");
#
# Parameters for ODEs
  Lambda_h=0.033;
  Psi_h=1.1e-04;
  Psi_v=0.13;
  sigma_v=0.50;
  sigma_h=19;
  beta_hv=0.022;
  beta_vh=0.48;
  beta_vhb=0.048;
  nu_h=0.10;
  nu_v=0.091;
  gamma_h=0.0035;
  delta_h=9.0e-05;
  rho_h=5.5e-04;
  mu_1h=1.6e-05;
  mu_2h=3.0e-07;
  mu_1v=0.033;
```

```
  mu_2v=2.0e-05;
#
# Parameters for PDEs
  id=1;
#
# No diffusion
  if(id==0){
    D_Sh=0;
    D_Eh=0;
    D_Ih=0;
    D_Rh=0;
    D_Sv=0;
    D_Ev=0;
    D_Iv=0;
  }
#
# Linear diffusion
  if(id==1){
    D_Sh=0.1;
    D_Eh=0.1;
    D_Ih=0.1;
    D_Rh=0.1;
    D_Sv=0.1;
    D_Ev=0.1;
    D_Iv=0.1;
  }
#
# Spatial grid (in r)
  nr=41;
  rl=0;ru=20;
  r=seq(from=rl,to=ru,by=0.5);
#
# Independent variable for ODE integration
  t0=0;tf=300;nout=7;
```

```
  tout=seq(from=t0,to=tf,by=50);
#
# Initial condition (t=0)
  ncase=1;
  u0=rep(0,7*nr);
  if(ncase==1){
    for(i in 1:nr){
      u0[i]      =500;
      u0[i+nr]   =10;
      u0[i+2*nr]=30;
      u0[i+3*nr]=0;
      u0[i+4*nr]=4000;
      u0[i+5*nr]=100;
      u0[i+6*nr]=50;
    }
  }
  if(ncase==2){
    for(i in 1:nr){
      u0[i]      =500;
      u0[i+nr]   =0;
      u0[i+2*nr]=30*exp(-0.1*r[i]^2);
      u0[i+3*nr]=0;
      u0[i+4*nr]=4000;
      u0[i+5*nr]=0;
      u0[i+6*nr]=50*exp(-0.1*r[i]^2);
    }
  }
  ncall=0;
#
# ODE integration
  out=lsodes(y=u0,times=tout,func=pde1a,
      sparsetype="sparseint",rtol=1e-6,
      atol=1e-6,maxord=5);
  nrow(out)
```

```
  ncol(out)
#
# Arrays for plotting numerical solution
  Sh=matrix(0,nrow=nr,ncol=nout);
  Eh=matrix(0,nrow=nr,ncol=nout);
  Ih=matrix(0,nrow=nr,ncol=nout);
  Rh=matrix(0,nrow=nr,ncol=nout);
  Sv=matrix(0,nrow=nr,ncol=nout);
  Ev=matrix(0,nrow=nr,ncol=nout);
  Iv=matrix(0,nrow=nr,ncol=nout);
  Nh=matrix(0,nrow=nr,ncol=nout);
  Nv=matrix(0,nrow=nr,ncol=nout);
  for(it in 1:nout){
    for(i in 1:nr){
      Sh[i,it]=out[it,i+1];
      Eh[i,it]=out[it,i+1+nr];
      Ih[i,it]=out[it,i+1+2*nr];
      Rh[i,it]=out[it,i+1+3*nr];
      Sv[i,it]=out[it,i+1+4*nr];
      Ev[i,it]=out[it,i+1+5*nr];
      Iv[i,it]=out[it,i+1+6*nr];
      Nh[i,it]=Sh[i,it]+Eh[i,it]+
               Ih[i,it]+Rh[i,it];
      Nv[i,it]=Sv[i,it]+Ev[i,it]+
               Iv[i,it];
    }
  }
#
# Display numerical solution
  for(it in 1:nout){
    if((it-1)*(it-4)*(it-nout)==0){
      cat(sprintf("\n"));
      cat(sprintf(
        "\n      t         Sh(r,t)       Eh(r,t)"));
```

```
      cat(sprintf(
        "\n                 Ih(r,t)        Rh(r,t)"));
      cat(sprintf(
        "\n                 Sv(r,t)        Ev(r,t)"));
      cat(sprintf(
        "\n                 Iv(r,t)"               ));
      cat(sprintf(
        "\n                 Nh(r,t)        Nv(r,t)"));
    for(i in 1:nr){
    if((i-1)*(i-21)*(i-nr)==0){
    cat(sprintf(
      "\n %6.0f %6.2f",tout[it],r[i]));
    cat(sprintf(
      "\n        %12.1f %12.1f",Sh[i,it],Eh[i,it]));
    cat(sprintf(
      "\n        %12.1f %12.1f",Ih[i,it],Rh[i,it]));
    cat(sprintf(
      "\n        %12.1f %12.1f",Sv[i,it],Ev[i,it]));
    cat(sprintf(
      "\n        %12.1f       ",Iv[i,it]));
    cat(sprintf(
      "\n        %12.1f %12.1f",Nh[i,it],Nv[i,it]));
    }
    }
    }
  }
#
# Calls to ODE routine
  cat(sprintf("\n\n ncall = %5d\n\n",ncall));
#
# Plot PDE solutions
#
# Sh
  par(mfrow=c(1,1));
```

```
  matplot(r,Sh,type="l",xlab="r",ylab="Sh(r,t)",
    lty=1,main="",lwd=2,col="black");
#
# Eh
  par(mfrow=c(1,1));
  matplot(r,Eh,type="l",xlab="r",ylab="Eh(r,t)",
    lty=1,main="",lwd=2,col="black");
#
# Ih
  par(mfrow=c(1,1));
  matplot(r,Ih,type="l",xlab="r",ylab="Ih(r,t)",
    lty=1,main="",lwd=2,col="black");
#
# Rh
  par(mfrow=c(1,1));
  matplot(r,Rh,type="l",xlab="r",ylab="Rh(r,t)",
    lty=1,main="",lwd=2,col="black");
#
# Sv
  par(mfrow=c(1,1));
  matplot(r,Sv,type="l",xlab="r",ylab="Sv(r,t)",
    lty=1,main="",lwd=2,col="black");
#
# Ev
  par(mfrow=c(1,1));
  matplot(r,Ev,type="l",xlab="r",ylab="Ev(r,t)",
    lty=1,main="",lwd=2,col="black");
#
# Iv
  par(mfrow=c(1,1));
  matplot(r,Iv,type="l",xlab="r",ylab="Iv(r,t)",
    lty=1,main="",lwd=2,col="black");
```

Listing 5.7: Main program for eqs. (5.6), (5.7), (5.8)

We can note the following details about Listing 5.7.

- Previous workspaces are deleted.

```
#
# SEIRV PDE malaria model
#
# Delete previous workspaces
  rm(list=ls(all=TRUE))
```

- The library integrator **deSolve** is accessed. Then the directory with the files for the solution·of eqs. (5.6), (5.7), (5.8) is designated. Note that **setwd** (set working directory) uses / rather than the usual \.

```
#
# Access ODE integrator
  library("deSolve");
#
# Access functions for numerical solution
  setwd("f:/infectious/chap5/sevenPDE");
  source("pde1a.R");
  source("dss004.R");
  source("dss044.R");
```

dss004 computes first derivatives. **dss044** does direct differentiation to second derivatives as discussed in Chapter 4 and Appendix A2, and next when the ODE/MOL **pde1a** routine is discussed.

- The parameters for high transmission from Table 5.2 are specified.

```
#
# Parameters for ODEs
  Lambda_h=0.033;
  Psi_h=1.1e-04;
  Psi_v=0.13;
```

```
    sigma_v=0.50;
    sigma_h=19;
    beta_hv=0.022;
    beta_vh=0.48;
    beta_vhb=0.048;
    nu_h=0.10;
    nu_v=0.091;
    gamma_h=0.0035;
    delta_h=9.0e-05;
    rho_h=5.5e-04;
    mu_1h=1.6e-05;
    mu_2h=3.0e-07;
    mu_1v=0.033;
    mu_2v=2.0e-05;
```

- The diffusivities in eqs. (5.6) are defined numerically. For id=0 they are zero so that eqs. (5.6) are ODEs as discussed previously.

```
#
# Parameters for PDEs
    id=1;
#
# No diffusion
    if(id==0){
      D_Sh=0;
      D_Eh=0;
      D_Ih=0;
      D_Rh=0;
      D_Sv=0;
      D_Ev=0;
      D_Iv=0;
    }
#
# Linear diffusion
```

```
if(id==1){
  D_Sh=0.1;
  D_Eh=0.1;
  D_Ih=0.1;
  D_Rh=0.1;
  D_Sv=0.1;
  D_Ev=0.1;
  D_Iv=0.1;
}
```

- A spatial grid of 41 points is defined for the interval $0 \leq r \leq 20$ so that r=0,0.5,...,20.

```
#
# Spatial grid (in r)
  nr=41;
  rl=0;ru=20;
  r=seq(from=rl,to=ru,by=0.5);
```

$r_u = 20$ was selected to demonstrate the use of a spatial scale that is not normalizd to $r_l = 0 \leq r \leq r_u = 1$. $r_u = 20$ could represent a circular domain with a radius of 20 km.
- An interval in t of 7 output points is defined for the interval $0 \leq t \leq 300$ so that tout=0,50,...,300.

```
#
# Independent variable for ODE integration
  t0=0;tf=300;nout=7;
  tout=seq(from=t0,to=tf,by=50);
```

$t_f = 300$ is in contrast with $t_f = 1200$ used for the high transmission ODE model discussed previously. This value of t_f was selected to give a series of 7 distinct solution curves plotted parametrically as discussed subsequently.

- ICs (5.7) are defined for two cases, `ncase=1,2`. The `for` steps through the grid in r (the ICs of eqs. (5.7) are functions of r).

```
#
# Initial condition (t=0)
  ncase=1;
  u0=rep(0,7*nr);
  if(ncase==1){
    for(i in 1:nr){
      u0[i]       =500;
      u0[i+nr]    =10;
      u0[i+2*nr]=30;
      u0[i+3*nr]=0;
      u0[i+4*nr]=4000;
      u0[i+5*nr]=100;
      u0[i+6*nr]=50;
    }
  }
  if(ncase==2){
    for(i in 1:nr){
      u0[i]       =500;
      u0[i+nr]    =0;
      u0[i+2*nr]=30*exp(-0.1*r[i]^2);
      u0[i+3*nr]=0;
      u0[i+4*nr]=4000;
      u0[i+5*nr]=0;
      u0[i+6*nr]=50*exp(-0.1*r[i]^2);
    }
  }
  ncall=0;
```

For `ncase=1`, the ICs are constant in r. For `ncase=2`, from ICs (5.7c,g), $I_h(r, t = 0) = I_{h0}(r) = e^{-0.1r^2}$, $I_v(r, t = 0) = I_{v0}(r) = e^{-0.1r^2}$ which initalizes a variation in r to which the

PDEs respond for $t > t_0 = 0$. In each case, $(7)(41) = 287$ ODE ICs are specified.

The number of calls to the MOL/ODE routine `pde1a` is also initialized.

- The integration of the $(7)(41) = 287$ ODEs is performed by `lsodes`. The arguments of `lsodes` are discussed in detail in Chapter 4. The MOL/ODE routine, `pde1a`, is discussed next.

```
#
# ODE integration
  out=lsodes(y=u0,times=tout,func=pde1a,
      sparsetype="sparseint",rtol=1e-6,
      atol=1e-6,maxord=5);
  nrow(out)
  ncol(out)
```

The sparse matrix facility of `lsodes` is used to good advantage since the ODE Jacobian matrix has $287^2 = 82369$ elements.

- The ODE solutions in `out` from `lsodes` are placed in seven arrays (matrices) for subsequent display.

```
#
# Arrays for plotting numerical solution
  Sh=matrix(0,nrow=nr,ncol=nout);
  Eh=matrix(0,nrow=nr,ncol=nout);
  Ih=matrix(0,nrow=nr,ncol=nout);
  Rh=matrix(0,nrow=nr,ncol=nout);
  Sv=matrix(0,nrow=nr,ncol=nout);
  Ev=matrix(0,nrow=nr,ncol=nout);
  Iv=matrix(0,nrow=nr,ncol=nout);
  Nh=matrix(0,nrow=nr,ncol=nout);
  Nv=matrix(0,nrow=nr,ncol=nout);
  for(it in 1:nout){
```

```
      for(i in 1:nr){
        Sh[i,it]=out[it,i+1];
        Eh[i,it]=out[it,i+1+nr];
        Ih[i,it]=out[it,i+1+2*nr];
        Rh[i,it]=out[it,i+1+3*nr];
        Sv[i,it]=out[it,i+1+4*nr];
        Ev[i,it]=out[it,i+1+5*nr];
        Iv[i,it]=out[it,i+1+6*nr];
        Nh[i,it]=Sh[i,it]+Eh[i,it]+
                 Ih[i,it]+Rh[i,it];
        Nv[i,it]=Sv[i,it]+Ev[i,it]+
                 Iv[i,it];
      }
    }
```

N_h, N_v are also computed and placed in two arrays. The offset +1 in out is required since each of the 7 solution vectors has the value of t as the first element. The ODE solutions are therefore in elements 2 to 287+1=288.

- The ODE solutions are displayed for $r = 0, 10, 20$ and $t = 0, 150, 300$.

```
#
# Display numerical solution
  for(it in 1:nout){
    if((it-1)*(it-4)*(it-nout)==0){
      cat(sprintf("\n"));
      cat(sprintf(
        "\n        t       Sh(r,t)        Eh(r,t)"));
      cat(sprintf(
        "\n                Ih(r,t)        Rh(r,t)"));
      cat(sprintf(
        "\n                Sv(r,t)        Ev(r,t)"));
      cat(sprintf(
        "\n                Iv(r,t)"                 ));
```

```
            cat(sprintf(
             "\n                  Nh(r,t)        Nv(r,t)"));
        for(i in 1:nr){
        if((i-1)*(i-21)*(i-nr)==0){
        cat(sprintf(
          "\n %6.0f %6.2f",tout[it],r[i]));
        cat(sprintf(
          "\n          %12.1f %12.1f",Sh[i,it],Eh[i,it]));
        cat(sprintf(
          "\n          %12.1f %12.1f",Ih[i,it],Rh[i,it]));
        cat(sprintf(
          "\n          %12.1f %12.1f",Sv[i,it],Ev[i,it]));
        cat(sprintf(
          "\n          %12.1f         ",Iv[i,it]));
        cat(sprintf(
          "\n          %12.1f %12.1f",Nh[i,it],Nv[i,it]));
        }
      }
    }
  }
```

Two ifs are used to make the selection of r and t.

- The total number of calls to pde1a is displayed at the end of the solution.

```
#
# Calls to ODE routine
  cat(sprintf("\n\n ncall = %5d\n\n",ncall));
```

- The seven PDE solutions (of eqs. (5.6)) are plotted with matplot.

```
#
# Plot PDE solutions
#
# Sh
```

```
   par(mfrow=c(1,1));
   matplot(r,Sh,type="l",xlab="r",ylab="Sh(r,t)",
     lty=1,main="",lwd=2,col="black");
```

            .   .

            .

            .   .

```
 #
 # Iv
   par(mfrow=c(1,1));
   matplot(r,Iv,type="l",xlab="r",ylab="Iv(r,t)",
     lty=1,main="",lwd=2,col="black");
```

This completes the discussion of the main program of Listing 5.7. The MOL/ODE routine `pde1a` is considered next.

(5.4.2) ODE/MOL routine

The ODE/MOL routine called by `lsodes` in Listing 5.7 follows.

```
   pde1a=function(t,u,parms){
 #
 # Function pde1a computes the t derivative
 # vectors of Sh(r,t),Eh(r,t),Ih(r,t),Rh(r,t),
 # Sv(r,t),Ev(r,t),Iv(r,t)
 #
 # One vector to seven vectors
   Sh=rep(0,nr);Eh=rep(0,nr);
   Ih=rep(0,nr);Rh=rep(0,nr);
   Sv=rep(0,nr);Ev=rep(0,nr);
   Iv=rep(0,nr);
   for(i in 1:nr){
     Sh[i]=u[i];
     Eh[i]=u[i+nr];
     Ih[i]=u[i+2*nr];
     Rh[i]=u[i+3*nr];
```

```
    Sv[i]=u[i+4*nr];
    Ev[i]=u[i+5*nr];
    Iv[i]=u[i+6*nr];
  }
#
# Algebra
  Nh=rep(0,nr);
  Nv=rep(0,nr);
  fhNh=rep(0,nr);
  fvNv=rep(0,nr);
  lambda_h=rep(0,nr);
  lambda_v=rep(0,nr);
  for(i in 1:nr){
  Nh[i]=Sh[i]+Eh[i]+Ih[i]+Rh[i];
  Nv[i]=Sv[i]+Ev[i]+Iv[i];
  fhNh[i]=mu_1h+mu_2h*Nh[i];
  fvNv[i]=mu_1v+mu_2v*Nv[i];
  lambda_h[i]=(sigma_v*Nv[i]*sigma_h)/
    (sigma_v*Nv[i]+sigma_h*Nh[i])*
      beta_hv*(Iv[i]/Nv[i]);
  lambda_v[i]=(sigma_v*Nh[i]*sigma_h)/
    (sigma_v*Nv[i]+sigma_h*Nh[i])*
    (beta_vh*(Ih[i]/Nh[i])+beta_vhb*
    (Rh[i]/Nh[i]));
  }
#
# Shr,Ehr,Ihr,Rhr
# Svr,Evr,Ivr
  Shr=dss004(rl,ru,nr,Sh);
  Ehr=dss004(rl,ru,nr,Eh);
  Ihr=dss004(rl,ru,nr,Ih);
  Rhr=dss004(rl,ru,nr,Rh);
  Svr=dss004(rl,ru,nr,Sv);
  Evr=dss004(rl,ru,nr,Ev);
```

```
  Ivr=dss004(rl,ru,nr,Iv);
#
# BCs
  Shr[1]=0;Shr[nr]=0;
  Ehr[1]=0;Ehr[nr]=0;
  Ihr[1]=0;Ihr[nr]=0;
  Rhr[1]=0;Rhr[nr]=0;
  Svr[1]=0;Svr[nr]=0;
  Evr[1]=0;Evr[nr]=0;
  Ivr[1]=0;Ivr[nr]=0;
#
# Shrr,Ehrr,Ihrr,Rhrr
# Svrr,Evrr,Ivrr
  nl=2;nu=2;
  Shrr=dss044(rl,ru,nr,Sh,Shr,nl=2,nu=2);
  Ehrr=dss044(rl,ru,nr,Eh,Ehr,nl=2,nu=2);
  Ihrr=dss044(rl,ru,nr,Ih,Ihr,nl=2,nu=2);
  Rhrr=dss044(rl,ru,nr,Rh,Rhr,nl=2,nu=2);
  Svrr=dss044(rl,ru,nr,Sv,Svr,nl=2,nu=2);
  Evrr=dss044(rl,ru,nr,Ev,Evr,nl=2,nu=2);
  Ivrr=dss044(rl,ru,nr,Iv,Ivr,nl=2,nu=2);
#
# PDEs
  Sht=rep(0,nr);Eht=rep(0,nr);
  Iht=rep(0,nr);Rht=rep(0,nr);
  Svt=rep(0,nr);Evt=rep(0,nr);
  Ivt=rep(0,nr);
#
# 0 le r le r0
  for(i in 1:nr){
#
# r=0
    if(i==1){
      Sht[i]=Lambda_h[i]+Psi_h*Nh[i]+rho_h*Rh[i]-
```

```
                lambda_h[i]*Sh[i]-fhNh[i]*Sh[i]+
                D_Sh*2*Shrr[i];
        Eht[i]=lambda_h[i]*Sh[i]-nu_h*Eh[i]-
                fhNh[i]*Eh[i]+
                D_Eh*2*Ehrr[i];
        Iht[i]=nu_h*Eh[i]-gamma_h*Ih[i]-
                fhNh[i]*Ih[i]-delta_h*Ih[i]+
                D_Ih*2*Ihrr[i];
        Rht[i]=gamma_h*Ih[i]-rho_h*Rh[i]-
                fhNh[i]*Rh[i]+
                D_Rh*2*Rhrr[i];
        Rht[i]=gamma_h*Ih[i]-rho_h*Rh[i]-fhNh[i]*Rh[i]+
                D_Rh*2*Rhrr[i];
        Svt[i]=Psi_v*Nv[i]-lambda_v[i]*Sv[i]-
                fvNv[i]*Sv[i]+D_Sv*2*Svrr[i];
        Evt[i]=lambda_v[i]*Sv[i]-nu_v*Ev[i]-
                fvNv[i]*Ev[i]+D_Ev*2*Evrr[i];
        Ivt[i]=nu_v*Ev[i]-fvNv[i]*Iv[i]+
                D_Iv*2*Ivrr[i];
    }
#
# r > 0
    if(i>1){
    ri=1/r[i];
    Sht[i]=Lambda_h+Psi_h*Nh[i]+rho_h*Rh[i]-
            lambda_h[i]*Sh[i]-fhNh[i]*Sh[i]+
            D_Sh*(Shrr[i]+ri*Shr[i]);
    Eht[i]=lambda_h[i]*Sh[i]-nu_h*Eh[i]-
            fhNh[i]*Eh[i]+
            D_Eh*(Ehrr[i]+ri*Ehr[i]);
    Iht[i]=nu_h*Eh[i]-gamma_h*Ih[i]-
            fhNh[i]*Ih[i]-delta_h*Ih[i]+
            D_Ih*(Ihrr[i]+ri*Ihr[i]);
    Rht[i]=gamma_h*Ih[i]-rho_h*Rh[i]-
```

```
                fhNh[i]*Rh[i]+
                D_Rh*(Rhrr[i]+ri*Rhr[i]);
        Svt[i]=Psi_v*Nv[i]-lambda_v[i]*Sv[i]-
                fvNv[i]*Sv[i]+
                D_Sv*(Svrr[i]+ri*Svr[i]);
        Evt[i]=lambda_v[i]*Sv[i]-nu_v*Ev[i]-
                fvNv[i]*Ev[i]+
                D_Ev*(Evrr[i]+ri*Evr[i]);
        Ivt[i]=nu_v*Ev[i]-fvNv[i]*Iv[i]+
                D_Iv*(Ivrr[i]+ri*Ivr[i]);
    }
#
# Next i
  }
#
# Seven vectors to one vector
  ut=rep(0,7*nr);
  for(i in 1:nr){
    ut[i]      =Sht[i];
    ut[i+nr]   =Eht[i];
    ut[i+2*nr]=Iht[i];
    ut[i+3*nr]=Rht[i];
    ut[i+4*nr]=Svt[i];
    ut[i+5*nr]=Evt[i];
    ut[i+6*nr]=Ivt[i];
  }
#
# Increment calls to pde1a
  ncall <<- ncall+1;
#
# Return derivative vector
  return(list(c(ut)));
  }
```

Listing 5.8: MOL/ODE routine `pde1a` for eqs. (5.6), (5.7), (5.8)

We can note the following details about Listing 5.8.

- The function is defined. u is the 287-vector of MOL/ODE dependent (state) variables. t is the corresponding value of *t*. parm is an argument for passing parameters to `pde1a` (unused, but required).

```
  pde1a=function(t,u,parms){
#
# Function pde1a computes the t derivative
# vectors of Sh(r,t),Eh(r,t),Ih(r,t),Rh(r,t),
# Sv(r,t),Ev(r,t),Iv(r,t)
```

- u is placed in seven 41-vectors, Sh to Iv, to facilitate the MOL programming of eqs. (5.6).

```
#
# One vector to seven vectors
  Sh=rep(0,nr);Eh=rep(0,nr);
  Ih=rep(0,nr);Rh=rep(0,nr);
  Sv=rep(0,nr);Ev=rep(0,nr);
  Iv=rep(0,nr);
  for(i in 1:nr){
    Sh[i]=u[i];
    Eh[i]=u[i+nr];
    Ih[i]=u[i+2*nr];
    Rh[i]=u[i+3*nr];
    Sv[i]=u[i+4*nr];
    Ev[i]=u[i+5*nr];
    Iv[i]=u[i+6*nr];
  }
```

- The algebra of eqs. (5.2) is programmed as a series of vectors, Nh to lambda_v.

```
#
# Algebra
  Nh=rep(0,nr);
  Nv=rep(0,nr);
  fhNh=rep(0,nr);
  fvNv=rep(0,nr);
  lambda_h=rep(0,nr);
  lambda_v=rep(0,nr);
  for(i in 1:nr){
  Nh[i]=Sh[i]+Eh[i]+Ih[i]+Rh[i];
  Nv[i]=Sv[i]+Ev[i]+Iv[i];
  fhNh[i]=mu_1h+mu_2h*Nh[i];
  fvNv[i]=mu_1v+mu_2v*Nv[i];
  lambda_h[i]=(sigma_v*Nv[i]*sigma_h)/
    (sigma_v*Nv[i]+sigma_h*Nh[i])*
      beta_hv*(Iv[i]/Nv[i]);
  lambda_v[i]=(sigma_v*Nh[i]*sigma_h)/
    (sigma_v*Nv[i]+sigma_h*Nh[i])*
    (beta_vh*(Ih[i]/Nh[i])+beta_vhb*
    (Rh[i]/Nh[i]));
  }
```

- The first derivatives in r are computed with dss004. The vectors for the derivatives are allocated by dss004, for example $\dfrac{\partial S_h}{\partial r} = $ Shr.

```
#
# Shr,Ehr,Ihr,Rhr
# Svr,Evr,Ivr
  Shr=dss004(rl,ru,nr,Sh);
  Ehr=dss004(rl,ru,nr,Eh);
  Ihr=dss004(rl,ru,nr,Ih);
  Rhr=dss004(rl,ru,nr,Rh);
  Svr=dss004(rl,ru,nr,Sv);
```

```
Evr=dss004(rl,ru,nr,Ev);
Ivr=dss004(rl,ru,nr,Iv);
```

- The homogeneous Neumann BCs, eqs. (5.8), are programmed.

```
#
# BCs
  Shr[1]=0;Shr[nr]=0;
  Ehr[1]=0;Ehr[nr]=0;
  Ihr[1]=0;Ihr[nr]=0;
  Rhr[1]=0;Rhr[nr]=0;
  Svr[1]=0;Svr[nr]=0;
  Evr[1]=0;Evr[nr]=0;
  Ivr[1]=0;Ivr[nr]=0;
```

The subscripts 1,nr correspond to $r = r_l = 0$ and $r = r_u = 20$, respectively.

- The second derivatives in r are computed, for example $\dfrac{\partial^2 S_h}{\partial r^2}$ = Shrr, by dss044.

```
#
# Shrr,Ehrr,Ihrr,Rhrr
# Svrr,Evrr,Ivrr
  nl=2;nu=2;
  Shrr=dss044(rl,ru,nr,Sh,Shr,nl=2,nu=2);
  Ehrr=dss044(rl,ru,nr,Eh,Ehr,nl=2,nu=2);
  Ihrr=dss044(rl,ru,nr,Ih,Ihr,nl=2,nu=2);
  Rhrr=dss044(rl,ru,nr,Rh,Rhr,nl=2,nu=2);
  Svrr=dss044(rl,ru,nr,Sv,Svr,nl=2,nu=2);
  Evrr=dss044(rl,ru,nr,Ev,Evr,nl=2,nu=2);
  Ivrr=dss044(rl,ru,nr,Iv,Ivr,nl=2,nu=2);
```

nl=2,nu=2 specify Neumann BCs. The first derivatives are inputs to dss044 from which the BC values are available (additional details about `dss044` are available in Appendix A2).

The second derivatives, for example, `Shrr` do not have to be allocated since this is done in `dss044`.

- The seven derivatives in t (LHSs of eqs. (5.6)) are allocated (declared).

```
#
# PDEs
  Sht=rep(0,nr);Eht=rep(0,nr);
  Iht=rep(0,nr);Rht=rep(0,nr);
  Svt=rep(0,nr);Evt=rep(0,nr);
  Ivt=rep(0,nr);
```

- The MOL/ODEs are programmed, starting with $r = 0$ for which the radial differential group $\dfrac{\partial^2}{\partial r^2} + \dfrac{1}{r}\dfrac{\partial}{\partial r}$ is regularized to $2\dfrac{\partial^2}{\partial r^2}$ as discussed in Chapter 4.

```
#
# 0 le r le r0
  for(i in 1:nr){
#
# r=0
    if(i==1){
      Sht[i]=Lambda_h[i]+Psi_h*Nh[i]+rho_h*Rh[i]-
             lambda_h[i]*Sh[i]-fhNh[i]*Sh[i]+
             D_Sh*2*Shrr[i];
      Eht[i]=lambda_h[i]*Sh[i]-nu_h*Eh[i]-
             fhNh[i]*Eh[i]+
             D_Eh*2*Ehrr[i];
      Iht[i]=nu_h*Eh[i]-gamma_h*Ih[i]-
             fhNh[i]*Ih[i]-delta_h*Ih[i]+
             D_Ih*2*Ihrr[i];
      Rht[i]=gamma_h*Ih[i]-rho_h*Rh[i]-
```

```
                fhNh[i]*Rh[i]+
                D_Rh*2*Rhrr[i];
        Svt[i]=Psi_v*Nv[i]-lambda_v[i]*Sv[i]-
                fvNv[i]*Sv[i]+D_Sv*2*Svrr[i];
        Evt[i]=lambda_v[i]*Sv[i]-nu_v*Ev[i]-
                fvNv[i]*Ev[i]+D_Ev*2*Evrr[i];
        Ivt[i]=nu_v*Ev[i]-fvNv[i]*Iv[i]+
                D_Iv*2*Ivrr[i];
    }
```

- The MOL/ODEs for $r > 0$ are programmed.

```
    #
    # r > 0
        if(i>1){
        ri=1/r[i];
        Sht[i]=Lambda_h+Psi_h*Nh[i]+rho_h*Rh[i]-
                lambda_h[i]*Sh[i]-fhNh[i]*Sh[i]+
                D_Sh*(Shrr[i]+ri*Shr[i]);
        Eht[i]=lambda_h[i]*Sh[i]-nu_h*Eh[i]-
                fhNh[i]*Eh[i]+
                D_Eh*(Ehrr[i]+ri*Ehr[i]);
        Iht[i]=nu_h*Eh[i]-gamma_h*Ih[i]-
                fhNh[i]*Ih[i]-delta_h*Ih[i]+
                D_Ih*(Ihrr[i]+ri*Ihr[i]);
        Rht[i]=gamma_h*Ih[i]-rho_h*Rh[i]-
                fhNh[i]*Rh[i]+
                D_Rh*(Rhrr[i]+ri*Rhr[i]);
        Svt[i]=Psi_v*Nv[i]-lambda_v[i]*Sv[i]-
                fvNv[i]*Sv[i]+
                D_Sv*(Svrr[i]+ri*Svr[i]);
        Evt[i]=lambda_v[i]*Sv[i]-nu_v*Ev[i]-
                fvNv[i]*Ev[i]+
                D_Ev*(Evrr[i]+ri*Evr[i]);
        Ivt[i]=nu_v*Ev[i]-fvNv[i]*Iv[i]+
```

```
                    D_Iv*(Ivrr[i]+ri*Ivr[i]);
      }
 #
 # Next i
  }
```

For example, $D_{\dot{S}h}\left(\dfrac{\partial^2}{\partial r^2}+\dfrac{1}{r}\dfrac{\partial}{\partial r}\right)$ = D_Sh*(Shrr[i]+ri*Shr

[i]) with $\dfrac{1}{r}$ = ri=1/r[i].

The concluding } completes the for in r (for(i in 1:nr)).

- The number of calls to pde1a is returned to the main program of Listing 5.7 by <<-.

```
 #
 # Increment calls to pde1a
   ncall <<- ncall+1;
```

- The derivative 287-vector is returned to lsodes as a list. c is the R vector utility.

```
 #
 # Return derivative vector
   return(list(c(ut)));
  }
```

The final } concludes pd1a.

This concludes the programming of eqs. (5.6), (5.7), (5.8). The output is considered next.

(5.4.3) Model output

The numerical output from the main program of Listing 5.7 follows for id=1, ncase=1.

[1] 7

[1] 288

t		Sh(r,t)	Eh(r,t)
		Ih(r,t)	Rh(r,t)
		Sv(r,t)	Ev(r,t)
		Iv(r,t)	
		Nh(r,t)	Nv(r,t)
0	0.00		
		500.0	10.0
		30.0	0.0
		4000.0	100.0
		50.0	
		540.0	4150.0
0	10.00		
		500.0	10.0
		30.0	0.0
		4000.0	100.0
		50.0	
		540.0	4150.0
0	20.00		
		500.0	10.0
		30.0	0.0
		4000.0	100.0
		50.0	
		540.0	4150.0

t		Sh(r,t)	Eh(r,t)
		Ih(r,t)	Rh(r,t)
		Sv(r,t)	Ev(r,t)
		Iv(r,t)	
		Nh(r,t)	Nv(r,t)
150	0.00		
		159.2	24.7
		282.5	71.1
		2718.5	1268.0

		863.5	
		537.6	4850.0
150	10.00		
		159.2	24.7
		282.5	71.1
		2718.5	1268.0
		863.5	
		537.6	4850.0
150	20.00		
		159.2	24.7
		282.5	71.1
		2718.5	1268.0
		863.5	
		537.6	4850.0

t		Sh(r,t)	Eh(r,t)
		Ih(r,t)	Rh(r,t)
		Sv(r,t)	Ev(r,t)
		Iv(r,t)	
		Nh(r,t)	Nv(r,t)
300	0.00		
		25.5	4.3
		285.6	217.6
		2600.4	1319.5
		930.1	
		533.0	4850.0
300	10.00		
		25.5	4.3
		285.6	217.6
		2600.4	1319.5
		930.1	
		533.0	4850.0
300	20.00		
		25.5	4.3

```
            285.6              217.6
           2600.4             1319.5
            930.1
            533.0             4850.0
```

```
ncall =    524
```

Table 5.6: Numerical output, id=1, ncase=1

We can note the following details about this output.

- The solution array out has the dimensions $nout = 7 \times 287 + 1 = 288$ as expected (the first element in each of the 7 solution vectors is for t.

```
[1] 7
```

```
[1] 288
```

- The ICs for $t = 0$ are confirmed. The verification of the ICs is important since if they are in error, the subsequent solution will also be in error.
- The solution is displayed at $t = 0, 150, 300, r = 0, 10, 20$ as implemented in the main program of Listing 5.7.
- There is no variation of the solution with r. For example, at $t = 300, r = 0, 10, 20$.

```
    300    0.00
                   25.5              4.3
                  285.6            217.6
                 2600.4           1319.5
                  930.1
                  533.0           4850.0
    300   10.00
                   25.5              4.3
                  285.6            217.6
```

		2600.4	1319.5
		930.1	
		533.0	4850.0
300	20.00		
		25.5	4.3
		285.6	217.6
		2600.4	1319.5
		930.1	
		533.0	4850.0

This invariance with r results from the constant ICs (in r) and the differentiation of the constants ICs with respect to r. For example, with $S_h(r, t = 300) = 25.5$, $\dfrac{\partial^2 S_h}{\partial r^2} = 0$, $0 \leq r \leq 20$. Also, $\dfrac{1}{r}\dfrac{\partial S_h}{\partial r} = 0$ for $r > 0$. The homogeneous Neumann BCs (5.8a) are consistent with these zero derivatives[1]. This invariance with r is an important check since if it is not observed, there is an error in the programming.

- The computational effort is modest, `ncall` = 524. That is, `lsodes` efficiently produced a solution to the 287 ODEs.

Selected graphical output is displayed in Figs. (5.5-1) and (5.5-5).

---

[1] If the BCs are not consistent with the PDE solutions at the interior points in r, they could introduce a discontinuity that would cause a variation of the solutions with r since the radial differentiation group would not be zero. For example, with homogeneous Neumann BCs, the solutions change with t at the boundaries (but not with r). Therefore, homogeneous Dirichlet BCs would be inconsistent with the PDE solutions since the solutions do not remain at constant values at the boundaries. In other words, the effect of homogeneous Dirichlet BCs would be to introduce a discontinuity at the boundaries, which would give apparent departures from solutions that are invariant in r.

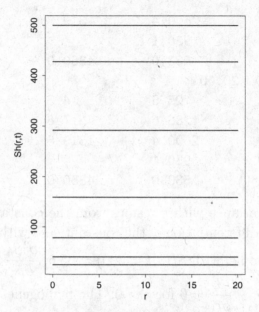

Figure 5.5-1: Numerical solution $S_h(r,t)$ from eq. (5.6a), id=1, ncase=1

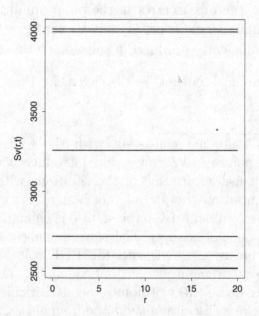

Figure 5.5-5: Numerical solution $S_v(r,t)$ from eq. (5.6e), id=1, ncase=1

The invariance of these solutions with r is clear.

With the verification of the solutions for constant ICs, variable ICs (in r) can now be considered with id=1, ncase=2 (the details for this case are given in the main program of Listing 5.7). The output for this case follows.

```
[1] 7

[1] 288
```

t		Sh(r,t)	Eh(r,t)
		Ih(r,t)	Rh(r,t)
		Sv(r,t)	Ev(r,t)
		Iv(r,t)	
		Nh(r,t)	Nv(r,t)
0	0.00		
		500.0	0.0
		30.0	0.0
		4000.0	0.0
		50.0	0.0
		530.0	4050.0
0	10.00		
		500.0	0.0
		0.0	0.0
		4000.0	0.0
		0.0	0.0
		500.0	4000.0
0	20.00		
		500.0	0.0
		0.0	0.0
		4000.0	0.0
		0.0	0.0
		500.0	4000.0

t	Sh(r,t)	Eh(r,t)
	Ih(r,t)	Rh(r,t)
	Sv(r,t)	Ev(r,t)
	Iv(r,t)	
	Nh(r,t)	Nv(r,t)
150	0.00	
	364.0	22.5
	102.4	15.6
	3814.6	638.0
	397.4	
	504.5	4850.0
150	10.00	
	458.3	8.5
	30.7	4.2
	4501.8	218.5
	129.6	
	501.6	4850.0
150	20.00	
	499.3	0.3
	1.1	0.1
	4837.4	7.9
	4.6	
	500.8	4850.0

t	Sh(r,t)	Eh(r,t)
	Ih(r,t)	Rh(r,t)
	Sv(r,t)	Ev(r,t)
	Iv(r,t)	
	Nh(r,t)	Nv(r,t)
300	0.00	
	84.3	15.8
	297.1	103.6
	2559.0	1353.5
	937.5	

```
                        500.9           4850.0
        300   10.00
                        148.7             23.8
                        258.7             69.4
                       2756.8           1246.9
                        846.3
                        500.6           4850.0
        300   20.00
                        277.5             28.1
                        165.2             30.0
                       3324.5            926.5
                        599.0
                        500.9           4850.0


    ncall =    556
```

Table 5.7: Numerical output, id=1, ncase=2

We can note the following details about this output.

- The dimensions of out are again 7×288.
- The ICs for ncase=2 are confirmed. For example,

$$S_h(r, t = 0) = 500, 500, 500; \quad r = 0, 10, 20$$

$$I_h(r, t = 0) = 30, 0, 0; \quad r = 0, 10, 20$$

$$S_v(r, t = 0) = 4000, 4000, 4000; \quad r = 0, 10, 20$$

$$I_v(r, t = 0) = 50, 0, 0; \quad r = 0, 10, 20$$

- The variations of the PDEs solutions with r and t is relatively complicated and can be better visualized graphically (figures that follow).

- The computatonal effort to compute a complete solution of the 287 ODEs is modest, `ncall = 556`. The sparse matrix facility of `lsodes` is effective in computing solutions efficiently.

Selected graphical output follows.

A significant reduction in the human susceptibles takes place (note the IC $S_h(r, t = 0) = 500$ for the beginning of the solution).

A significant increase in the human infecteds takes place (note the IC $I_h(r, t = 0) = 30e^{-0.1r^2}$ for the beginning of the solution at the bottom of the plot).

A significant increase in the human recovereds takes place (note the IC $R_h(r, t = 0) = 0$ for the beginning of the solution at the bottom of the plot).

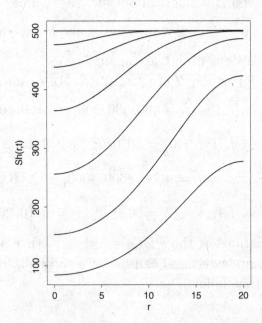

Figure 5.6-1: Numerical solution $S_h(r, t)$ from eq. (5.6a), `id=1`, `ncase=2`

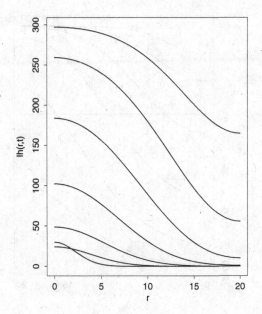

Figure 5.6-3: Numerical solution $I_h(r,t)$ from eq. (5.6c), `id=1`, `ncase=2`

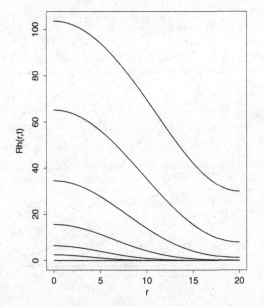

Figure 5.6-4: Numerical solution $R_h(r,t)$ from eq. (5.6d), `id=1`, `ncase=2`

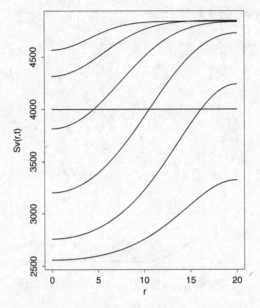

Figure 5.6-5: Numerical solution $S_v(r,t)$ from eq. (5.6e), id=1, ncase=2

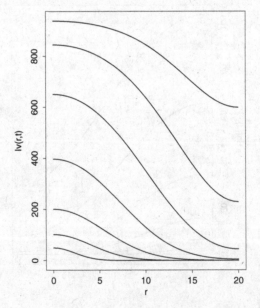

Figure 5.6-7: Numerical solution $I_v(r,t)$ from eq. (5.6g), id=1, ncase=2

A significant decrease in the mosquito susceptibles takes place (note the IC $S_v(r, t = 0) = 4000$ for the beginning of the solution).

A significant increase in the mosquito infecteds takes place (note the IC $I_v(r, t = 0) = 50e^{-0.1r^2}$ for the beginning of the solution at the bottom of the plot).

The concluding malaria model is based on eqs. (5.6) with cross diffusion added to selected PDEs.

(5.5) PDE Malaria Model, Cross Diffusion

Additional interaction between (1) $E_h(r, t)$ and $I_v(r, t)$ through the product function $E_h(r, t)I_v(r, t)$ and (2) $E_v(r, t)$ and $I_v(r, t)$ through the product function $E_v(r, t)I_v(r, t)$ is added to eqs. (5.6b,c,f,g) as cross diffusion.

$$\frac{\partial E_h}{\partial t} = \lambda_h(t)S_h - \nu_h E_h - f_h(N_h)E_h + D_{Eh}\left(\frac{\partial^2 E_h}{\partial r^2} + \frac{1}{r}\frac{\partial E_h}{\partial r}\right) +$$

$$D_{EhIv}\left(\frac{\partial^2 E_h I_v}{\partial r^2} + \frac{1}{r}\frac{\partial E_h I_v}{\partial r}\right) \qquad (5.9a)$$

$$\frac{\partial I_h}{\partial t} = \nu_h E_h - \gamma_h I_h - f_h(N_h)I_h - \delta_h I_h + D_{Ih}\left(\frac{\partial^2 I_h}{\partial r^2} + \frac{1}{r}\frac{\partial I_h}{\partial r}\right) +$$

$$D_{EhIv}\left(\frac{\partial^2 E_h I_v}{\partial r^2} + \frac{1}{r}\frac{\partial E_h I_v}{\partial r}\right) \qquad (5.9b)$$

$$\frac{\partial E_v}{\partial t} = \lambda_v(t)S_v - \nu_v E_v - f_v(N_v)E_v + D_{Ev}\left(\frac{\partial^2 E_v}{\partial r^2} + \frac{1}{r}\frac{\partial E_v}{\partial r}\right) +$$

$$D_{EvIv}\left(\frac{\partial^2 E_v I_v}{\partial r^2} + \frac{1}{r}\frac{\partial E_v I_v}{\partial r}\right) \qquad (5.9c)$$

$$\frac{\partial I_v}{\partial t} = \nu_v E_v - f_v(N_v)I_v + D_{Iv}\left(\frac{\partial^2 I_v}{\partial r^2} + \frac{1}{r}\frac{\partial I_v}{\partial r}\right) +$$

$$D_{EvIv}\left(\frac{\partial^2 E_v I_v}{\partial r^2} + \frac{1}{r}\frac{\partial E_v I_v}{\partial r}\right) \tag{5.9d}$$

where D_{EhIv}, D_{EvIv} are cross diffusivities. Eqs. (5.9) are then combined with the previous eqs. (5.6a,d,e) to constitute a 7×7 PDE system.

BCs are added to eqs. (5.9) for the radial derivatives of the cross diffusion terms.

$$\frac{\partial E_h I_v(r = r_l, t)}{\partial r} = \frac{\partial E_h I_v(r = r_u, t)}{\partial r} = 0 \tag{5.10a}$$

$$\frac{\partial E_v I_v(r = r_l, t)}{\partial r} = \frac{\partial E_v I_v(r = r_u, t)}{\partial r} = 0 \tag{5.10b}$$

Routines for the addition of eqs. (5.9), (5.10) follow.

(5.5.1) Main program

```
#
# SEIRV PDE malaria model
#
# Delete previous workspaces
  rm(list=ls(all=TRUE))
#
# Access ODE integrator
  library("deSolve");
#
# Access functions for numerical solution
  setwd("f:/infectious/chap5/sevenPDE");
  source("pde1b.R");
  source("dss004.R");
```

```
  source("dss044.R");
#
# Parameters for ODEs
  Lambda_h=0.033;
  Psi_h=1.1e-04;
  Psi_v=0.13;
  sigma_v=0.50;
  sigma_h=19;
  beta_hv=0.022;
  beta_vh=0.48;
  beta_vhb=0.048;
  nu_h=0.10;
  nu_v=0.091;
  gamma_h=0.0035;
  delta_h=9.0e-05;
  rho_h=5.5e-04;
  mu_1h=1.6e-05;
  mu_2h=3.0e-07;
  mu_1v=0.033;
  mu_2v=2.0e-05;
#
# Parameters for PDEs
  id=1;
#
# Linear diffusion
  if(id==0){
    D_Sh=0.1;
    D_Eh=0.1;
    D_Ih=0.1;
    D_Rh=0.1;
    D_Sv=0.1;
    D_Ev=0.1;
    D_Iv=0.1;
    D_EhIv=0;
```

```
      D_EvIv=0;
  }
#
# Linear + cross diffusion
  if(id==1){
    D_Sh=0.1;
    D_Eh=0.1;
    D_Ih=0.1;
    D_Rh=0.1;
    D_Sv=0.1;
    D_Ev=0.1;
    D_Iv=0.1;
    D_EhIv=0.001;
    D_EvIv=0.001;
  }
#
# Spatial grid (in r)
  nr=41;
  rl=0;ru=20;
  r=seq(from=rl,to=ru,by=0.5);
#
# Independent variable for ODE integration
  t0=0;tf=300;nout=7;
  tout=seq(from=t0,to=tf,by=50);
#
# Initial condition (t=0)
  ncase=2;
  u0=rep(0,7*nr);
  if(ncase==1){
    for(i in 1:nr){
      u0[i]      =500;
      u0[i+nr]   =10;
      u0[i+2*nr]=30;
      u0[i+3*nr]=0;
```

```
      u0[i+4*nr]=4000;
      u0[i+5*nr]=100;
      u0[i+6*nr]=50;
    }
  }
  if(ncase==2){
    for(i in 1:nr){
      u0[i]      =500;
      u0[i+nr]   =0;
      u0[i+2*nr]=30*exp(-0.1*r[i]^2);
      u0[i+3*nr]=0;
      u0[i+4*nr]=4000;
      u0[i+5*nr]=0;
      u0[i+6*nr]=50*exp(-0.1*r[i]^2);
    }
  }
  ncall=0;
#
# ODE integration
  out=lsodes(y=u0,times=tout,func=pde1b,
      sparsetype="sparseint",rtol=1e-6,
      atol=1e-6,maxord=5);
  nrow(out)
  ncol(out)
#
# Arrays for plotting numerical solution
  Sh=matrix(0,nrow=nr,ncol=nout);
  Eh=matrix(0,nrow=nr,ncol=nout);
  Ih=matrix(0,nrow=nr,ncol=nout);
  Rh=matrix(0,nrow=nr,ncol=nout);
  Sv=matrix(0,nrow=nr,ncol=nout);
  Ev=matrix(0,nrow=nr,ncol=nout);
  Iv=matrix(0,nrow=nr,ncol=nout);
  Nh=matrix(0,nrow=nr,ncol=nout);
```

```
  Nv=matrix(0,nrow=nr,ncol=nout);
EhIv=matrix(0,nrow=nr,ncol=nout);
EvIv=matrix(0,nrow=nr,ncol=nout);
  for(it in 1:nout){
    for(i in 1:nr){
      Sh[i,it]=out[it,i+1];
      Eh[i,it]=out[it,i+1+nr];
      Ih[i,it]=out[it,i+1+2*nr];
      Rh[i,it]=out[it,i+1+3*nr];
      Sv[i,it]=out[it,i+1+4*nr];
      Ev[i,it]=out[it,i+1+5*nr];
      Iv[i,it]=out[it,i+1+6*nr];
      Nh[i,it]=Sh[i,it]+Eh[i,it]+
               Ih[i,it]+Rh[i,it];
      Nv[i,it]=Sv[i,it]+Ev[i,it]+
               Iv[i,it];
    EhIv[i,it]=Eh[i,it]*Ih[i,it];
    EvIv[i,it]=Ev[i,it]*Iv[i,it];
    }
  }
#
# Display numerical solution
  for(it in 1:nout){
    if((it-1)*(it-4)*(it-nout)==0){
      cat(sprintf("\n"));
      cat(sprintf(
        "\n        t       Sh(r,t)       Eh(r,t)"));
      cat(sprintf(
        "\n                Ih(r,t)       Rh(r,t)"));
      cat(sprintf(
        "\n                Sv(r,t)       Ev(r,t)"));
      cat(sprintf(
        "\n                Iv(r,t)               "));
      cat(sprintf(
```

```
        "\n                Nh(r,t)        Nv(r,t)"));
    cat(sprintf(
        "\n            EhIv(r,t)      EvIv(r,t)"));
  for(i in 1:nr){
    if((i-1)*(i-21)*(i-nr)==0){
    cat(sprintf(
      "\n %6.0f %6.2f",tout[it],r[i]));
    cat(sprintf(
      "\n %12.1f %12.1f",Sh[i,it],Eh[i,it]));
    cat(sprintf(
      "\n %12.1f %12.1f",Ih[i,it],Rh[i,it]));
    cat(sprintf(
      "\n %12.1f %12.1f",Sv[i,it],Ev[i,it]));
    cat(sprintf(
      "\n %12.1f        ",Iv[i,it]));
    cat(sprintf(
      "\n %12.1f %12.1f",Nh[i,it],Nv[i,it]));
    cat(sprintf(
      "\n %12.1f %12.1f",EhIv[i,it],EvIv[i,it]));
    }
  }
  }
}
#
# Calls to ODE routine
  cat(sprintf("\n\n ncall = %5d\n\n",ncall));
#
# Plot PDE solutions
#
# Sh
  par(mfrow=c(1,1));
  matplot(r,Sh,type="l",xlab="r",ylab="Sh(r,t)",
    lty=1,main="",lwd=2,col="black");
#
```

```
# Eh
  par(mfrow=c(1,1));
  matplot(r,Eh,type="l",xlab="r",ylab="Eh(r,t)",
    lty=1,main="",lwd=2,col="black");
#
# Ih
  par(mfrow=c(1,1));
  matplot(r,Ih,type="l",xlab="r",ylab="Ih(r,t)",
    lty=1,main="",lwd=2,col="black");
#
# Rh
  par(mfrow=c(1,1));
  matplot(r,Rh,type="l",xlab="r",ylab="Rh(r,t)",
    lty=1,main="",lwd=2,col="black");
#
# Sv
  par(mfrow=c(1,1));
  matplot(r,Sv,type="l",xlab="r",ylab="Sv(r,t)",
    lty=1,main="",lwd=2,col="black");
#
# Ev
  par(mfrow=c(1,1));
  matplot(r,Ev,type="l",xlab="r",ylab="Ev(r,t)",
    lty=1,main="",lwd=2,col="black");
#
# Iv
  par(mfrow=c(1,1));
  matplot(r,Iv,type="l",xlab="r",ylab="Iv(r,t)",
    lty=1,main="",lwd=2,col="black");
#
# EhIv
  par(mfrow=c(1,1));
  matplot(
    r,EhIv,type="l",xlab="r",ylab="EhIv(r,t)",
```

```
    lty=1,main="",lwd=2,col="black");
#
# EvIv
  par(mfrow=c(1,1));
  matplot(
    r,EvIv,type="l",xlab="r",ylab="EvIv(r,t)",
    lty=1,main="",lwd=2,col="black");
```

Listing 5.9: Main program for the cross diffusion model

The main program of Listing 5.9 is similar to the main program of Listing 5.7. Therefore, the differences are emphasized in the following discussion.

- The MOL/ODE routine is pde1b (discussed subsequently).

```
  #
  # Access functions for numerical solution
    setwd("f:/infectious/chap5/sevenPDE");
    source("pde1b.R");
    source("dss004.R");
    source("dss044.R");
```

- Parameters for the high transmission case (Table 5.2) are used.
- Two cases of diffusion are programmed. For id=0, linear (Fickian) diffusion is used, but cross diffusion is not (D_EhIv=D_EvIv=0). For id=1, both linear and cross diffusion are used. Thus, a comparison of the solutions for id=0,1 gives an indication of the contribution of cross diffusion.

```
  #
  # Parameters for PDEs
    id=1;
  #
  # Linear diffusion
    if(id==0){
```

```
    D_Sh=0.1;
    D_Eh=0.1;
    D_Ih=0.1;
    D_Rh=0.1;
    D_Sv=0.1;
    D_Ev=0.1;
    D_Iv=0.1;
    D_EhIv=0;
    D_EvIv=0;
  }
#
# Linear + cross diffusion
  if(id==1){
    D_Sh=0.1;
    D_Eh=0.1;
    D_Ih=0.1;
    D_Rh=0.1;
    D_Sv=0.1;
    D_Ev=0.1;
    D_Iv=0.1;
    D_EhIv=0.001;
    D_EvIv=0.001;
  }
```

The values of D_EhIv, D_EvIv were selected to give a balance of linear and cross diffusion. For larger values (0.01), the radial profiles were essentially flat in r. For smaller values (0.0001), the effect of cross diffusion was essentially negligible.

- The same intervals in r and t as in Listing 5.7 are used.
- The same cases for the ICs, ncase=1,2, as in Listing 5.7 are used.
- The integration of the 287 ODEs is by lsodes with the MOL/ODE routine pde1b.

```
#
# ODE integration
  out=lsodes(y=u0,times=tout,func=pde1b,
      sparsetype="sparseint",rtol=1e-6,
      atol=1e-6,maxord=5);
  nrow(out)
  ncol(out)
```

- Additional matrices are allocated for the product functions EhIv, EvIv.

```
  EhIv=matrix(0,nrow=nr,ncol=nout);
  EvIv=matrix(0,nrow=nr,ncol=nout);
```

- The product functions are placed in the matrices for each r (index i) and t (index it).

```
    EhIv[i,it]=Eh[i,it]*Iv[i,it];
    EvIv[i,it]=Ev[i,it]*Iv[i,it];
```

- Display of the product functions is added.

```
  Heading
      cat(sprintf(
        "\n                EhIv(r,t)      EvIv(r,t)"));

  Numerical values
      cat(sprintf(
        "\n %12.1f %12.1f",EhIv[i,it],EvIv[i,it]));
```

- Plotting of the product functions is added.

```
  #
  # EhIv
  par(mfrow=c(1,1));
  matplot(
    r,EhIv,type="l",xlab="r",ylab="EhIv(r,t)",
    lty=1,main="",lwd=2,col="black");
```

```
#
# EvIv
  par(mfrow=c(1,1));
  matplot(
    r,EvIv,type="l",xlab="r",ylab="EvIv(r,t)",
    lty=1,main="",lwd=2,col="black");
```

Thus, the graphical output is `Sh,Eh,Ih,Rh,Sv,Ev,Iv` (seven plots) plus `EhIv,EvIv` (two plots) for a total of nine plots.

The ODE/MOL routine `pde1b` is considered next.

(5.5.2) ODE/MOL routine

```
  pde1b=function(t,u,parms){
#
# Function pde1b computes the t derivative
# vectors of Sh(r,t),Eh(r,t),Ih(r,t),Rh(r,t),
# Sv(r,t),Ev(r,t),Iv(r,t)
#
# One vector to seven vectors
  Sh=rep(0,nr);Eh=rep(0,nr);
  Ih=rep(0,nr);Rh=rep(0,nr);
  Sv=rep(0,nr);Ev=rep(0,nr);
  Iv=rep(0,nr);
  for(i in 1:nr){
    Sh[i]=u[i];
    Eh[i]=u[i+nr];
    Ih[i]=u[i+2*nr];
    Rh[i]=u[i+3*nr];
    Sv[i]=u[i+4*nr];
    Ev[i]=u[i+5*nr];
    Iv[i]=u[i+6*nr];
  }
```

```
#
# Algebra
  Nh=rep(0,nr);
  Nv=rep(0,nr);
  fhNh=rep(0,nr);
  fvNv=rep(0,nr);
  lambda_h=rep(0,nr);
  lambda_v=rep(0,nr);
  for(i in 1:nr){
  Nh[i]=Sh[i]+Eh[i]+Ih[i]+Rh[i];
  Nv[i]=Sv[i]+Ev[i]+Iv[i];
  fhNh[i]=mu_1h+mu_2h*Nh[i];
  fvNv[i]=mu_1v+mu_2v*Nv[i];
  lambda_h[i]=(sigma_v*Nv[i]*sigma_h)/
    (sigma_v*Nv[i]+sigma_h*Nh[i])*
      beta_hv*(Iv[i]/Nv[i]);
  lambda_v[i]=(sigma_v*Nh[i]*sigma_h)/
      (sigma_v*Nv[i]+sigma_h*Nh[i])*
      (beta_vh*(Ih[i]/Nh[i])+beta_vhb*
      (Rh[i]/Nh[i]));
  }
#
# Shr,Ehr,Ihr,Rhr
# Svr,Evr,Ivr
  Shr=dss004(rl,ru,nr,Sh);
  Ehr=dss004(rl,ru,nr,Eh);
  Ihr=dss004(rl,ru,nr,Ih);
  Rhr=dss004(rl,ru,nr,Rh);
  Svr=dss004(rl,ru,nr,Sv);
  Evr=dss004(rl,ru,nr,Ev);
  Ivr=dss004(rl,ru,nr,Iv);
#
# BCs
  Shr[1]=0;Shr[nr]=0;
```

```
  Ehr[1]=0;Ehr[nr]=0;
  Ihr[1]=0;Ihr[nr]=0;
  Rhr[1]=0;Rhr[nr]=0;
  Svr[1]=0;Svr[nr]=0;
  Evr[1]=0;Evr[nr]=0;
  Ivr[1]=0;Ivr[nr]=0;
#
# Shrr,Ehrr,Ihrr,Rhrr
# Svrr,Evrr,Ivrr
  nl=2;nu=2;
  Shrr=dss044(rl,ru,nr,Sh,Shr,nl=2,nu=2);
  Ehrr=dss044(rl,ru,nr,Eh,Ehr,nl=2,nu=2);
  Ihrr=dss044(rl,ru,nr,Ih,Ihr,nl=2,nu=2);
  Rhrr=dss044(rl,ru,nr,Rh,Rhr,nl=2,nu=2);
  Svrr=dss044(rl,ru,nr,Sv,Svr,nl=2,nu=2);
  Evrr=dss044(rl,ru,nr,Ev,Evr,nl=2,nu=2);
  Ivrr=dss044(rl,ru,nr,Iv,Ivr,nl=2,nu=2);
#
# Product funtions
  EhIv=rep(0,nr);EvIv=rep(0,nr);
  for(i in 1:nr){
    EhIv[i]=Eh[i]*Iv[i];
    EvIv[i]=Ev[i]*Iv[i];
  }
#
# First derivatives
  EhIvr=dss004(rl,ru,nr,EhIv);
  EvIvr=dss004(rl,ru,nr,EvIv);
#
# BCs
  EhIvr[1]=0;EhIvr[nr]=0;
  EvIvr[1]=0;EvIvr[nr]=0;
#
# Second derivatives
```

```
  nl=2;nu=2;
  EhIvrr=dss044(rl,ru,nr,EhIv,EhIvr,nl,nu);
  EvIvrr=dss044(rl,ru,nr,EvIv,EvIvr,nl,nu);
#
# PDEs
  Sht=rep(0,nr);Eht=rep(0,nr);
  Iht=rep(0,nr);Rht=rep(0,nr);
  Svt=rep(0,nr);Evt=rep(0,nr);
  Ivt=rep(0,nr);
#
# 0 le r le r0
  for(i in 1:nr){
#
# r=0
    if(i==1){
      Sht[i]=Lambda_h[i]+Psi_h*Nh[i]+rho_h*Rh[i]-
             lambda_h[i]*Sh[i]-fhNh[i]*Sh[i]+
             D_Sh*2*Shrr[i];
      Eht[i]=lambda_h[i]*Sh[i]-nu_h*Eh[i]-
             fhNh[i]*Eh[i]+
             D_Eh*2*Ehrr[i]+D_EhIv*2*EhIvrr[i];
      Iht[i]=nu_h*Eh[i]-gamma_h*Ih[i]-fhNh[i]*Ih[i]-
             delta_h*Ih[i]+D_Ih*2*Ihrr[i]+
             D_EhIv*2*EhIvrr[i];
      Rht[i]=gamma_h*Ih[i]-rho_h*Rh[i]-fhNh[i]*Rh[i]+
             D_Rh*2*Rhrr[i];
      Svt[i]=Psi_v*Nv[i]-lambda_v[i]*Sv[i]-
             fvNv[i]*Sv[i]+D_Sv*2*Svrr[i];
      Evt[i]=lambda_v[i]*Sv[i]-nu_v*Ev[i]-
             fvNv[i]*Ev[i]+
             D_Ev*2*Evrr[i]+D_EvIv*2*EvIvrr[i];
      Ivt[i]=nu_v*Ev[i]-fvNv[i]*Iv[i]+
             D_Iv*2*Ivrr[i]+D_EhIv*2*EhIvrr[i]+
                           D_EvIv*2*EvIvrr[i];
```

```
    }
#
# r > 0
    if(i>1){
      ri=1/r[i];
      Sht[i]=Lambda_h+Psi_h*Nh[i]+rho_h*Rh[i]-
             lambda_h[i]*Sh[i]-fhNh[i]*Sh[i]+
             D_Sh*(Shrr[i]+ri*Shr[i]);
      Eht[i]=lambda_h[i]*Sh[i]-nu_h*Eh[i]-
             fhNh[i]*Eh[i]+
             D_Eh*(Ehrr[i]+ri*Ehr[i])+
             D_EhIv*(EhIvrr[i]+ri*EhIvr[i]);
      Iht[i]=nu_h*Eh[i]-gamma_h*Ih[i]-fhNh[i]*Ih[i]-
             delta_h*Ih[i]+
             D_Ih*(Ihrr[i]+ri*Ihr[i])+
             D_EhIv*(EhIvrr[i]+ri*EhIvr[i]);
      Rht[i]=gamma_h*Ih[i]-rho_h*Rh[i]-fhNh[i]*Rh[i]+
             D_Rh*(Rhrr[i]+ri*Rhr[i]);
      Svt[i]=Psi_v*Nv[i]-lambda_v[i]*Sv[i]-
             fvNv[i]*Sv[i]+
             D_Sv*(Svrr[i]+ri*Svr[i]);
      Evt[i]=lambda_v[i]*Sv[i]-nu_v*Ev[i]-
             fvNv[i]*Ev[i]+
             D_Ev*(Evrr[i]+ri*Evr[i])+
             D_EvIv*(EvIvrr[i]+ri*EvIvr[i]);
      Ivt[i]=nu_v*Ev[i]-fvNv[i]*Iv[i]+
             D_Iv*(Ivrr[i]+ri*Ivr[i])+
             D_EhIv*(EhIvrr[i]+ri*EhIvr[i])+
             D_EvIv*(EvIvrr[i]+ri*EvIvr[i]);
    }
#
# Next i
    }
#
```

```
# Seven vectors to one vector
  ut=rep(0,7*nr);
  for(i in 1:nr){
    ut[i]      =Sht[i];
    ut[i+nr]   =Eht[i];
    ut[i+2*nr]=Iht[i];
    ut[i+3*nr]=Rht[i];
    ut[i+4*nr]=Svt[i];
    ut[i+5*nr]=Evt[i];
    ut[i+6*nr]=Ivt[i];
  }
#
# Increment calls to pde1b
  ncall <<- ncall+1;
#
# Return derivative vector
  return(list(c(ut)));
  }
```

Listing 5.10: MOL/ODE routine `pde1b` for the cross diffusion model

`pde1b` is similar to `pde1a` of Listing 5.8 so only the differences are considered.

- The function is defined (with the name change).

  ```
  pde1b=function(t,u,parms){
  #
  # Function pde1b computes the t derivative
  # vectors of Sh(r,t),Eh(r,t),Ih(r,t),Rh(r,t),
  # Sv(r,t),Ev(r,t),Iv(r,t)
  ```

- The input ODE 287-vector u is placed in seven 41-vectors to facilitate subsequent programming.
- The derivatives in r are computed as in Listing 5.7.

- The product functions are added.

```
#
# Product funtions
  EhIv=rep(0,nr);EvIv=rep(0,nr);
  for(i in 1:nr){
    EhIv[i]=Eh[i]*Iv[i];
    EvIv[i]=Ev[i]*Iv[i];
  }
```

- The first derivatives in r of the product functions are computed.

```
#
# First derivatives
  EhIvr=dss004(rl,ru,nr,EhIv);
  EvIvr=dss004(rl,ru,nr,EvIv);
```

Again, the vectors with the derivatives are allocated in dss004.

- Homogeneous Neumann BCs are applied to the product functions.

```
#
# BCs
  EhIvr[1]=0;EhIvr[nr]=0;
  EvIvr[1]=0;EvIvr[nr]=0;
```

Subscripts 1,nr correspond to $r = r_l = 0, r = r_u = 20$.

- The second derivatives of the product functions are computed with dss044.

```
#
# Second derivatives
  nl=2;nu=2;
  EhIvrr=dss044(rl,ru,nr,EhIv,EhIvv,nl,nu);
  EvIvrr=dss044(rl,ru,nr,EvIv,EvIvr,nl,nu);
```

- Cross diffusion is added to the ODEs for E_h, E_v, I_v at $r = 0$.

```
Eht[i]=lambda_h[i]*Sh[i]-nu_h*Eh[i]-
       fhNh[i]*Eh[i]+
       D_Eh*2*Ehrr[i]+
       D_EhIv*2*EhIvrr[i];
Evt[i]=lambda_v[i]*Sv[i]-nu_v*Ev[i]-
       fvNv[i]*Ev[i]+
       D_Ev*2*Evrr[i]+
       D_EvIv*2*EvIvrr[i];
Ivt[i]=nu_v*Ev[i]-fvNv[i]*Iv[i]+
       D_Iv*2*Ivrr[i]+D_EhIv*2*EhIvrr[i]+
                      D_EvIv*2*EvIvrr[i];
```

- Cross diffusion is added to the ODEs for E_h, E_v, I_v for $r > 0$.

```
Eht[i]=lambda_h[i]*Sh[i]-nu_h*Eh[i]-
       fhNh[i]*Eh[i]+
       D_Eh*(Ehrr[i]+ri*Ehr[i])+
       D_EhIv*(EhIvrr[i]+ri*EhIvr[i]);
Evt[i]=lambda_v[i]*Sv[i]-nu_v*Ev[i]-
       fvNv[i]*Ev[i]+
       D_Ev*(Evrr[i]+ri*Evr[i])+
       D_EvIv*(EvIvrr[i]+ri*EvIvr[i]);
Ivt[i]=nu_v*Ev[i]-fvNv[i]*Iv[i]+
       D_Iv*(Ivrr[i]+ri*Ivr[i])+
       D_EhIv*(EhIvrr[i]+ri*EhIvr[i])+
       D_EvIv*(EvIvrr[i]+ri*EvIvr[i]);
```

- The seven derivative (in t) 41-vectors are placed in a single derivative vector ut.
- The number of calls to pde1b is returned to the main program of Listing 5.9, and the derivative 287-vector is returned to lsodes as a list

The output from the routines in Listings 5.9, 5.10 is considered next

(5.5.3) Model output

The output from the routines of Listings 5.9, 5.10 follows.

[1] 7

[1] 288

```
        t        Sh(r,t)        Eh(r,t)
                 Ih(r,t)        Rh(r,t)
                 Sv(r,t)        Ev(r,t)
                 Iv(r,t)
                 Nh(r,t)        Nv(r,t)
                 EhIv(r,t)      EvIv(r,t)
    0    0.00
                  500.0            0.0
                   30.0            0.0
                 4000.0            0.0
                   50.0
                  530.0         4050.0
                    0.0            0.0
    0   10.00
                  500.0            0.0
                    0.0            0.0
                 4000.0            0.0
                    0.0
                  500.0         4000.0
                    0.0            0.0
    0   20.00
                  500.0            0.0
                    0.0            0.0
                 4000.0            0.0
```

	0.0	
	500.0	4000.0
	0.0	0.0
t	Sh(r,t)	Eh(r,t)
	Ih(r,t)	Rh(r,t)
	Sv(r,t)	Ev(r,t)
	Iv(r,t)	
	Nh(r,t)	Nv(r,t)
	EhIv(r,t)	EvIv(r,t)
150	0.00	
	391.8	15.5
	72.8	12.4
	4019.3	474.4
	266.6	
	492.5	4760.3
	4135.8	126454.6
150	10.00	
	451.8	9.9
	36.0	4.7
	4447.6	254.3
	152.9	
	502.4	4854.8
	1514.2	38875.4
150	20.00	
	498.3	0.6
	1.9	0.2
	4828.7	14.2
	8.6	
	501.0	4851.5
	5.2	121.9
t	Sh(r,t)	Eh(r,t)
	Ih(r,t)	Rh(r,t)

		Sv(r,t)	Ev(r,t)
		Iv(r,t)	
		Nh(r,t)	Nv(r,t)
		EhIv(r,t)	EvIv(r,t)
300	0.00		
		104.3	19.3
		272.0	87.3
		2609.7	1289.6
		868.1	
		482.9	4767.4
		16793.7	1119460.6
300	10.00		
		140.7	23.3
		258.5	69.7
		2724.9	1248.2
		840.5	
		492.1	4813.6
		19543.8	1049087.3
300	20.00		
		190.6	27.6
		242.4	51.0
		2893.1	1192.9
		811.6	
		511.7	4897.6
		22436.3	968209.1

```
ncall =   1120
```

Table 5.8: Numerical output, id=1, ncase=2, with cross diffusion

We can note the following details about this output.

- The dimensions of out are again 7 × 288.

- The ICs correspond to `id=1, ncase=2`. Specifically, $E_h(r, t = 0) = E_v(r, t = 0) = 0$ so that the product functions are $E_h I_v(r, t = 0) = E_v I_v(r, t = 0) = 0$.
- The product functions increase rapidly with t so that, for example, at $t = 300$, $E_h(r, t = 300)I_v(r, t = 300) = 22436.3$, $E_v(r, t = 0)I_v(r, t = 300) = 968209.1$.

    We would therefore expect that cross diffusion would have a significant effect on the solutions. This is confirmed by comparing, for example, Fig. 5.6-3 with Fig. 5.7-3, and Fig. 5.6-7 with Fig. 5.7-7.
- The computational effort is acceptable, `ncall = 1120`.

Selected graphical output follows.

The changes in the solutions with the addition of cross diffusion can be observed by using `id=0` but the corresponding figures are not presented to conserve space.

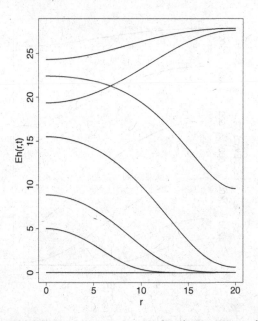

Figure 5.7-2: Numerical solution $E_h(r, t)$ from eq. (5.9a), `id=1`, `ncase=2`

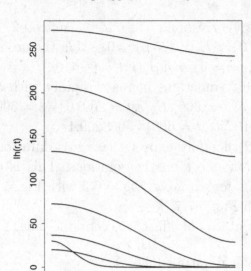

Figure 5.7-3: Numerical solution $I_h(r,t)$ from eq. (5.9b), `id=1`, `ncase=2`

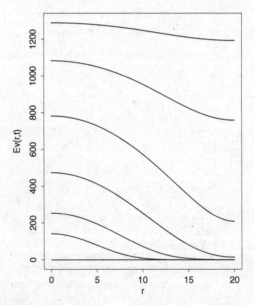

Figure 5.7-6: Numerical solution $E_v(r,t)$ from eq. (5.9c), `id=1`, `ncase=2`

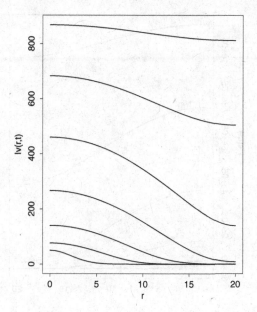

Figure 5.7-7: Numerical solution $I_v(r,t)$ from eq. (5.9d), `id=1`, `ncase=2`

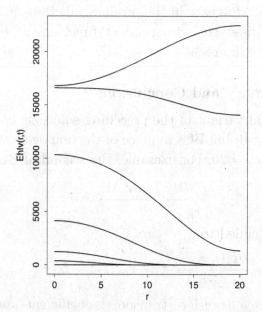

Figure 5.7-8: Numerical solution $E_h I_v(r,t)$, `id=1`, `ncase=2`

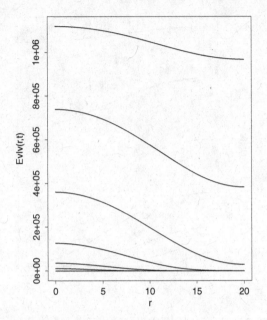

Figure 5.7-9: Numerical solution $E_v I_v(r,t)$, id=1, ncase=2

The rapid increase in the product functions in Figs. 5.7-8,9 is clear (consider the zero product functions at $t = 0$ at the bottom of the figures).

(5.6) Summary and Conclusions

An additional variant of the preceding solutions can be considered by using Robin BCs in place of the homogeneous Neumann BCs at $r = r_u = 20$. For example, the second of BCs (5.8c)

$$\frac{\partial I_h(r = r_u, t)}{\partial r} = 0 \qquad (5.8c)$$

could be extended to

$$D_{Ih}\frac{\partial I_h(r = r_u, t)}{\partial r} = k_{Ih}\left(I_{ha} - I_h(r = r_u, t)\right)$$

where k_{Ih} is a transfer (transport) coefficient and I_{ha} is the infected human population outside the radial domain with the outer boundary at $r = r_u = 20$. This Robin BC can be easily implemented, for example, in `pde1a` of Listing 5.8. A special case of particular interest would be for $I_{ha} = 0$ to study the migration of infected humans to beyond the radial domain $r = r_l = 0 \le r \le r = r_u = 20$ (this extension is left as an exercise for the reader).

In the previous analysis of the ODE and PDE malaria models, an analytical solution was not used to verify the numerical solutions (primarily because an analytical solution is probably not available). This leaves the question of the accuracy of the numerical solutions. This can be addressed in three ways: (1) the accuracy of the ODE integration in t can be studied by varying the error tolerances in the calls to `lsodes`, (2) the number of grid points in r can be varied, a form of h refinement, and (3) the order of the finite difference (FD) approximations of the derivatives in r can be varied, a form of p refinement.

For (3), the order of the FD approximations can easily be changed, for example, by using `dss046` ($O(h^6)$) in place of `dss044` ($O(h^4)$) and observing the changes in the numerical solution.

For (2), the number of grid points in r can be varied, and this number does not necessarily have to be increased to observe changes in the solution (since for `nr=41`, the number of ODEs is already large, 287). For example, `nr=31` would provide an inferred accuracy of the numerical solutions.

The use of (1), (2) and (3) is left as excerises for the reader to study the accuracy of the numerical solutions without having to use an analytical solution.

The PDE model of eqs. (5.6), (5.7), (5.8) illustrates the selection of space and time scales in two ways:

(1) For a given set of model parameters (constants), the space and time scales are selected to give distinct solutions (when plotted), e.g., $r = r_l = 0 \le r \le r = r_u = 20$, $t = t_0 = 0 \le$

$t \leq t = t_f = 300$. If t_f is too small, the solutions essentially remain at the ICs. If t_f is too large, the solutions essentially go immediately to the final (equilibrium) solutions.

(2) For given space and time scales, the parameters are selected to give distinct solutions. This might be a step in parameter estimation, that is, the solutions correspond to observed distributions (data) in space and time through the selection of parameter values.

Additional interactions between PDE dependent variables pairs through cross diffusion (beyond the product functions $E_h I_v$ and $E_v I_v$) can be readily studied by the methods discussed previously. Nonlinear functions other than (multiplication) product functions can also be studied numerically.

In conclusion, the ODE and PDE malaria models can be conveniently studied numerically, with the assignment of numerical values to the parameters as a principal requirement. The preceding analysis is next repeated in the concluding chapter for the dynamics of the Zika virus.

References

[1] Carter, R. (2002) Spatial simulation of malaria transmission and its control by malaria transmission blocking vaccination, *International Journal for Parasitology*, **32**, pp 1617-1624

[2] Chitnis, N., J.M. Hyman and J.M Cushing (2008), Determining important parameters in the spread of malaria through sensitivity analysis of a mathematical model, *Bulletin of Mathematical Biology*, **70**, pp 1272-1298

[3] Macdonald, G. (1956), Theory of the eradication of malaria, *Bulletin World Health Organization*, **15**, pp 369-387

[4] Macdonald, G., C.B. Cuellar and C.V. Foll (1968), The dynamics of malaria, *Bulletin World Health Organization*, **38**, pp 743-755

Chapter 6

Vector-Borne Diseases, Zika Virus

(6.1) Introduction

The application of the preceding ODE/PDE analysis to Zika is considered in this chapter. A distinguishing feature of Zika, as with malaria, is that it is vector-borne and the vector is a mosquito. Therefore, the models that are considered include human and mosquito dynamics.

(6.2) ODE Zika Model

The model is from [1] stated as ODEs in t. The ODE model is then extended to PDEs to include spatial effects, that is, a spatiotemporal model.

The model is a 15×15 (15 equations in 15 unknowns[1]) ODE system.

$$\frac{dS_B}{dt} = \pi_B - q_A \pi_B A_W - q_l \pi_B I_W - q_R \pi_B R_w -$$

$$\lambda_B(I_V, N_B) S_b - (\alpha + \mu_B) S_B \qquad (6.1\text{-}1)$$

---

[1]For this concluding chapter, because of the number of differential equations in each set, generally 15, numeric labeling of the equations is used in place of the alphanumeric labeling of the previous chapters.

353

$$\frac{dE_B}{dt} = \lambda_B(I_V, N_B)S_B - (\alpha + \sigma_B + \mu_B)E_B \qquad (6.1\text{-}2)$$

$$\frac{dA_B}{dt} = q_A \pi_B A_W + (1 - p)\sigma_B E_B - (\alpha + \gamma_B + \mu_B)A_B \qquad (6.1\text{-}3)$$

$$\frac{dI_B}{dt} = q_I \pi_B I_W + p\sigma_B E_B - (\alpha + \gamma_B + \mu_B)I_B \qquad (6.1\text{-}4)$$

$$\frac{dI_{BM}}{dt} = r q_R \pi_B R_W - (\alpha + \mu_B)I_{BM} \qquad (6.1\text{-}5)$$

$$\frac{dR_B}{dt} = (1 - r)q_R \pi_B R_W + \gamma_B A_B + \gamma_B I_B - (\alpha + \mu_B)R_B \qquad (6.1\text{-}6)$$

$$\frac{dS_W}{dt} = \alpha S_B - \lambda_W(I_V, N_W)S_W - \mu_W S_W \qquad (6.1\text{-}7)$$

$$\frac{dE_W}{dt} = \lambda_W(I_V, N_W)S_W - (\sigma_W + \mu_W)E_W \qquad (6.1\text{-}8)$$

$$\frac{dA_W}{dt} = (1 - p)\sigma_W E_W - (\gamma_W + \mu_W)A_W \qquad (6.1\text{-}9)$$

$$\frac{dI_W}{dt} = p\sigma_W E_W - (\gamma_W + \mu_W)I_W \qquad (6.1\text{-}10)$$

$$\frac{dI_{WM}}{dt} = \alpha I_{BM} - \mu_W I_{WM} \qquad (6.1\text{-}11)$$

$$\frac{dR_W}{dt} = \alpha R_B + \gamma_W A_W + \gamma_W I_W - \mu_W R_W \qquad (6.1\text{-}12)$$

$$\frac{dS_V}{dt} = \pi_V - \lambda_V(A_B, I_B, A_W, I_W, N_B, N_W)S_V - \mu_V S_V \quad (6.1\text{-}13)$$

$$\frac{dE_V}{dt} = \lambda_V(A_B, I_B, A_W, I_W, N_B, N_W)S_V - (\mu_V + \sigma_V)E_V$$
$$(6.1\text{-}14)$$

$$\frac{dI_V}{dt} = \sigma_V E_V - \mu_V I_V \quad (6.1\text{-}15)$$

with the associated algebra ([1], eqs. 2.1)

$$N_B = S_B + E_B + A_B + I_B + I_{BM} + R_B \quad (6.1\text{-}16)$$

$$N_W = S_W + E_W + A_W + I_W + I_{WM} + R_W \quad (6.1\text{-}17)$$

$$N_V = S_V + E_V + I_V \quad (6.1\text{-}18)$$

$$\lambda_W(I_V, N_W) = \frac{\beta_W b_V I_V}{N_W} \quad (6.1\text{-}19)$$

$$\lambda_B(I_V, N_B) = \frac{\eta \beta_B b_V I_V}{N_B} \quad (6.1\text{-}20)$$

$$\lambda_V(A_B, I_B, A_W, I_W, N_B, N_W) =$$
$$\beta_V b_V \left[\frac{I_W + \rho_W A_W + \eta(I_B + \rho_B A_B)}{N_W + \eta N_B} \right] \quad (6.1\text{-}21)$$

The ODE dependent variables follow.

- $S_B(t), S_W(t)$: susceptible newly born babies and adults
- $E_B(t), E_W(t)$: exposed newly born babies and adults

- $A_B(t), A_W(t)$: asymptomatic newly born babies and adults
- $I_B(t), I_W(t)$: symptomatic newly born without microcephaly and adults
- $I_{BM}(t), I_{WM}(t)$: microcephalic newly born babies and adults
- $R_B(t), R_W(t)$: recovered newly born babies and adults
- $S_V(t)$: susceptible female mosquitoes
- $E_V(t)$: exposed female mosquitoes
- $I_V(t)$: infected female mosquitoes

Table 6.1: Dependent (state) variables of eqs. (6.1) ([1], Table 1)

The parameters in eqs. (6.1) follow.

- π_B: birth rate newly born babies
- p: fraction of adults and newly born babies who are asymptomatic
- $1 - p$: remaining fraction of adults and newly born babies who are infectious
- α: maturation rate
- r, q_A, q_I, q_R: fractions of newly born babies who are infected and have microcephaly
- $1 - r$: remaining fraction of newly born babies who have microcephaly
- η: modification parameter
- β_W, β_B: transmission probability per contact of adults and newly born babies
- ρ_W, ρ_B: infectivity modification parameters in asymptomatic adults and newly born babies
- σ_W, σ_B: progression rate of exposed adults and newly born babies
- γ_W, γ_B: recovery rate of asymptomatic and symptomatic adults and newly born babies

- μ_W, μ_B: natural death rate of adults and newly born babies
- π_V: recruitment rate of mosquitoes
- β_V: transmission probability per contact of susceptible mosquitoes
- b_V: mosquito biting rate
- σ_V: progression rate of exposed mosquitoes
- μ_V: natural death rate of mosquitoes

Table 6.2: Parameters of eqs. (6.1) ([1], Table 1)

The numerical values of the parameters in eqs. (6.1) (time units are days) follow.

Parameter	Value
α	$1/(16 \times 365)$
η	1
ρ_B, ρ_W	0.5
p, r, q_A, q_I, q_R	0.5
β_W	0.33
σ_W	$1/7.5$
γ_W	$1/8.5$
μ_W	$1/(70 \times 365)$
π_B	$1/(15 \times 365)$
β_B	0.33
σ_B	$1/7.5$
γ_B	$1/8.5$
μ_B	$1/(1860 \times 365)$
π_V	500
β_V	0.33
b_V	0.5
σ_V	$1/3.5$
μ_V	$1/21$

Table 6.3: Numerical parameter values ([1], Table 3)

Eqs. (6.1-1) to (6.1-15) are first order in t so that each requires one initial condition (IC)[2].

$$S_B(t = 0) = S_{B0} = 5000; \quad E_B(t = 0) = E_{B0} = 200$$

$$A_B(t = 0) = A_{B0} = 200 \tag{6.2-1,2,3}$$

$$I_B(t = 0) = I_{B0} = 50; \quad I_{BM}(t = 0) = I_{BM0} = 20$$

$$RB(t = 0) = R_{B0} = 10 \tag{6.2-4,5,6}$$

$$S_W(t = 0) = S_{W0} = 10000; \quad E_W(t = 0) = E_{W0} = 220$$

$$A_W(t = 0) = A_{W0} = 400 \tag{6.2-7,8,9}$$

$$I_W(t = 0) = I_{W0} = 100; \quad I_{WM}(t = 0) = I_{WM0} = 120$$

$$R_W(t = 0) = R_{W0} = 200 \tag{6.2-10,11,12}$$

$$S_V(t = 0) = S_{V0} = 500; \quad E_V(t = 0) = E_{V0} = 100$$

$$I_V(t = 0) = I_{V0} = 100 \tag{6.2-13,14,15}$$

Eqs. (6.1) and (6.2) with the parameters in Table 6.3 constitute the ODE Zika model. The model is implemented in the R routines that follow.

---

[2]The ICs were provided by F.B. Agusto ([1]).

(6.2.1) Main program

The main program for eqs. (6.1), (6.2) follows.

```
#
# SEIRV ODE Zika model
#
# Delete previous workspaces
  rm(list=ls(all=TRUE))
#
# Access ODE integrator
  library("deSolve");
#
# Access functions for numerical solution
  setwd("f:/infectious/chap6/fifteenODE");
  source("ode1a.R");
#
# Parameters
  alpha=1/(16*365);    b_V=0.5;
  beta_B=0.33;         beta_V=0.33;
  beta_W=0.33;         eta=1;
  gamma_B=1/8.5;       gamma_W=1/8.5;
  mu_B=1/(18.60*365);  mu_V=1/21;
  mu_W=1/(70*365);     p=0.5;
  pi_B=1/(15*365);     pi_V=500;
  q_A=0.5;             q_I=0.5;
  q_R=0.5;             r=0.5;
  rho_B=0.5;           rho_W=0.5;
  sigma_B=1/7.5;       sigma_V=1/3.5;
  sigma_W=1/7.5;
#
# Independent variable for ODE integration
  t0=0;tf=250;
  tout=seq(from=t0,to=tf,by=250/40);
# print(tout);
```

```
#
# Initial conditions (t=0)
  ncase=1;
  u0=rep(0,15);
  S_B0=5000;   E_B0=200;  A_B0=200;
  I_B0=50;     I_BM0=20;  R_B0=10;
  S_W0=10000;  E_W0=220;  A_W0=400;
  I_W0=100;    I_WM0=120; R_W0=200;
  S_V0=500;    E_V0=100;  I_V0=100;
  if(ncase==1){
    u0[1]=S_B0;    u0[2]=E_B0;   u0[3]=A_B0;
    u0[4]=I_B0;    u0[5]=I_BM0;  u0[6]=R_B0;
    u0[7]=S_W0;    u0[8]=E_W0;   u0[9]=A_W0;
   u0[10]=I_W0;  u0[11]=I_WM0;  u0[12]=R_W0;
   u0[13]=S_V0;   u0[14]=E_V0;  u0[15]=I_V0;
  }
 ncall=0;
#
# ODE integration
  out=lsodes(y=u0,times=tout,func=ode1a,
      sparsetype="sparseint",rtol=1e-6,
      atol=1e-6,maxord=5);
  nrow(out)
  ncol(out)
#
# Arrays for plotting numerical solutions
  nout=41;
  S_B=rep(0,nout); E_B=rep(0,nout);
  A_B=rep(0,nout); I_B=rep(0,nout);
 I_BM=rep(0,nout); R_B=rep(0,nout);
  S_W=rep(0,nout); E_W=rep(0,nout);
  A_W=rep(0,nout); I_W=rep(0,nout);
 I_WM=rep(0,nout); R_W=rep(0,nout);
  S_V=rep(0,nout); E_V=rep(0,nout);
```

```
I_V=rep(0,nout); N_B=rep(0,nout);
N_W=rep(0,nout); N_V=rep(0,nout);
for(it in 1:nout){
  S_B[it]=out[it,2];
  E_B[it]=out[it,3];
  A_B[it]=out[it,4];
  I_B[it]=out[it,5];
 I_BM[it]=out[it,6];
  R_B[it]=out[it,7];
  S_W[it]=out[it,8];
  E_W[it]=out[it,9];
  A_W[it]=out[it,10];
  I_W[it]=out[it,11];
 I_WM[it]=out[it,12];
  R_W[it]=out[it,13];
  S_V[it]=out[it,14];
  E_V[it]=out[it,15];
  I_V[it]=out[it,16];
  N_B[it]=S_B[it]+E_B[it]+A_B[it]+I_B[it]+
          I_BM[it]+R_B[it];
  N_W[it]=S_W[it]+E_W[it]+A_W[it]+I_W[it]+
          I_WM[it]+R_W[it];
  N_V[it]=S_V[it]+E_V[it]+I_V[it];
}
#
# Display numerical solution
  for(it in 1:nout){
    if((it-1)*(it-21)*(it-nout)==0){
      cat(sprintf("\n"));
      cat(sprintf(
        "\n        t      S_B(t)       E_B(t)"));
      cat(sprintf(
        "\n              A_B(t)       I_B(t)"));
      cat(sprintf(
```

```
          "\n              I_BM(t)      R_B(t)"));
    cat(sprintf(
          "\n              S_W(t)       E_W(t)"));
    cat(sprintf(
          "\n              A_W(t)       I_W(t)"));
    cat(sprintf(
          "\n              I_WM(t)      R_W(t)"));
    cat(sprintf(
          "\n              S_V(t)       E_V(t)"));
    cat(sprintf(
          "\n              I_V(t)       N_B(t)"));
    cat(sprintf(
          "\n              N_W(t)       N_V(t)"));
    cat(sprintf(
          "\n %6.0f %10.0f %10.0f",
          tout[it],S_B[it],E_B[it]));
    cat(sprintf("\n
          %10.0f %10.0f",A_B[it],I_B[it]));
    cat(sprintf("\n
          %10.0f %10.0f",I_BM[it],R_B[it]));
    cat(sprintf("\n
          %10.0f %10.0f",S_W[it],E_W[it]));
    cat(sprintf("\n
          %10.0f %10.0f",A_W[it],I_W[it]));
    cat(sprintf("\n
          %10.0f %10.0f",I_WM[it],R_W[it]));
    cat(sprintf("\n
          %10.0f %10.0f",S_V[it],E_V[it]));
    cat(sprintf("\n
          %10.0f %10.0f",I_V[it],N_B[it]));
    cat(sprintf("\n
          %10.0f %10.0f",N_W[it],N_V[it]));
  }
}
```

```
#
# Calls to ODE routine
  cat(sprintf("\n\n ncall = %5d\n\n",ncall));
#
# Plot ODE solutions
#
# S_B
  par(mfrow=c(1,1));
  matplot(r,S_B,type="l",xlab="r",
    ylab="S_B(r,t)",lty=1,main="",
    lwd=2,col="black");
#
# E_B
  par(mfrow=c(1,1));
  matplot(r,E_B,type="l",xlab="r",
    ylab="E_B(r,t)",lty=1,main="",
    lwd=2,col="black");
#
# A_B
  par(mfrow=c(1,1));
  matplot(r,A_B,type="l",xlab="r",
    ylab="A_B(r,t)",lty=1,main="",
    lwd=2,col="black");
#
# I_B
  par(mfrow=c(1,1));
  matplot(r,I_B,type="l",xlab="r",
    ylab="I_B(r,t)",lty=1,main="",
    lwd=2,col="black");
#
# I_BM
  par(mfrow=c(1,1));
  matplot(r,I_BM,type="l",xlab="r",
    ylab="I_BM(r,t)",lty=1,main="",
```

```
    lwd=2,col="black");
#
# R_B
  par(mfrow=c(1,1));
  matplot(r,R_B,type="l",xlab="r",
    ylab="R_B(r,t)",lty=1,main="",
    lwd=2,col="black");
#
# S_W
  par(mfrow=c(1,1));
  matplot(r,S_W,type="l",xlab="r",
    ylab="S_W(r,t)",lty=1,main="",
    lwd=2,col="black");
#
# E_W
  par(mfrow=c(1,1));
  matplot(r,E_W,type="l",xlab="r",
    ylab="E_W(r,t)",lty=1,main="",
    lwd=2,col="black");
#
# A_W
  par(mfrow=c(1,1));
  matplot(r,A_W,type="l",xlab="r",
    ylab="A_W(r,t)",lty=1,main="",
    lwd=2,col="black");
#
# I_W
  par(mfrow=c(1,1));
  matplot(r,I_W,type="l",xlab="r",
    ylab="I_W(r,t)",lty=1,main="",
    lwd=2,col="black");
#
# I_WM
  par(mfrow=c(1,1));
```

```
  matplot(r,I_WM,type="l",xlab="r",
    ylab="I_WM(r,t)",lty=1,main="",
    lwd=2,col="black");
#
# R_W
  par(mfrow=c(1,1));
  matplot(r,R_W,type="l",xlab="r",
    ylab="R_W(r,t)",lty=1,main="",
    lwd=2,col="black");
#
# S_V
  par(mfrow=c(1,1));
  matplot(r,S_V,type="l",xlab="r",
    ylab="S_V(r,t)",lty=1,main="",
    lwd=2,col="black");
#
# E_V
  par(mfrow=c(1,1));
  matplot(r,E_V,type="l",xlab="r",
    ylab="E_V(r,t)",lty=1,main="",
    lwd=2,col="black");
#
# I_V
  par(mfrow=c(1,1));
  matplot(r,I_V,type="l",xlab="r",
    ylab="I_V(r,t)",lty=1,main="",
    lwd=2,col="black");
#
# N_B
  par(mfrow=c(1,1));
  matplot(r,N_B,type="l",xlab="r",
    ylab="N_B(r,t)",lty=1,main="",
    lwd=2,col="black");
#
```

```
# N_W
  par(mfrow=c(1,1));
  matplot(r,N_W,type="l",xlab="r",
    ylab="N_W(r,t)",lty=1,main="",
    lwd=2,col="black");
#
# N_V
  par(mfrow=c(1,1));
  matplot(r,N_V,type="l",xlab="r",
    ylab="N_V(r,t)",lty=1,main="",
    lwd=2,col="black");
```

Listing 6.1: Main program for eqs. (6.1), (6.2)

We can note the following details about Listing 6.1.

- The R ODE integrator library `deSolve` is accessed. Then the directory with the files for the solution of eqs. (6.1), (6.2), is designated. Note that `setwd` (set working directory) uses / rather than the usual \.

```
#
# SEIRV ODE Zika model
#
# Delete previous workspaces
  rm(list=ls(all=TRUE))
#
# Access ODE integrator
  library("deSolve");
#
# Access functions for numerical solution
  setwd("f:/infectious/chap6/fifteenODE");
  source("ode1a.R");
```

The MOL/ODE routine is `ode1a`.

- The parameters of Table 6.3 are specified.

```
#
# Parameters
  alpha=1/(16*365);    b_V=0.5;
  beta_B=0.33;         beta_V=0.33;
  beta_W=0.33;         eta=1;
  gamma_B=1/8.5;       gamma_W=1/8.5;
  mu_B=1/(18.60*365);  mu_V=1/21;
  mu_W=1/(70*365);     p=0.5;
  pi_B=1/(15*365);     pi_V=500;
  q_A=0.5;             q_I=0.5;
  q_R=0.5;             r=0.5;
  rho_B=0.5;           rho_W=0.5;
  sigma_B=1/7.5;       sigma_V=1/3.5;
  sigma_W=1/7.5;
```

- The interval in t, $0 \leq t \leq 250$, is defined with nout=26 output points so that tout=0,10,...,250 (the print statement indicates how numerical values can be displayed for initial testing).

```
#
# Independent variable for ODE integration
  t0=0;tf=250;nout=26;
  tout=seq(from=t0,to=tf,by=250/(nout-1));
# print(tout);
```

- ICs (6.2) are placed in a vector u0.

```
#
# Initial conditions (t=0)
  ncase=1;
  u0=rep(0,15);
  S_B0=5000;  E_B0=200; A_B0=200;
  I_B0=50;    I_BM0=20; R_B0=10;
  S_W0=10000; E_W0=220; A_W0=400;
  I_W0=100;   I_WM0=120; R_W0=200;
```

```
S_V0=500;    E_V0=100; I_V0=100;
if(ncase==1){
  u0[1]=S_B0;    u0[2]=E_B0;    u0[3]=A_B0;
  u0[4]=I_B0;    u0[5]=I_BM0;   u0[6]=R_B0;
  u0[7]=S_W0;    u0[8]=E_W0;    u0[9]=A_W0;
  u0[10]=I_W0; u0[11]=I_WM0; u0[12]=R_W0;
  u0[13]=S_V0;   u0[14]=E_V0;   u0[15]=I_V0;
}
ncall=0;
```

The counter for the number of calls to the MOL/ODE routine, ode1a (discussed subsequently), is also set numerically.

- Integration of the 15 ODEs is by lsodes. The ODE/MOL routine is ode1a. IC vector u0 informs lsodes of the number of ODEs to be integrated (15).

```
#
# ODE integration
  out=lsodes(y=u0,times=tout,func=ode1a,
      sparsetype="sparseint",rtol=1e-6,
      atol=1e-6,maxord=5);
  nrow(out)
  ncol(out)
```

- Arrays for the 15 ODE solutions returned by lsodes in out are declared (allocated), plus arrays for the totals N_B,N_W,N_V.

```
#
# Arrays for plotting numerical solutions
  S_B=rep(0,nout); E_B=rep(0,nout);
  A_B=rep(0,nout); I_B=rep(0,nout);
 I_BM=rep(0,nout); R_B=rep(0,nout);
  S_W=rep(0,nout); E_W=rep(0,nout);
  A_W=rep(0,nout); I_W=rep(0,nout);
```

```
I_WM=rep(0,nout); R_W=rep(0,nout);
S_V=rep(0,nout); E_V=rep(0,nout);
I_V=rep(0,nout); N_B=rep(0,nout);
N_W=rep(0,nout); N_V=rep(0,nout);
```

- The $15 + 3 = 18$ solution variables are placed in the vectors for subsequent display. out[it,1] is the value of t, so the indexing for the ODEs starts at out[it,2].

```
for(it in 1:nout){
  S_B[it]=out[it,2];
  E_B[it]=out[it,3];
  A_B[it]=out[it,4];
  I_B[it]=out[it,5];
  I_BM[it]=out[it,6];
  R_B[it]=out[it,7];
  S_W[it]=out[it,8];
  E_W[it]=out[it,9];
  A_W[it]=out[it,10];
  I_W[it]=out[it,11];
  I_WM[it]=out[it,12];
  R_W[it]=out[it,13];
  S_V[it]=out[it,14];
  E_V[it]=out[it,15];
  I_V[it]=out[it,16];
  N_B[it]=S_B[it]+E_B[it]+A_B[it]+I_B[it]+
          I_BM[it]+R_B[it];
  N_W[it]=S_W[it]+E_W[it]+A_W[it]+I_W[it]+
          I_WM[it]+R_W[it];
  N_V[it]=S_V[it]+E_V[it]+I_V[it];
}
```

- The numerical solutions are displayed numerically at $t = 0, 125, 250$.

```
#
```

```
# Display numerical solution
  for(it in 1:nout){
    if((it-1)*(it-13)*(it-nout)==0){
      cat(sprintf("\n"));
      cat(sprintf(
        "\n        t       S_B(t)        E_B(t)"));
      cat(sprintf(
        "\n              A_B(t)        I_B(t)"));
      cat(sprintf(
        "\n            I_BM(t)        R_B(t)"));
      cat(sprintf(
        "\n            S_W(t)        E_W(t)"));
      cat(sprintf(
        "\n            A_W(t)        I_W(t)"));
      cat(sprintf(
        "\n            I_WM(t)        R_W(t)"));
      cat(sprintf(
        "\n            S_V(t)        E_V(t)"));
      cat(sprintf(
        "\n            I_V(t)        N_B(t)"));
      cat(sprintf(
        "\n            N_W(t)        N_V(t)"));
      cat(sprintf(
        "\n %6.0f %10.0f %10.0f",
        tout[it],S_B[it],E_B[it]));
      cat(sprintf("\n
        %10.0f %10.0f",A_B[it],I_B[it]));
      cat(sprintf("\n
        %10.0f %10.0f",I_BM[it],R_B[it]));
      cat(sprintf("\n
        %10.0f %10.0f",S_W[it],E_W[it]));
      cat(sprintf("\n
        %10.0f %10.0f",A_W[it],I_W[it]));
      cat(sprintf("\n
```

```
         %10.0f %10.0f",I_WM[it],R_W[it]));
      cat(sprintf("\n
         %10.0f %10.0f",S_V[it],E_V[it]));
      cat(sprintf("\n
         %10.0f %10.0f",I_V[it],N_B[it]));
      cat(sprintf("\n
         %10.0f %10.0f",N_W[it],N_V[it]));
    }
  }
```

- The number of calls to `ode1a` is displayed at the end of the solution.

```
#
# Calls to ODE routine
  cat(sprintf("\n\n ncall = %5d\n\n",ncall));
```

- The solutions are displayed graphically with `plot` (a total of 18 plots).

```
#
# Plot ODE solutions
#
# S_B
  par(mfrow=c(1,1));
  matplot(r,S_B,type="l",xlab="r",
    ylab="S_B(r,t)",lty=1,main="",
    lwd=2,col="black");
```

```
#
# N_V
  par(mfrow=c(1,1));
  matplot(r,N_V,type="l",xlab="r",
    ylab="N_V(r,t)",lty=1,main="",
```

```
              lwd=2,col="black");
```

This completes the programming of the main program. The
MOL/ODE routine ode1a is considered next.

(6.2.2) ODE/MOL routine

ODE/MOL routine ode1a called by lsodes follows.

```
  ode1a=function(t,u,parms){
#
# Function ode1a computes the t derivative
# vectors of S_B(t) to I_V(t)
#
# One vector to fifteen scalars
  S_B=rep(0,1);  E_B=rep(0,1);A_B=rep(0,1);
  I_B=rep(0,1);I_BM=rep(0,1);R_B=rep(0,1);
  S_W=rep(0,1);  E_W=rep(0,1);A_W=rep(0,1);
  I_W=rep(0,1);I_WM=rep(0,1);R_W=rep(0,1);
  S_V=rep(0,1);  E_V=rep(0,1);I_V=rep(0,1);
  S_B[1]=u[1];
  E_B[1]=u[2];
  A_B[1]=u[3];
  I_B[1]=u[4];
 I_BM[1]=u[5];
  R_B[1]=u[6];
  S_W[1]=u[7];
  E_W[1]=u[8];
  A_W[1]=u[9];
  I_W[1]=u[10];
 I_WM[1]=u[11];
  R_W[1]=u[12];
  S_V[1]=u[13];
  E_V[1]=u[14];
  I_V[1]=u[15];
```

```
#
# Algebra
  N_B=rep(0,1);N_W=rep(0,1);N_V=rep(0,1);
  N_B[1]=S_B[1]+E_B[1]+A_B[1]+I_B[1]+I_BM[1]+R_B[1];
  N_W[1]=S_W[1]+E_W[1]+A_W[1]+I_W[1]+I_WM[1]+R_W[1];
  N_V[1]=S_V[1]+E_V[1]+I_V[1];
  lambda_W=beta_W*b_V*I_V[1]/N_W[1];
  lambda_B=eta*beta_B*b_V*I_V[1]/N_B[1];
  lambda_V=beta_V*b_V*(I_W[1]+rho_W*A_W[1]+
    eta*(I_B[1]+rho_B*A_B[1]))/(N_W[1]+eta*N_B[1]);
#
# ODEs
  S_Bt=rep(0,1); E_Bt=rep(0,1);A_Bt=rep(0,1);
  I_Bt=rep(0,1);I_BMt=rep(0,1);R_Bt=rep(0,1);
  S_Wt=rep(0,1); E_Wt=rep(0,1);A_Wt=rep(0,1);
  I_Wt=rep(0,1);I_WMt=rep(0,1);R_Wt=rep(0,1);
  S_Vt=rep(0,1); E_Vt=rep(0,1);I_Vt=rep(0,1);
  S_Bt[1]=pi_B-q_A*pi_B*A_W[1]-q_I*pi_B*
    I_W[1]-q_R*pi_B*R_W[1]-lambda_B*S_B[1]-
    (alpha+mu_B)*S_B[1];
  E_Bt[1]=lambda_B*S_B[1]-(alpha+sigma_B+
    mu_B)*E_B[1];
  A_Bt[1]=q_A*pi_B*A_W[1]+(1-p)*sigma_B*
    E_B[1]-(alpha+gamma_B+mu_B)*A_B[1];
  I_Bt[1]=q_I*pi_B*I_W[1]+p*sigma_B*E_B[1]-
    (alpha+gamma_B+mu_B)*I_B[1];
  I_BMt[1]=r*q_R*pi_B*R_W[1]-(alpha+mu_B)*
    I_BM[1];
  R_Bt[1]=(1-r)*q_R*pi_B*R_W[1]+gamma_B*
    A_B[1]+gamma_B*I_B[1]-(alpha+mu_B)*
    R_B[1];
  S_Wt[1]=alpha*S_B[1]-lambda_W*S_W[1]-
    mu_W*S_W[1];
  E_Wt[1]=lambda_W*S_W[1]-(sigma_W+mu_W)*
```

```
   E_W[1];
  A_Wt[1]=(1-p)*sigma_W*E_W[1]-(gamma_W+
    mu_W)*A_W[1];
  I_Wt[1]=p*sigma_W*E_W[1]-(gamma_W+mu_W)*
    I_W[1];
  I_WMt[1]=alpha*I_BM[1]-mu_W*I_WM[1];
  R_Wt[1]=alpha*R_B[1]+gamma_W*A_W[1]+
    gamma_W*I_W[1]-
    mu_W*R_W[1];
  S_Vt[1]=pi_V-lambda_V*S_V[1]-mu_V*S_V[1];
  E_Vt[1]=lambda_V*S_V[1]-(mu_V+sigma_V)*
    E_V[1];
  I_Vt[1]=sigma_V*E_V[1]-mu_V*I_V[1];
#
# Positive solutions
  if(S_B[1]<0)S_Bt[1]=0;
#
# Fifteen vectors to one vector
  ut=rep(0,15);
    ut[1]=S_Bt[1];
    ut[2]=E_Bt[1];
    ut[3]=A_Bt[1];
    ut[4]=I_Bt[1];
    ut[5]=I_BMt[1];
    ut[6]=R_Bt[1];
    ut[7]=S_Wt[1];
    ut[8]=E_Wt[1];
    ut[9]=A_Wt[1];
   ut[10]=I_Wt[1];
   ut[11]=I_WMt[1];
   ut[12]=R_Wt[1];
   ut[13]=S_Vt[1];
   ut[14]=E_Vt[1];
   ut[15]=I_Vt[1];
```

```
#
# Increment calls to ode1a
  ncall <<- ncall+1;
#
# Return derivative vector
  return(list(c(ut)));
  }
```

Listing 6.2: MOL/ODE routine ode1a for eqs. (6.1), (6.2)

We can note the following details about Listing 6.2.

- The function is defined.

```
ode1a=function(t,u,parms){
#
# Function ode1a computes the t derivative
# vectors of S_B(t) to I_V(t)
```

t is the current value of t in eqs. (6.1). u the 15-vector of ODE dependent variables. parm is an argument to pass parameters to ode1a (unused, but required in the argument list). The arguments must be listed in the order stated to properly interface with lsodes called in the main program of Listing 6.1. The derivative vector of the LHS of eqs. (6.1) is calculated next and returned to lsodes.

- u is placed in 15 1-vectors (scalars) to facilitate the programming of eqs. (6.1). One-element vectors are used to facilitate the programming of the subsequent PDE versions of eqs. (6.1).

```
#
# One vector to fifteen vectors
  S_B=rep(0,1); E_B=rep(0,1);A_B=rep(0,1);
  I_B=rep(0,1);I_BM=rep(0,1);R_B=rep(0,1);
  S_W=rep(0,1); E_W=rep(0,1);A_W=rep(0,1);
```

```
   I_W=rep(0,1);I_WM=rep(0,1);R_W=rep(0,1);
   S_V=rep(0,1); E_V=rep(0,1);I_V=rep(0,1);
   S_B[1]=u[1];
   E_B[1]=u[2];
   A_B[1]=u[3];
   I_B[1]=u[4];
 I_BM[1]=u[5];
   R_B[1]=u[6];
   S_W[1]=u[7];
   E_W[1]=u[8];
   A_W[1]=u[9];
   I_W[1]=u[10];
 I_WM[1]=u[11];
   R_W[1]=u[12];
   S_V[1]=u[13];
   E_V[1]=u[14];
   I_V[1]=u[15];
```

- Associated algebra of eqs. (6.1-16) to (6.1-21) is programmed.

```
   #
   # Algebra
   N_B=rep(0,1);N_W=rep(0,1);N_V=rep(0,1);
   N_B[1]=S_B[1]+E_B[1]+A_B[1]+I_B[1]+
          I_BM[1]+R_B[1];
   N_W[1]=S_W[1]+E_W[1]+A_W[1]+I_W[1]+
          I_WM[1]+R_W[1];
   N_V[1]=S_V[1]+E_V[1]+I_V[1];
   lambda_W=beta_W*b_V*I_V[1]/N_W[1];
   lambda_B=eta*beta_B*b_V*I_V[1]/N_B[1];
   lambda_V=beta_V*b_V*(I_W[1]+rho_W*A_W[1]+
     eta*(I_B[1]+rho_B*A_B[1]))/(N_W[1]+
     eta*N_B[1]);
```

Again, one-element arrays are used to faciliate the subsequent programming of PDEs.

- Eqs. (6.1) are programmed.

```
#
# ODEs
  S_Bt=rep(0,1); E_Bt=rep(0,1);A_Bt=rep(0,1);
  I_Bt=rep(0,1);I_BMt=rep(0,1);R_Bt=rep(0,1);
  S_Wt=rep(0,1); E_Wt=rep(0,1);A_Wt=rep(0,1);
  I_Wt=rep(0,1);I_WMt=rep(0,1);R_Wt=rep(0,1);
  S_Vt=rep(0,1); E_Vt=rep(0,1);I_Vt=rep(0,1);
  S_Bt[1]=pi_B-q_A*pi_B*A_W[1]-q_I*pi_B*
    I_W[1]-q_R*pi_B*R_W[1]-lambda_B*S_B[1]-
    (alpha+mu_B)*S_B[1];
  E_Bt[1]=lambda_B*S_B[1]-(alpha+sigma_B+
    mu_B)*E_B[1];
  A_Bt[1]=q_A*pi_B*A_W[1]+(1-p)*sigma_B*
    E_B[1]-(alpha+gamma_B+mu_B)*A_B[1];
  I_Bt[1]=q_I*pi_B*I_W[1]+p*sigma_B*E_B[1]-
    (alpha+gamma_B+mu_B)*I_B[1];
  I_BMt[1]=r*q_R*pi_B*R_W[1]-(alpha+mu_B)*
    I_BM[1];
  R_Bt[1]=(1-r)*q_R*pi_B*R_W[1]+gamma_B*
    A_B[1]+gamma_B*I_B[1]-(alpha+mu_B)*
    R_B[1];
  S_Wt[1]=alpha*S_B[1]-lambda_W*S_W[1]-
    mu_W*S_W[1];
  E_Wt[1]=lambda_W*S_W[1]-(sigma_W+mu_W)*
    E_W[1];
  A_Wt[1]=(1-p)*sigma_W*E_W[1]-(gamma_W+
    mu_W)*A_W[1];
  I_Wt[1]=p*sigma_W*E_W[1]-(gamma_W+mu_W)*
    I_W[1];
  I_WMt[1]=alpha*I_BM[1]-mu_W*I_WM[1];
```

```
R_Wt[1]=alpha*R_B[1]+gamma_W*A_W[1]+
  gamma_W*i_W[1]-mu_W*R_W[1];
S_Vt[1]=pi_V-lambda_V*S_V[1]-mu_V*S_V[1];
E_Vt[1]=lambda_V*S_V[1]-(mu_V+sigma_V)*
  E_V[1];
I_Vt[1]=sigma_V*E_V[1]-mu_V*I_V[1];
```

The 15 one-element t derivative vectors are the final result (the LHSs of eqs. (6.1)). For example, S_Bt $= \dfrac{dS_B}{dt}$ in eq. (6.1-1).

- $S_B(t)$ was observed to eventually have slightly negative values which is physically impossible. In order to prevent this, the following statement was added to zero the derivative, S_Bt[1]=0.

```
#
# Positive solutions
  if(S_B[1]<0)S_Bt[1]=0;
```

The question remains why $S_B(t)$ acquired negative values. This can occur if $S_B(t)$ has a positive IC (which it does, $S_B(t = 0) = 5000$), and the derivative $\dfrac{dS_B}{dt} < 0$ (which is expected if $S_B(t)$ decays with t), but the derivative remains negative long enough for $S_B(t) < 0$. Therefore, an examination of the RHS terms of eq. (6.1-1) is required to observe and explain why $\dfrac{dS_B}{dt} < 0$ leads to $S_B(t) < 0$.

This is an example of the importance of studying the RHSs of ODEs (and PDEs) as well as their solutions to understand the features of the solutions. The use of ode1a without if(S_B[1]<0)S_Bt[1]=0 is left as an exercise. Also, this can be extended to examine the RHS of eq. (6.1-1) in detail.

- The 15 1-vectors are placed in a vector of t derivatives, ut.

```
#
# Fifteen vectors to one vector
  ut=rep(0,15);
    ut[1]=S_Bt[1];
    ut[2]=E_Bt[1];
    ut[3]=A_Bt[1];
    ut[4]=I_Bt[1];
    ut[5]=I_BMt[1];
    ut[6]=R_Bt[1];
    ut[7]=S_Wt[1];
    ut[8]=E_Wt[1];
    ut[9]=A_Wt[1];
   ut[10]=I_Wt[1];
   ut[11]=I_WMt[1];
   ut[12]=R_Wt[1];
   ut[13]=S_Vt[1];
   ut[14]=E_Vt[1];
   ut[15]=I_Vt[1];
```

- The number of calls to ode1a is incremented and returned to the main program of Listing 6.1 by <<-.

```
#
# Increment calls to ode1a
  ncall <<- ncall+1;
```

-

- The derivative vector ut is returned to lsodes as a list. c is the R vector utility.

```
#
# Return derivative vector
  return(list(c(ut)));
```

```
    }
```

The final } concludes ode1a.

The output from the routines in Listings 6.1, 6.2 follows.

(6.2.3) Model output

The numerical output from the main program of Listing 6.1 is in Table 6.4.

[1] 26

[1] 16

t	S_B(t)	E_B(t)
	A_B(t)	I_B(t)
	I_BM(t)	R_B(t)
	S_W(t)	E_W(t)
	A_W(t)	I_W(t)
	I_WM(t)	R_W(t)
	S_V(t)	E_V(t)
	I_V(t)	N_B(t)
	N_W(t)	N_V(t)
0	5000	200
	200	50
	20	10
	10000	220
	400	100
	120	200
	500	100
	100	5480
	11040	700

t	S_B(t)	E_B(t)
	A_B(t)	I_B(t)
	I_BM(t)	R_B(t)
	S_W(t)	E_W(t)
	A_W(t)	I_W(t)
	I_WM(t)	R_W(t)
	S_V(t)	E_V(t)
	I_V(t)	N_B(t)
	N_W(t)	N_V(t)
120	347	140
	110	110
	35	4532
	2874	454
	294	294
	120	7050
	9088	176
	1203	5275
	11086	10468

t	S_B(t)	E_B(t)
	A_B(t)	I_B(t)
	I_BM(t)	R_B(t)
	S_W(t)	E_W(t)
	A_W(t)	I_W(t)
	I_WM(t)	R_W(t)
	S_V(t)	E_V(t)
	I_V(t)	N_B(t)
	N_W(t)	N_V(t)
250	-0	0
	0	0
	87	5002
	1094	10
	8	8
	121	9902

```
         10430              4
            66           5089
         11143          10500
```

```
ncall =    629
```

Table 6.4: Numerical output for eqs. (6.1), (6.2)

We can note the following details about this output.

- The dimensions of the solution matrix out are 26×16 for 26 output points (programmed in Listing 6.1) and $15 + 1 = 16$ for 15 ODEs and one place at the beginning of each solution vector for t.

```
[1] 26
```

```
[1] 16
```

- The ICs of eqs. (6.2) are confirmed. This check is important since if the ICs are not correct, the subsequent solution will not be correct.
- The output is for $t = 0, 120, 250$ as programmed in Listing 6.1.
- $S_B(t = 250)$ appears to have come from the constraint discussed previously S_B = -0.
- The computational effort for a complete solution is modest, ncall = 629.

The graphical output includes 18 plots. A subset follows.

Without the nonnegativity constraint, the solution is slightly negative at $t = 250$ (-27) which is imperceptible on the plot compared to the IC of 5000.

```
    t      S_B(t)        E_B(t)
           A_B(t)        I_B(t)
          I_BM(t)        R_B(t)
```

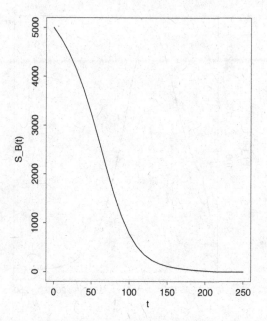

Figure 6.1-1: Numerical solution $S_B(t)$ from eq. (6.1-1)

250	-27	-0
	-0	-0

The infected babies drops from 50 initially to essentially zero at $t = 250$. So the Zika is stable in the long term. The curve has a slight gridding (nonsmooth) effect. This could be reduced by increasing the number of output points (above 26). This is left as an exercise.

The infected humans drops from 100 initially to 8 at $t = 250$. So again, Zika is stable in the long term.

The infected mosquito population goes through a maximum as indicated in Table 6.4.

t	I_V(t)
0	100

t	I_V(t)

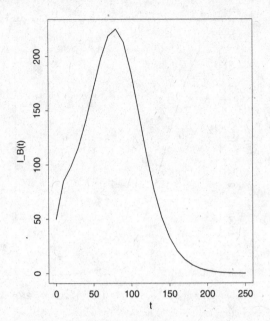

Figure 6.1-4: Numerical solution $I_B(t)$ from eq. (6.1-4)

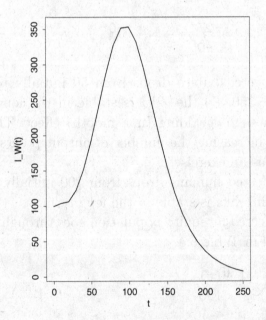

Figure 6.1-10: Numerical solution $I_W(t)$ from eq. (6.1-10)

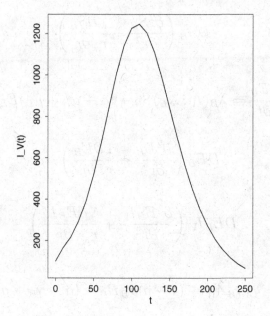

Figure 6.1-15: Numerical solution $I_V(t)$ from eq. (6.1-15)

```
  120          1203


   t         I_V(t)
  250           66
```

so the infected mosquitoes have a lower population at the end of the solution than at the beginning.

The model of eqs. (6.1) does not include spatial effects, which are considered next by extending the ODEs to PDEs.

(6.3) PDE Zika Model

The model equations follow.

$$\frac{\partial S_B}{\partial t} = \pi_B - q_A \pi_B A_W - q_l \pi_B I_W - q_R \pi_B R_w -$$

$$\lambda_B(I_V, N_B) S_b - (\alpha + \mu_B) S_B +$$

$$DS_B \left(\frac{\partial^2 S_B}{\partial r^2} + \frac{1}{r} \frac{\partial S_B}{\partial r} \right) \tag{6.3-1}$$

$$\frac{\partial E_B}{\partial t} = \lambda_B(I_V, N_B)S_B - (\alpha + \sigma_B + \mu_B)E_B +$$

$$DE_B \left(\frac{\partial^2 E_B}{\partial r^2} + \frac{1}{r} \frac{\partial E_B}{\partial r} \right) +$$

$$DE_B I_V \left(\frac{\partial^2 E_B I_V}{\partial r^2} + \frac{1}{r} \frac{\partial E_B I_V}{\partial r} \right) \tag{6.3-2}$$

$$\frac{\partial A_B}{\partial t} = q_A \pi_B A_W + (1-p)\sigma_B E_B - (\alpha + \gamma_B + \mu_B)A_B +$$

$$DA_B \left(\frac{\partial^2 A_B}{\partial r^2} + \frac{1}{r} \frac{\partial A_B}{\partial r} \right) \tag{6.3-3}$$

$$\frac{\partial I_B}{\partial t} = q_l \pi_B I_W + p\sigma_B E_B - (\alpha + \gamma_B + \mu_B)I_B +$$

$$DI_B \left(\frac{\partial^2 I_B}{\partial r^2} + \frac{1}{r} \frac{\partial I_B}{\partial r} \right) \tag{6.3-4}$$

$$\frac{\partial I_{BM}}{\partial t} = rq_R \pi_B R_W - (\alpha + \mu_B)I_{BM} +$$

$$DI_{BM} \left(\frac{\partial^2 I_{BM}}{\partial r^2} + \frac{1}{r} \frac{\partial I_{BM}}{\partial r} \right) \tag{6.3-5}$$

$$\frac{\partial R_B}{\partial t} = (1-r)q_R \pi_B R_W + \gamma_B A_B + \gamma_B I_B - (\alpha + \mu_B)R_B +$$

$$DR_B \left(\frac{\partial^2 R_B}{\partial r^2} + \frac{1}{r} \frac{\partial R_B}{\partial r} \right) \tag{6.3-6}$$

$$\frac{\partial S_W}{\partial t} = \alpha S_B - \lambda_W(I_V, N_W) S_W - \mu_W S_W +$$

$$DS_W \left(\frac{\partial^2 S_W}{\partial r^2} + \frac{1}{r} \frac{\partial S_W}{\partial r} \right) \tag{6.3-7}$$

$$\frac{\partial E_W}{\partial t} = \lambda_W(I_V, N_W) S_W - (\sigma_W + \mu_W) E_W +$$

$$DE_W \left(\frac{\partial^2 E_W}{\partial r^2} + \frac{1}{r} \frac{\partial E_W}{\partial r} \right) +$$

$$DE_W I_V \left(\frac{\partial^2 E_W I_V}{\partial r^2} + \frac{1}{r} \frac{\partial E_W I_V}{\partial r} \right) \tag{6.3-8}$$

$$\frac{\partial A_W}{\partial t} = (1 - p)\sigma_W E_W - (\gamma_W + \mu_W) A_W +$$

$$DA_W \left(\frac{\partial^2 A_W}{\partial r^2} + \frac{1}{r} \frac{\partial A_W}{\partial r} \right) \tag{6.3-9}$$

$$\frac{\partial I_W}{\partial t} = p\sigma_W E_W - (\gamma_W + \mu_W) I_W +$$

$$DE_W \left(\frac{\partial^2 E_W}{\partial r^2} + \frac{1}{r} \frac{\partial E_W}{\partial r} \right) \tag{6.3-10}$$

$$\frac{\partial I_{WM}}{\partial t} = \alpha I_{BM} - \mu_W I_{WM} +$$

$$DI_{BM} \left(\frac{\partial^2 I_{BM}}{\partial r^2} + \frac{1}{r} \frac{\partial I_{BM}}{\partial r} \right) \tag{6.3-11}$$

$$\frac{\partial R_W}{\partial t} = \alpha R_B + \gamma_W A_W + \gamma_W I_W - \mu_W R_W +$$

$$DR_W \left(\frac{\partial^2 R_W}{\partial r^2} + \frac{1}{r} \frac{\partial R_W}{\partial r} \right) \tag{6.3-12}$$

$$\frac{\partial S_V}{\partial t} = \pi_V - \lambda_V (A_B, I_B, A_W, I_W, N_B, N_W) S_V - \mu_V S_V +$$

$$DS_V \left(\frac{\partial^2 S_V}{\partial r^2} + \frac{1}{r} \frac{\partial S_V}{\partial r} \right) \tag{6.3-13}$$

$$\frac{\partial E_V}{\partial t} = \lambda_V (A_B, I_B, A_W, I_W, N_B, N_W) S_V - (\mu_V + \sigma_V) E_V +$$

$$DE_V \left(\frac{\partial^2 E_V}{\partial r^2} + \frac{1}{r} \frac{\partial E_V}{\partial r} \right) \tag{6.3-14}$$

$$\frac{\partial I_V}{\partial t} = \sigma_V E_V - \mu_V I_V +$$

$$DI_V \left(\frac{\partial^2 I_V}{\partial r^2} + \frac{1}{r} \frac{\partial I_V}{\partial r} \right) +$$

$$DE_B I_V \left(\frac{\partial^2 E_B I_V}{\partial r^2} + \frac{1}{r} \frac{\partial E_B I_V}{\partial r} \right) +$$

$$DE_W I_V \left(\frac{\partial^2 E_W I_V}{\partial r^2} + \frac{1}{r} \frac{\partial E_W I_V}{\partial r} \right) \tag{6.3-15}$$

We can note the following details of eqs. (6.3).

- A linear (Fickian) diffusion term in radial coordinates has been added to each ODE of eqs. (6.1).
- Eqs. (6.3-2), (6.3-8), (6.3-15) for $E_B(r,t), E_W(r,t),$ $I_V(r,t)$ have a cross diffusion term.

The ICs for eqs. (6.3) follow.

$$S_B(r,t=0) = S_{B0}(r) = 5000; \ E_B(r,t=0) = E_{B0}(r) = 200$$
$$(6.4\text{-}1,2)$$

$$A_B(r,t=0) = A_{B0}(r) = 20; \ I_B(r,t=0) = I_{B0}(r) = 50$$
$$(6.4\text{-}3,4)$$

$$I_{BM}(r,t=0) = I_{BM0}(r) = 20; \ R_B(r,t=0) = R_{B0}(r) = 10$$
$$(6.4\text{-}5,6)$$

$$S_W(r,t=0) = S_{W0}(r) = 10000; \ E_W(r,t=0) = E_{W0}(r) = 220$$
$$(6.4\text{-}7,8)$$

$$A_W(r,t=0) = A_{W0}(r) = 400; \ I_W(r,t=0) = I_{W0}(r) = 100$$
$$(6.4\text{-}9,10)$$

$$I_{WM}(r,t=0) = I_{WM0}(r) = 120; \ R_W(r,t=0) = R_{W0}(r) = 200$$
$$(6.4\text{-}11,12)$$

$$S_V(r,t=0) = S_{V0}(r) = 500; \ E_V(r,t=0) = E_{V0}(r) = 100$$
$$(6.4\text{-}13,14)$$

$$I_V(r,t=0) = I_{V0}(r) = 100 \qquad (6.4\text{-}15)$$

The BCs for eqs. (6.3-1) to (6.3-15) are (with $r_l = 0, r_u = 1$)

$$\frac{\partial S_B(r = r_l, t)}{\partial r} = \frac{\partial S_B(r = r_u, t)}{\partial r} = 0 \qquad (6.5\text{-}1)$$

$$\frac{\partial E_B(r = r_l, t)}{\partial r} = \frac{\partial E_B(r = r_u, t)}{\partial r} = 0 \qquad (6.5\text{-}2)$$

$$\frac{\partial A_B(r = r_l, t)}{\partial r} = \frac{\partial A_B(r = r_u, t)}{\partial r} = 0 \qquad (6.5\text{-}3)$$

$$\frac{\partial I_B(r = r_l, t)}{\partial r} = \frac{\partial I_B(r = r_u, t)}{\partial r} = 0 \qquad (6.5\text{-}4)$$

$$\frac{\partial R_{BM}(r = r_l, t)}{\partial r} = \frac{\partial R_{BM}(r = r_u, t)}{\partial r} = 0 \qquad (6.5\text{-}5)$$

$$\frac{\partial R_B(r = r_l, t)}{\partial r} = \frac{\partial R_B(r = r_u, t)}{\partial r} = 0 \qquad (6.5\text{-}6)$$

$$\frac{\partial S_W(r = r_l, t)}{\partial r} = \frac{\partial S_W(r = r_u, t)}{\partial r} = 0 \qquad (6.5\text{-}7)$$

$$\frac{\partial E_W(r = r_l, t)}{\partial r} = \frac{\partial E_W(r = r_u, t)}{\partial r} = 0 \qquad (6.5\text{-}8)$$

$$\frac{\partial A_W(r = r_l, t)}{\partial r} = \frac{\partial A_W(r = r_u, t)}{\partial r} = 0 \qquad (6.5\text{-}9)$$

$$\frac{\partial I_W(r = r_l, t)}{\partial r} = \frac{\partial I_W(r = r_u, t)}{\partial r} = 0 \qquad (6.5\text{-}10)$$

$$\frac{\partial I_{WM}(r=r_l,t)}{\partial r} = \frac{\partial I_{WM}(r=r_u,t)}{\partial r} = 0 \qquad (6.5\text{-}11)$$

$$\frac{\partial R_W(r=r_l,t)}{\partial r} = \frac{\partial R_W(r=r_u,t)}{\partial r} = 0 \qquad (6.5\text{-}12)$$

$$\frac{\partial S_V(r=r_l,t)}{\partial r} = \frac{\partial S_V(r=r_u,t)}{\partial r} = 0 \qquad (6.5\text{-}13)$$

$$\frac{\partial E_V(r=r_l,t)}{\partial r} = \frac{\partial E_V(r=r_u,t)}{\partial r} = 0 \qquad (6.5\text{-}14)$$

$$\frac{\partial I_V(r=r_l,t)}{\partial r} = \frac{\partial I_V(r=r_u,t)}{\partial r} = 0 \qquad (6.5\text{-}15)$$

Eqs. (6.3), (6.4), (6.5) constitute the PDE Zika model. The routines for the solution of these equations are considered next.

(6.3.1) Main program

The main program for eqs. (6.3), (6.4), (6.5) is listed next.

```
#
# SEIRV PDE Zika model
#
# Delete previous workspaces
  rm(list=ls(all=TRUE))
#
# Access ODE integrator
  library("deSolve");
#
# Access functions for numerical solution
  setwd("f:/infectious/chap6/fifteenPDE");
  source("pde1a.R");
  source("dss004.R");
```

```
  source("dss044.R");
#
# Parameters
  alpha=1/(16*365);        b_V=0.5;
  beta_B=0.33;             beta_V=0.33;
  beta_W=0.33;             eta=1;
  gamma_B=1/8.5;           gamma_W=1/8.5;
  mu_B=1/(18.60*365);      u_V=1/21;
  mu_W=1/(70*365);p=0.5;   pi_B=1/(15*365);
  pi_V=500;                q_A=0.5;
  q_I=0.5;                 q_R=0.5;
  rg=0.5;                  rho_B=0.5;
  rho_W=0.5;               sigma_B=1/7.5;
  sigma_V=1/3.5;           sigma_W=1/7.5;
#
# Diffusivities
  DS_B=1.0e-02;  DE_B=1.0e-02;DA_B=1.0e-02;
  DI_B=1.0e-02;DI_BM=1.0e-02;DR_B=1.0e-02;
  DS_W=1.0e-02;  DE_W=1.0e-02;DA_W=1.0e-02;
  DI_W=1.0e-02;DI_WM=1.0e-02;DR_W=1.0e-02;
  DS_V=1.0e-02;  DE_V=1.0e-02;DI_V=1.0e-02;
  DE_BI_V=1.0e-04;DE_WI_V=1.0e-04;
#
# Spatial grid
  nr=21;rl=0;ru=1;
  r=seq(from=rl,to=ru,by=(ru-rl)/(nr-1));
#
# Independent variable for ODE integration
  t0=0;tf=25;nout=6;
  tout=seq(from=t0,to=tf,by=(tf-t0)/(nout-1));
#
# Initial conditions
  S_B0=5000;   E_B0=200; A_B0=200;
  I_B0=50;     I_BM0=20; R_B0=10;
```

```
  S_W0=10000; E_W0=220; A_W0=400;
  I_W0=100;   I_WM0=120; R_W0=200;
  S_V0=500;    E_V0=100; I_V0=100;
  u0=rep(0,15*nr);
  for(i in 1:nr){
    u0[i]=S_B0;          u0[i+nr]=E_B0;
    u0[i+2*nr]=A_B0;     u0[i+3*nr]=I_B0;
    u0[i+4*nr]=I_BM0;    u0[i+5*nr]=R_B0;
    u0[i+6*nr]=S_W0;     u0[i+7*nr]=E_W0;
    u0[i+8*nr]=A_W0;     u0[i+9*nr]=I_W0;
    u0[i+10*nr]=I_WM0;   u0[i+11*nr]=R_W0;
    u0[i+12*nr]=S_V0;    u0[i+13*nr]=E_V0;
    u0[i+14*nr]=I_V0;
  }
  for(i in 1:nr){
    u0[i]        =S_B0*exp(-10*r[i]^2);
    u0[i+6*nr]  =S_W0*exp(-10*r[i]^2);
    u0[i+12*nr]=S_V0*exp(-10*r[i]^2);
  }
  ncall=0;
#
# ODE integration
  out=lsodes(y=u0,times=tout,func=pde1a,
      sparsetype ="sparseint",rtol=1e-6,
      atol=1e-6,maxord=5);
  nrow(out)
  ncol(out)
#
# Arrays for plotting numerical solutions
  S_B=matrix(0,nrow=nr,ncol=nout);
  E_B=matrix(0,nrow=nr,ncol=nout);
  A_B=matrix(0,nrow=nr,ncol=nout);
  I_B=matrix(0,nrow=nr,ncol=nout);
 I_BM=matrix(0,nrow=nr,ncol=nout);
```

```
  R_B=matrix(0,nrow=nr,ncol=nout);
  S_W=matrix(0,nrow=nr,ncol=nout);
  E_W=matrix(0,nrow=nr,ncol=nout);
  A_W=matrix(0,nrow=nr,ncol=nout);
  I_W=matrix(0,nrow=nr,ncol=nout);
 I_WM=matrix(0,nrow=nr,ncol=nout);
  R_W=matrix(0,nrow=nr,ncol=nout);
  S_V=matrix(0,nrow=nr,ncol=nout);
  E_V=matrix(0,nrow=nr,ncol=nout);
  I_V=matrix(0,nrow=nr,ncol=nout);
  N_B=matrix(0,nrow=nr,ncol=nout);
  N_W=matrix(0,nrow=nr,ncol=nout);
  N_V=matrix(0,nrow=nr,ncol=nout);
  for(it in 1:nout){
  for(i in 1:nr){
    S_B[i,it]=out[it,i+1];
    E_B[i,it]=out[it,i+1+nr];
    A_B[i,it]=out[it,i+1+2*nr];
    I_B[i,it]=out[it,i+1+3*nr];
   I_BM[i,it]=out[it,i+1+4*nr];
    R_B[i,it]=out[it,i+1+5*nr];
    S_W[i,it]=out[it,i+1+6*nr];
    E_W[i,it]=out[it,i+1+7*nr];
    A_W[i,it]=out[it,i+1+8*nr];
    I_W[i,it]=out[it,i+1+9*nr];
   I_WM[i,it]=out[it,i+1+10*nr];
    R_W[i,it]=out[it,i+1+11*nr];
    S_V[i,it]=out[it,i+1+12*nr];
    E_V[i,it]=out[it,i+1+13*nr];
    I_V[i,it]=out[it,i+1+14*nr];
    N_B[i,it]=S_B[i,it]+E_B[i,it]+A_B[i,it]+
              I_B[i,it]+I_BM[i,it]+R_B[i,it];
    N_W[i,it]=S_W[i,it]+E_W[i,it]+A_W[i,it]+
              I_W[i,it]+I_WM[i,it]+R_W[i,it];
```

```
   N_V[i,it]=S_V[i,it]+E_V[i,it]+I_V[i,it];
  }
 }
#
# Display numerical solution
  for(it in 1:nout){
    if((it-1)*(it-nout)==0){
    for(i in 1:nr){
      if((i-1)*(i-nr)==0){
      cat(sprintf("\n"));
  cat(sprintf(
        "\n               t              r"));
      cat(sprintf(
        "\n  %10.0f %10.0f",tout[it],r[i]));
      cat(sprintf(
        "\n       S_B(t)        E_B(t)"));
      cat(sprintf(
        "\n       A_B(t)        I_B(t)"));
      cat(sprintf(
        "\n      I_BM(t)        R_B(t)"));
      cat(sprintf(
        "\n       S_W(t)        E_W(t)"));
      cat(sprintf(
        "\n       A_W(t)        I_W(t)"));
      cat(sprintf(
        "\n      I_WM(t)        R_W(t)"));
      cat(sprintf(
        "\n       S_V(t)        E_V(t)"));
      cat(sprintf(
        "\n       I_V(t)        N_B(t)"));
      cat(sprintf(
        "\n       N_W(t)        N_V(t)"));
      cat(sprintf(
        "\n  %10.0f %10.0f",S_B[i,it],E_B[i,it]));
```

```
      cat(sprintf(
        "\n  %10.0f %10.0f",A_B[i,it],I_B[i,it]));
      cat(sprintf(
        "\n  %10.0f %10.0f",I_BM[i,it],R_B[i,it]));
      cat(sprintf(
        "\n  %10.0f %10.0f",S_W[i,it],E_W[i,it]));
      cat(sprintf(
        "\n  %10.0f %10.0f",A_W[i,it],I_W[i,it]));
      cat(sprintf(
        "\n  %10.0f %10.0f",I_WM[i,it],R_W[i,it]));
      cat(sprintf(
        "\n  %10.0f %10.0f",S_V[i,it],E_V[i,it]));
      cat(sprintf(
        "\n  %10.0f %10.0f",I_V[i,it],N_B[i,it]));
      cat(sprintf(
        "\n  %10.0f %10.0f",N_W[i,it],N_V[i,it]));
      }
    }
    }
  }
#
# Calls to ODE routine
  cat(sprintf("\n\n ncall = %5d\n\n",ncall));
#
# Plot PDE solutions
#
# S_B
  par(mfrow=c(1,1));
  matplot(r,S_B,type="l",xlab="r",
    ylab="S_B(r,t)",lty=1,main="",
    lwd=2,col="black");
#
# E_B
  par(mfrow=c(1,1));
```

```
  matplot(r,E_B,type="l",xlab="r",
    ylab="E_B(r,t)",lty=1,main="",
    lwd=2,col="black");
#
# A_B
  par(mfrow=c(1,1));
  matplot(r,A_B,type="l",xlab="r",
    ylab="A_B(r,t)",lty=1,main="",
    lwd=2,col="black");
#
# I_B
  par(mfrow=c(1,1));
  matplot(r,I_B,type="l",xlab="r",
    ylab="I_B(r,t)",lty=1,main="",
    lwd=2,col="black");
#
# I_BM
  par(mfrow=c(1,1));
  matplot(r,I_BM,type="l",xlab="r",
    ylab="I_BM(r,t)",lty=1,main="",
    lwd=2,col="black");
#
# R_B
  par(mfrow=c(1,1));
  matplot(r,R_B,type="l",xlab="r",
    ylab="R_B(r,t)",lty=1,main="",
    lwd=2,col="black");
#
# S_W
  par(mfrow=c(1,1));
  matplot(r,S_W,type="l",xlab="r",
    ylab="S_W(r,t)",lty=1,main="",
    lwd=2,col="black");
#
```

```
# E_W
  par(mfrow=c(1,1));
  matplot(r,E_W,type="l",xlab="r",
    ylab="E_W(r,t)",lty=1,main="",
    lwd=2,col="black");
#
# A_W
  par(mfrow=c(1,1));
  matplot(r,A_W,type="l",xlab="r",
    ylab="A_W(r,t)",lty=1,main="",
    lwd=2,col="black");
#
# I_W
  par(mfrow=c(1,1));
  matplot(r,I_W,type="l",xlab="r",
    ylab="I_W(r,t)",lty=1,main="",
    lwd=2,col="black");
#
# I_WM
  par(mfrow=c(1,1));
  matplot(r,I_WM,type="l",xlab="r",
    ylab="I_WM(r,t)",lty=1,main="",
    lwd=2,col="black");
#
# R_W
  par(mfrow=c(1,1));
  matplot(r,R_W,type="l",xlab="r",
    ylab="R_W(r,t)",lty=1,main="",
    lwd=2,col="black");
#
# S_V
  par(mfrow=c(1,1));
  matplot(r,S_V,type="l",xlab="r",
    ylab="S_V(r,t)",lty=1,main="",
```

```
    lwd=2,col="black");
#
# E_V
  par(mfrow=c(1,1));
  matplot(r,E_V,type="l",xlab="r",
    ylab="E_V(r,t)",lty=1,main="",
    lwd=2,col="black");
#
# I_V
  par(mfrow=c(1,1));
  matplot(r,I_V,type="l",xlab="r",
    ylab="I_V(r,t)",lty=1,main="",
    lwd=2,col="black");
#
# N_B
  par(mfrow=c(1,1));
  matplot(r,N_B,type="l",xlab="r",
    ylab="N_B(r,t)",lty=1,main="",
    lwd=2,col="black");
#
# N_W
  par(mfrow=c(1,1));
  matplot(r,N_W,type="l",xlab="r",
    ylab="N_W(r,t)",lty=1,main="",
    lwd=2,col="black");
#
# N_V
  par(mfrow=c(1,1));
  matplot(r,N_V,type="l",xlab="r",
    ylab="N_V(r,t)",lty=1,main="",
    lwd=2,col="black");
```

Listing 6.3: Main program for eqs. (6.3), (6.4), (6.5)

We can note the following details about Listing 6.3.

- The R ODE integrator library `deSolve` is accessed. Then the directory with the files for the solution of eqs. (6.3), (6.4), (6.5) is designated.

```
#
# SEIRV PDE Zika model
#
# Delete previous workspaces
  rm(list=ls(all=TRUE))
#
# Access ODE integrator
  library("deSolve");
#
# Access functions for numerical solution
  setwd("f:/infectious/chap6/fifteenPDE");
  source("pde1a.R");
  source("dss004.R");
  source("dss044.R");
```

The ODE/MOL routine is `pde1a`. `dss004`, `dss044` are library routines for the calcualtion of first and second derivatives in r, respectively.

- The model parameters in Table 6.3 are defined numerically.

```
#
# Parameters
  alpha=1/(16*365);        b_V=0.5;
  beta_B=0.33;             beta_V=0.33;
  beta_W=0.33;             eta=1;
  gamma_B=1/8.5;           gamma_W=1/8.5;
  mu_B=1/(18.60*365);      u_V=1/21;
  mu_W=1/(70*365);p=0.5;   pi_B=1/(15*365);
  pi_V=500;                q_A=0.5;
  q_I=0.5;                 q_R=0.5;
```

```
rg=0.5;                    rho_B=0.5;
rho_W=0.5;                 sigma_B=1/7.5;
sigma_V=1/3.5;             sigma_W=1/7.5;
```

- The diffusivities in eqs. (6.3) are defined numerically.

```
#
# Diffusivities
  DS_B=1.0e-02; DE_B=1.0e-02;DA_B=1.0e-02;
  DI_B=1.0e-02;DI_BM=1.0e-02;DR_B=1.0e-02;
  DS_W=1.0e-02; DE_W=1.0e-02;DA_W=1.0e-02;
  DI_W=1.0e-02;DI_WM=1.0e-02;DR_W=1.0e-02;
  DS_V=1.0e-02; DE_V=1.0e-02;DI_V=1.0e-02;
  DE_BI_V=1.0e-04;DE_WI_V=1.0e-04;
```

The cross diffusivities, DE_BI_V, DE_WI_V, were selected to give additional smoothing to the solutions with linear (Fickian) diffusion.

- A spatial grid of nr=21 points is defined for the interval $0 \leq r \leq 1$ so that $r = 0, 0.05, ..., 1$.

```
#
# Spatial grid
  nr=21;rl=0;ru=1;
  r=seq(from=rl,to=ru,by=(ru-rl)/(nr-1));
```

nr=21 was selected so that the number of ODEs is $(15)(21) = 315$ which is about the same number of ODEs as for the 7×7 model of Chapter 5, $(7)(41) = 287$, and gives solutions to the PDE Zika model with acceptable computation.

- The interval in t, $0 \leq t \leq 25$, is defined with nout=6 output points so that tout=0,5,...,25 which gives plots of the solutions against r with six parametric curves in t.

```
#
# Independent variable for ODE integration
```

```
t0=0;tf=25;nout=6;
tout=seq(from=t0,to=tf,by=(tf-t0)/(nout-1));
```

- The ICs of eqs. (6.4) are defined as constants so that the solutions would not vary with r.

```
#
# Initial conditions
  S_B0=5000;    E_B0=200; A_B0=200;
  I_B0=50;      I_BM0=20; R_B0=10;
  S_W0=10000;   E_W0=220; A_W0=400;
  I_W0=100;     I_WM0=120; R_W0=200;
  S_V0=500;     E_V0=100; I_V0=100;
  u0=rep(0,15*nr);
  for(i in 1:nr){
    u0[i]=S_B0;          u0[i+nr]=E_B0;
    u0[i+2*nr]=A_B0;     u0[i+3*nr]=I_B0;
    u0[i+4*nr]=I_BM0;    u0[i+5*nr]=R_B0;
    u0[i+6*nr]=S_W0;     u0[i+7*nr]=E_W0;
    u0[i+8*nr]=A_W0;     u0[i+9*nr]=I_W0;
    u0[i+10*nr]=I_WM0;   u0[i+11*nr]=R_W0;
    u0[i+12*nr]=S_V0;    u0[i+13*nr]=E_V0;
    u0[i+14*nr]=I_V0;
  }
```

Then variation in r is added as Gaussian functions for $S_B(r, t = 0), S_W(r, t = 0), S_V(r, t = 0)$.

```
  for(i in 1:nr){
    u0[i]        =S_B0*exp(-10*r[i]^2);
    u0[i+6*nr]  =S_W0*exp(-10*r[i]^2);
    u0[i+12*nr]=S_V0*exp(-10*r[i]^2);
  }
  ncall=0;
```

The number of calls to pde1a is also initialized.

- The $(15)(21) = 315$ MOL/ODEs (the length of u0), are integrated by `lsodes`. `pde1a` is the MOL/ODE routine discussed subsequently.

```
#
# ODE integration
  out=lsodes(y=u0,times=tout,func=pde1a,
      sparsetype="sparseint",rtol=1e-6,
      atol=1e-6,maxord=5);
  nrow(out)
  ncol(out)
```

- Arrays are defined for the numerical solutions to eqs. (6.3-1) to (6.3-15) and the population sums of eqs. (6.1-16) to (6.1-18).

```
#
# Arrays for plotting numerical solutions
  S_B=matrix(0,nrow=nr,ncol=nout);
  E_B=matrix(0,nrow=nr,ncol=nout);
  A_B=matrix(0,nrow=nr,ncol=nout);
  I_B=matrix(0,nrow=nr,ncol=nout);
 I_BM=matrix(0,nrow=nr,ncol=nout);
  R_B=matrix(0,nrow=nr,ncol=nout);
  S_W=matrix(0,nrow=nr,ncol=nout);
  E_W=matrix(0,nrow=nr,ncol=nout);
  A_W=matrix(0,nrow=nr,ncol=nout);
  I_W=matrix(0,nrow=nr,ncol=nout);
 I_WM=matrix(0,nrow=nr,ncol=nout);
  R_W=matrix(0,nrow=nr,ncol=nout);
  S_V=matrix(0,nrow=nr,ncol=nout);
  E_V=matrix(0,nrow=nr,ncol=nout);
  I_V=matrix(0,nrow=nr,ncol=nout);
  N_B=matrix(0,nrow=nr,ncol=nout);
  N_W=matrix(0,nrow=nr,ncol=nout);
```

```
N_V=matrix(0,nrow=nr,ncol=nout);
```

- The solutions to eqs. (6.3-1) to (6.3-15) and the sums of eqs. (6.1-16) to (6.1-18) are placed in the allocated arrays. The offset i+1 in the second subscript of out reflects the value of t at the beginning of each solution vector returned by lsodes.

```
for(it in 1:nout){
for(i in 1:nr){
  S_B[i,it]=out[it,i+1];
  E_B[i,it]=out[it,i+1+nr];
  A_B[i,it]=out[it,i+1+2*nr];
  I_B[i,it]=out[it,i+1+3*nr];
 I_BM[i,it]=out[it,i+1+4*nr];
  R_B[i,it]=out[it,i+1+5*nr];
  S_W[i,it]=out[it,i+1+6*nr];
  E_W[i,it]=out[it,i+1+7*nr];
  A_W[i,it]=out[it,i+1+8*nr];
  I_W[i,it]=out[it,i+1+9*nr];
 I_WM[i,it]=out[it,i+1+10*nr];
  R_W[i,it]=out[it,i+1+11*nr];
  S_V[i,it]=out[it,i+1+12*nr];
  E_V[i,it]=out[it,i+1+13*nr];
  I_V[i,it]=out[it,i+1+14*nr];
  N_B[i,it]=S_B[i,it]+E_B[i,it]+A_B[i,it]+
            I_B[i,it]+I_BM[i,it]+R_B[i,it];
  N_W[i,it]=S_W[i,it]+E_W[i,it]+A_W[i,it]+
            I_W[i,it]+I_WM[i,it]+R_W[i,it];
  N_V[i,it]=S_V[i,it]+E_V[i,it]+I_V[i,it];
}
}
```

- The ODE solutions at $r = r_l = 0, r = r_u = 1$ and $t = 0$, 250 are displayed numerically.

```
#
# Display numerical solution
  for(it in 1:nout){
    if((it-1)*(it-nout)==0){
    for(i in 1:nr){
      if((i-1)*(i-nr)==0){
      cat(sprintf("\n"));
      cat(sprintf(
        "\n              t              r"));
      cat(sprintf(
        "\n %10.0f %10.0f",tout[it],r[i]));
      cat(sprintf(
        "\n        S_B(t)        E_B(t)"));
      cat(sprintf(
        "\n        A_B(t)        I_B(t)"));
      cat(sprintf(
        "\n       I_BM(t)        R_B(t)"));
      cat(sprintf(
        "\n        S_W(t)        E_W(t)"));
      cat(sprintf(
        "\n        A_W(t)        I_W(t)"));
      cat(sprintf(
        "\n       I_WM(t)        R_W(t)"));
      cat(sprintf(
        "\n        S_V(t)        E_V(t)"));
      cat(sprintf(
        "\n        I_V(t)        N_B(t)"));
      cat(sprintf(
        "\n        N_W(t)        N_V(t)"));
      cat(sprintf("\n
        %10.0f %10.0f",S_B[i,it],E_B[i,it]));
      cat(sprintf("\n
        %10.0f %10.0f",A_B[i,it],I_B[i,it]));
      cat(sprintf("\n
```

```
            %10.0f %10.0f",I_BM[i,it],R_B[i,it]));
        cat(sprintf("\n
            %10.0f %10.0f",S_W[i,it],E_W[i,it]));
        cat(sprintf("\n
            %10.0f %10.0f",A_W[i,it],I_W[i,it]));
        cat(sprintf("\n
            %10.0f %10.0f",I_WM[i,it],R_W[i,it]));
        cat(sprintf("\n
            %10.0f %10.0f",S_V[i,it],E_V[i,it]));
        cat(sprintf("\n
            %10.0f %10.0f",I_V[i,it],N_B[i,it]));
        cat(sprintf("\n
            %10.0f %10.0f",N_W[i,it],N_V[i,it]));
        }
    }
    }
    }
```

- The number of calls to pde1a is displayed at the end of the solution.

```
#
# Calls to ODE routine
    cat(sprintf("\n\n ncall = %5d\n\n",ncall));
```

- The 15 PDE solutions and 3 population sums are plotted with matplot (a total of 18 plots).

```
#
# Plot PDE solutions
#
# S_B
    par(mfrow=c(1,1));
    matplot(r,S_B,type="l",xlab="r",
        ylab="S_B(r,t)",lty=1,main="",
        lwd=2,col="black");
```

```
#
# N_V
  par(mfrow=c(1,1));
  matplot(r,N_V,type="l",xlab="r",
    ylab="N_V(r,t)",lty=1,main="",
    lwd=2,col="black");
```

This completes the discussion of the main program of Listing 6.3. pde1a called by the main program is listed next.

(6.3.2) ODE/MOL routine

The ODE/MOL routine for eqs. (6.3), (6.4), (6.5) follows.

```
pde1a=function(t,u,parms){
#
# Function pde1a computes the t derivative
# vectors of S_B(t) to I_V(t)
#
# One vector to fifteen vectors
  S_B=rep(0,nr);  E_B=rep(0,nr);A_B=rep(0,nr);
  I_B=rep(0,nr);I_BM=rep(0,nr);R_B=rep(0,nr);
  S_W=rep(0,nr);  E_W=rep(0,nr);A_W=rep(0,nr);
  I_W=rep(0,nr);I_WM=rep(0,nr);R_W=rep(0,nr);
  S_V=rep(0,nr);  E_V=rep(0,nr);I_V=rep(0,nr);
  for (i in 1:nr){
    S_B[i]=u[i];
    E_B[i]=u[i+nr];
    A_B[i]=u[i+2*nr];
    I_B[i]=u[i+3*nr];
   I_BM[i]=u[i+4*nr];
    R_B[i]=u[i+5*nr];
```

```
      S_W[i]=u[i+6*nr];
      E_W[i]=u[i+7*nr];
      A_W[i]=u[i+8*nr];
      I_W[i]=u[i+9*nr];
     I_WM[i]=u[i+10*nr];
      R_W[i]=u[i+11*nr];
      S_V[i]=u[i+12*nr];
      E_V[i]=u[i+13*nr];
      I_V[i]=u[i+14*nr];
    }
#
# Algebra
  N_B=rep(0,nr);N_W=rep(0,nr);N_V=rep(0,nr);
  lambda_W=rep(0,nr);
  lambda_B=rep(0,nr);
  lambda_V=rep(0,nr);
  for (i in 1:nr){
    N_B[i]=S_B[i]+E_B[i]+A_B[i]+I_B[i]+
           I_BM[i]+R_B[i];
    N_W[i]=S_W[i]+E_W[i]+A_W[i]+I_W[i]+
           I_WM[i]+R_W[i];
    N_V[i]=S_V[i]+E_V[i]+I_V[i];
    lambda_W[i]=beta_W*b_V*I_V[i]/
                N_W[i];
    lambda_B[i]=eta*beta_B*b_V*I_V[i]/
                N_B[i];
    lambda_V[i]=beta_V*b_V*(I_W[i]+
      rho_W*A_W[i]+eta*(I_B[i]+
      rho_B*A_B[i]))/(N_W[i]+
      eta*N_B[i]);
    }
#
# First derivatives
  S_Br=dss004(rl,ru,nr,S_B);
```

```
  E_Br=dss004(rl,ru,nr,E_B);
  A_Br=dss004(rl,ru,nr,A_B);
  I_Br=dss004(rl,ru,nr,I_B);
 I_BMr=dss004(rl,ru,nr,I_BM);
  R_Br=dss004(rl,ru,nr,R_B);
  S_Wr=dss004(rl,ru,nr,S_W);
  E_Wr=dss004(rl,ru,nr,E_W);
  A_Wr=dss004(rl,ru,nr,A_W);
  I_Wr=dss004(rl,ru,nr,I_W);
 I_WMr=dss004(rl,ru,nr,I_WM);
  R_Wr=dss004(rl,ru,nr,R_W);
  S_Vr=dss004(rl,ru,nr,S_V);
  E_Vr=dss004(rl,ru,nr,E_V);
  I_Vr=dss004(rl,ru,nr,I_V);
#
# BCs
  S_Br[1]=0;S_Br[nr]=0;
  E_Br[1]=0;E_Br[nr]=0;
  A_Br[1]=0;A_Br[nr]=0;
  I_Br[1]=0;I_Br[nr]=0;
 I_BMr[1]=0;I_BMr[nr]=0;
  R_Br[1]=0;R_Br[nr]=0;
  S_Wr[1]=0;S_Wr[nr]=0;
  E_Wr[1]=0;E_Wr[nr]=0;
  A_Wr[1]=0;A_Wr[nr]=0;
  I_Wr[1]=0;I_Wr[nr]=0;
 I_WMr[1]=0;I_WMr[nr]=0;
  R_Wr[1]=0;R_Wr[nr]=0;
  S_Vr[1]=0;S_Vr[nr]=0;
  E_Vr[1]=0;E_Vr[nr]=0;
  I_Vr[1]=0;I_Vr[nr]=0;
#
# Second derivatives
  nl=2;nu=2;
```

```
  S_Brr=dss044(rl,ru,nr,S_B,S_Br,nl,nu);
  E_Brr=dss044(rl,ru,nr,E_B,E_Br,nl,nu);
  A_Brr=dss044(rl,ru,nr,A_B,A_Br,nl,nu);
  I_Brr=dss044(rl,ru,nr,I_B,I_Br,nl,nu);
 I_BMrr=dss044(rl,ru,nr,I_BM,I_BMr,nl,nu);
  R_Brr=dss044(rl,ru,nr,R_B,R_Br,nl,nu);
  S_Wrr=dss044(rl,ru,nr,S_W,S_Wr,nl,nu);
  E_Wrr=dss044(rl,ru,nr,E_W,E_Wr,nl,nu);
  A_Wrr=dss044(rl,ru,nr,A_W,A_Wr,nl,nu);
  I_Wrr=dss044(rl,ru,nr,I_W,I_Wr,nl,nu);
 I_WMrr=dss044(rl,ru,nr,I_WM,I_WMr,nl,nu);
  R_Wrr=dss044(rl,ru,nr,R_W,R_Wr,nl,nu);
  S_Vrr=dss044(rl,ru,nr,S_V,S_Vr,nl,nu);
  E_Vrr=dss044(rl,ru,nr,E_V,E_Vr,nl,nu);
  I_Vrr=dss044(rl,ru,nr,I_V,I_Vr,nl,nu);
#
# Product functions
  E_BI_V=rep(0,nr);
  E_WI_V=rep(0,nr);
  for(i in 1:nr){
    E_BI_V[i]=E_B[i]*I_V[i];
    E_WI_V[i]=E_W[i]*I_V[i]
  }
#
# First derivatives
  E_BI_Vr=dss004(rl,ru,nr,E_BI_V);
  E_WI_Vr=dss004(rl,ru,nr,E_WI_V);
#
# BCs
  E_BI_Vr[1]=0;E_BI_Vr[nr]=0;
  E_WI_Vr[1]=0;E_WI_Vr[nr]=0;
#
# Second derivatives
  nl=2;nu=2;
```

```
  E_BI_Vrr=
    dss044(rl,ru,nr,E_BI_V,E_BI_Vr,nl,nu);
  E_WI_Vrr=
    dss044(rl,ru,nr,E_WI_V,E_WI_Vr,nl,nu);
#
# PDEs
  S_Bt=rep(0,nr); E_Bt=rep(0,nr);
  A_Bt=rep(0,nr); I_Bt=rep(0,nr);
 I_BMt=rep(0,nr); R_Bt=rep(0,nr);
  S_Wt=rep(0,nr); E_Wt=rep(0,nr);
  A_Wt=rep(0,nr); I_Wt=rep(0,nr);
 I_WMt=rep(0,nr); R_Wt=rep(0,nr);
  S_Vt=rep(0,nr); E_Vt=rep(0,nr);
  I_Vt=rep(0,nr);
  for(i in 1:nr){
#
# r=0
    if(i==1){
    S_Bt[i]=pi_B-q_A*pi_B*A_W[i]-
      q_I*pi_B*I_W[i]-q_R*pi_B*R_W[i]-
      lambda_B[i]*S_B[i]-(alpha+mu_B)*
      S_B[i]+DS_B*2*S_Brr[i];
    E_Bt[i]=lambda_B[i]*S_B[i]-(alpha+
      sigma_B+mu_B)*E_B[i]+DE_B*2*
      E_Brr[i]+DE_BI_V*2*E_BI_Vrr[i];
    A_Bt[i]=q_A*pi_B*A_W[i]+(1-p)*
      sigma_B*E_B[i]-(alpha+gamma_B+
      mu_B)*A_B[i]+
      DA_B*2*A_Brr[i];
    I_Bt[i]=q_I*pi_B*I_W[i]+p*sigma_B*
      E_B[i]-(alpha+gamma_B+mu_B)*
      I_B[i]+DI_B*2*I_Brr[i];
   I_BMt[i]=rg*q_R*pi_B*R_W[i]-
      (alpha+mu_B)*I_BM[i]+DI_BM*
```

```
      2*I_BMrr[i];
    R_Bt[i]=(1-rg)*q_R*pi_B*R_W[i]+
      gamma_B*A_B[i]+gamma_B*I_B[i]-
      (alpha+mu_B)*R_B[i]+DR_B*
      2*R_Brr[i];
   S_Wt[i]=alpha*S_B[i]-lambda_W[i]*
      S_W[i]-mu_W*S_W[i]+DS_W*2*S_Wrr[i];
   E_Wt[i]=lambda_W[i]*S_W[i]-(sigma_W+
      mu_W)*E_W[i]+DE_W*2*E_Wrr[i]+
      DE_WI_V*2*E_WI_Vrr[i];
   A_Wt[i]=(1-p)*sigma_W*E_W[i]-
      (gamma_W+mu_W)*A_W[i]+DA_W*
      2*A_Wrr[i];
   I_Wt[i]=p*sigma_W*E_W[i]-(gamma_W+
      mu_W)*I_W[i]+DI_W*2*I_Wrr[i];
 I_WMt[i]=alpha*I_BM[i]-mu_W*I_WM[i]+
      DI_WM*2*I_WMrr[i];
   R_Wt[i]=alpha*R_B[i]+gamma_W*A_W[i]+
      gamma_W*I_W[i]-mu_W*R_W[i]+
      DR_W*2*R_Wrr[i];
   S_Vt[i]=pi_V-lambda_V[i]*S_V[i]-
      mu_V*S_V[i]+DS_V*2*S_Vrr[i];
   E_Vt[i]=lambda_V[i]*S_V[i]-
      (mu_V+sigma_V)*E_V[i]+
      DE_V*2*E_Vrr[i];
   I_Vt[i]=sigma_V*E_V[i]-
      mu_V*I_V[i]+
      DI_V*2*I_Vrr[i]+DE_BI_V*
      2*E_BI_Vrr[i]+DE_WI_V*
      2*E_WI_Vrr[i];
   }
#
# r > 0
   if(i>1){
```

```
    ri=1/r[i];
S_Bt[i]=pi_B-q_A*pi_B*A_W[i]-
    q_I*pi_B*I_W[i]-q_R*pi_B*R_W[i]-
    lambda_B[i]*S_B[i]-(alpha+mu_B)*
    S_B[i]+DS_B*(S_Brr[i]+ri*S_Br[i]);
E_Bt[i]=lambda_B[i]*S_B[i]-(alpha+
    sigma_B+mu_B)*E_B[i]+DE_B*
    (E_Brr[i]+ri*E_Br[i])+
    DE_BI_V*(E_BI_Vrr[i]+
    ri*E_BI_Vr[i]);
A_Bt[i]=q_A*pi_B*A_W[i]+(1-p)*
    sigma_B*E_B[i]-(alpha+gamma_B+
    mu_B)*A_B[i]+DA_B*(A_Brr[i]+
    ri*A_Br[i]);
I_Bt[i]=q_I*pi_B*I_W[i]+p*sigma_B*
    E_B[i]-(alpha+gamma_B+mu_B)*
    I_B[i]+DI_B*(I_Brr[i]+ri*I_Br[i]);
I_BMt[i]=rg*q_R*pi_B*R_W[i]-(alpha+
    mu_B)*I_BM[i]+DI_BM*(I_BMrr[i]+
    ri*I_BMr[i]);
R_Bt[i]=(1-rg)*q_R*pi_B*R_W[i]+
    gamma_B*A_B[i]+gamma_B*I_B[i]-
    (alpha+mu_B)*R_B[i]+DR_B*
    (R_Brr[i]+ri*R_Br[i]);
S_Wt[i]=alpha*S_B[i]-lambda_W[i]*
    S_W[i]-mu_W*S_W[i]+DS_W*(S_Wrr[i]+
    ri*S_Wr[i]);
E_Wt[i]=lambda_W[i]*S_W[i]-(sigma_W+
    mu_W)*E_W[i]+DE_W*(E_Wrr[i]+
    ri*E_Wr[i])+DE_WI_V*(E_WI_Vrr[i]+
    ri*E_WI_Vr[i]);
A_Wt[i]=(1-p)*sigma_W*E_W[i]-
    (gamma_W+mu_W)*A_W[i]+DA_W*
    (A_Wrr[i]+ri*A_Wr[i]);
```

```
      I_Wt[i]=p*sigma_W*E_W[i]-
         (gamma_W+mu_W)*I_W[i]+
         DI_W*(I_Wrr[i]+ri*I_Wr[i]);
    I_WMt[i]=alpha*I_BM[i]-mu_W*I_WM[i]+
         DI_WM*(I_WMrr[i]+ri*I_WMr[i]);
    R_Wt[i]=alpha*R_B[i]+gamma_W*A_W[i]+
         gamma_W*I_W[i]-mu_W*R_W[i]+
         DR_W*(R_Wrr[i]+ri*R_Wr[i]);
    S_Vt[i]=pi_V-lambda_V[i]*S_V[i]-
         mu_V*S_V[i]+DS_V*(S_Vrr[i]+
         ri*S_Vr[i]);
    E_Vt[i]=lambda_V[i]*S_V[i]-
         (mu_V+sigma_V)*E_V[i]+
         DE_V*(E_Vrr[i]+ri*E_Vr[i]);
    I_Vt[i]=sigma_V*E_V[i]-mu_V*
         I_V[i]+DI_V*(I_Vrr[i]+ri*
         I_Vr[i])+DE_BI_V*(E_BI_Vrr[i]+
         ri*E_BI_Vr[i])+DE_WI_V*
         (E_WI_Vrr[i]+ri*E_WI_Vr[i]);
    }
  }
#
# Fifteen vectors to one vector
  ut=rep(0,15*nr);
  for (i in 1:nr){
    ut[i]      =S_Bt[i];
    ut[i+nr]   =E_Bt[i];
    ut[i+2*nr]=A_Bt[i];
    ut[i+3*nr]=I_Bt[i];
    ut[i+4*nr]=I_BMt[i];
    ut[i+5*nr]=R_Bt[i];
    ut[i+6*nr]=S_Wt[i];
    ut[i+7*nr]=E_Wt[i];
    ut[i+8*nr]=A_Wt[i];
```

```
  ut[i+9*nr]=I_Wt[i];
  ut[i+10*nr]=I_WMt[i];
  ut[i+11*nr]=R_Wt[i];
  ut[i+12*nr]=S_Vt[i];
  ut[i+13*nr]=E_Vt[i];
  ut[i+14*nr]=I_Vt[i];
  }
#
# Increment calls to pde1a
  ncall <<- ncall+1;
#
# Return derivative vector
  return(list(c(ut)));
  }
```

Listing 6.4: ODE/MOL program for eqs. (6.3), (6.4), (6.5)

We can note the following details about Listing 6.4.

- The function is defined. u is the 315-vector of MOL/ODE dependent variables for eqs. (6.3-1) to (6.3-15). t is the current value of t. parm to pass parameters to pde1a is unused, but is required.

```
  pde1a=function(t,u,parms){
#
# Function pde1a computes the t derivative
# vectors of S_B(t) to I_V(t)
```

- u is placed in 15 21-vectors to facilitate the MOL programming of eqs. (6.3-1) to (6.3-15).

```
#
# One vector to fifteen vectors
  S_B=rep(0,nr); E_B=rep(0,nr);A_B=rep(0,nr);
  I_B=rep(0,nr);I_BM=rep(0,nr);R_B=rep(0,nr);
  S_W=rep(0,nr); E_W=rep(0,nr);A_W=rep(0,nr);
```

```
        I_W=rep(0,nr);I_WM=rep(0,nr);R_W=rep(0,nr);
        S_V=rep(0,nr); E_V=rep(0,nr);I_V=rep(0,nr);
        for (i in 1:nr){
          S_B[i]=u[i];
          E_B[i]=u[i+nr];
          A_B[i]=u[i+2*nr];
          I_B[i]=u[i+3*nr];
         I_BM[i]=u[i+4*nr];
          R_B[i]=u[i+5*nr];
          S_W[i]=u[i+6*nr];
          E_W[i]=u[i+7*nr];
          A_W[i]=u[i+8*nr];
          I_W[i]=u[i+9*nr];
         I_WM[i]=u[i+10*nr];
          R_W[i]=u[i+11*nr];
          S_V[i]=u[i+12*nr];
          E_V[i]=u[i+13*nr];
          I_V[i]=u[i+14*nr];
        }
```

- The algebra of eqs. (6.1-16) to (6.1-21) is programmed.

```
#
# Algebra
N_B=rep(0,nr);N_W=rep(0,nr);N_V=rep(0,nr);
lambda_W=rep(0,nr);
lambda_B=rep(0,nr);
lambda_V=rep(0,nr);
for (i in 1:nr){
  N_B[i]=S_B[i]+E_B[i]+A_B[i]+I_B[i]+
          I_BM[i]+R_B[i];
  N_W[i]=S_W[i]+E_W[i]+A_W[i]+I_W[i]+
          I_WM[i]+R_W[i];
  N_V[i]=S_V[i]+E_V[i]+I_V[i];
  lambda_W[i]=beta_W*b_V*I_V[i]/
```

```
                N_W[i];
       lambda_B[i]=eta*beta_B*b_V*I_V[i]/
                N_B[i];
       lambda_V[i]=beta_V*b_V*(I_W[i]+
         rho_W*A_W[i]+eta*(I_B[i]+
         rho_B*A_B[i]))/(N_W[i]+
         eta*N_B[i]);
     }
```

- The first derivatives in r are computed with dss004, for example, $\dfrac{\partial S_B(r,t)}{\partial r} = $ S_Br.

```
#
# First derivatives
  S_Br=dss004(rl,ru,nr,S_B);
  E_Br=dss004(rl,ru,nr,E_B);
  A_Br=dss004(rl,ru,nr,A_B);
  I_Br=dss004(rl,ru,nr,I_B);
 I_BMr=dss004(rl,ru,nr,I_BM);
  R_Br=dss004(rl,ru,nr,R_B);
  S_Wr=dss004(rl,ru,nr,S_W);
  E_Wr=dss004(rl,ru,nr,E_W);
  A_Wr=dss004(rl,ru,nr,A_W);
  I_Wr=dss004(rl,ru,nr,I_W);
 I_WMr=dss004(rl,ru,nr,I_WM);
  R_Wr=dss004(rl,ru,nr,R_W);
  S_Vr=dss004(rl,ru,nr,S_V);
  E_Vr=dss004(rl,ru,nr,E_V);
  I_Vr=dss004(rl,ru,nr,I_V);
```

- Homogeneous Neumann BCs (6.5-1) to (6.5-15) are implemented.

```
#
# BCs
```

```
   S_Br[1]=0;S_Br[nr]=0;
   E_Br[1]=0;E_Br[nr]=0;
   A_Br[1]=0;A_Br[nr]=0;
   I_Br[1]=0;I_Br[nr]=0;
  I_BMr[1]=0;I_BMr[nr]=0;
   R_Br[1]=0;R_Br[nr]=0;
   S_Wr[1]=0;S_Wr[nr]=0;
   E_Wr[1]=0;E_Wr[nr]=0;
   A_Wr[1]=0;A_Wr[nr]=0;
   I_Wr[1]=0;I_Wr[nr]=0;
  I_WMr[1]=0;I_WMr[nr]=0;
   R_Wr[1]=0;R_Wr[nr]=0;
   S_Vr[1]=0;S_Vr[nr]=0;
   E_Vr[1]=0;E_Vr[nr]=0;
   I_Vr[1]=0;I_Vr[nr]=0;
```

Subscripts 1,nr correspond to $r = r_l = 0, r = r_u = 1$.

- The second derivatives in r are computed with dss044, for example, $\dfrac{\partial^2 S_B(r,t)}{\partial r^2} = $ S_Brr.

```
#
# Second derivatives
  nl=2;nu=2;
  S_Brr=dss044(rl,ru,nr,S_B,S_Br,nl,nu);
  E_Brr=dss044(rl,ru,nr,E_B,E_Br,nl,nu);
  A_Brr=dss044(rl,ru,nr,A_B,A_Br,nl,nu);
  I_Brr=dss044(rl,ru,nr,I_B,I_Br,nl,nu);
 I_BMrr=dss044(rl,ru,nr,I_BM,I_BMr,nl,nu);
  R_Brr=dss044(rl,ru,nr,R_B,R_Br,nl,nu);
  S_Wrr=dss044(rl,ru,nr,S_W,S_Wr,nl,nu);
  E_Wrr=dss044(rl,ru,nr,E_W,E_Wr,nl,nu);
  A_Wrr=dss044(rl,ru,nr,A_W,A_Wr,nl,nu);
  I_Wrr=dss044(rl,ru,nr,I_W,I_Wr,nl,nu);
 I_WMrr=dss044(rl,ru,nr,I_WM,I_WMr,nl,nu);
```

```
R_Wrr=dss044(rl,ru,nr,R_W,R_Wr,nl,nu);
S_Vrr=dss044(rl,ru,nr,S_V,S_Vr,nl,nu);
E_Vrr=dss044(rl,ru,nr,E_V,E_Vr,nl,nu);
I_Vrr=dss044(rl,ru,nr,I_V,I_Vr,nl,nu);
```

- The product functions used in the cross derivatives, $E_B(r,t)I_V(r,t), E_W(r,t)I_V(r,t)$, are computed.

```
#
# Product functions
  E_BI_V=rep(0,nr);
  E_WI_V=rep(0,nr);
  for(i in 1:nr){
    E_BI_V[i]=E_B[i]*I_V[i];
    E_WI_V[i]=E_W[i]*I_V[i]
  }
```

- The first derivatives of the product functions are computed, for example, $\dfrac{\partial E_B I_V}{\partial r} = \text{E\_BI\_Vr}$.

```
#
# First derivatives
  E_BI_Vr=dss004(rl,ru,nr,E_BI_V);
  E_WI_Vr=dss004(rl,ru,nr,E_WI_V);
```

- The BCs for the product functions are computed, for example, $\dfrac{\partial E_B I_V(r=r_l,t)}{\partial r} = \text{E\_BI\_Vr[1]} = 0$.

```
#
# BCs
  E_BI_Vr[1]=0;E_BI_Vr[nr]=0;
  E_WI_Vr[1]=0;E_WI_Vr[nr]=0;
```

- The second derivatives of the product functions are computed, for example, $\dfrac{\partial^2 E_B I_V}{\partial r^2} = \text{E\_BI\_Vrr}$.

```
#
# Second derivatives
  nl=2;nu=2;
  E_BI_Vrr=
    dss044(rl,ru,nr,E_BI_V,E_BI_Vr,nl,nu);
  E_WI_Vrr=
    dss044(rl,ru,nr,E_WI_V,E_WI_Vr,nl,nu);
```

nl=2;nu=2; specifies (homogeneous) Neumann BCs.

- Eqs. (6.3-1) to (6.3-15) are programmed, starting with the declaration of the derivatives in t, for example $\dfrac{\partial S_B}{\partial t}$ = S_Bt

```
#
# PDEs
  S_Bt=rep(0,nr); E_Bt=rep(0,nr);
  A_Bt=rep(0,nr); I_Bt=rep(0,nr);
 I_BMt=rep(0,nr); R_Bt=rep(0,nr);
  S_Wt=rep(0,nr); E_Wt=rep(0,nr);
  A_Wt=rep(0,nr); I_Wt=rep(0,nr);
 I_WMt=rep(0,nr); R_Wt=rep(0,nr);
  S_Vt=rep(0,nr); E_Vt=rep(0,nr);
  I_Vt=rep(0,nr);
  for(i in 1:nr){
```

- Eqs. (6.3-1) to (6.3-15) are programmed at $r = 0$. For example, eq. (6.3-1) is programmed as

```
S_Bt[i]=pi_B-q_A*pi_B*A_W[i]-
q_I*pi_B*I_W[i]-q_R*pi_B*R_W[i]-
lambda_B[i]*S_B[i]-(alpha+mu_B)*
S_B[i]+DS_B*(S_Brr[i]+ri*S_Br[i]);
```

with $DS_B \left(\dfrac{\partial^2 S_B}{\partial r^2} + \dfrac{1}{r} \dfrac{\partial S_B}{\partial r} \right) = DS_B 2 \dfrac{\partial^2 S_B}{\partial r^2}$ is programmed as DS_B*2*S_Brr[i].

The cross diffusion term in eq. (6.3-2),

$$DE_BI_V\left(\frac{\partial^2 E_BI_V}{\partial r^2} + \frac{1}{r}\frac{\partial E_BI_V}{\partial r}\right) = DE_BI_V2\frac{\partial^2 E_VI_V}{\partial r^2}$$

is programmed as DE_BI_V*2*E_BI_Vrr[i] (in the eq. for
E_Bt[i]).

```
#
# r=0
    if(i==1){
    S_Bt[i]=pi_B-q_A*pi_B*A_W[i]-
      q_I*pi_B*I_W[i]-q_R*pi_B*R_W[i]-
      lambda_B[i]*S_B[i]-(alpha+mu_B)*
      S_B[i]+DS_B*2*S_Brr[i];
    E_Bt[i]=lambda_B[i]*S_B[i]-(alpha+
      sigma_B+mu_B)*E_B[i]+DE_B*2*
      E_Brr[i]+DE_BI_V*2*E_BI_Vrr[i];
    A_Bt[i]=q_A*pi_B*A_W[i]+(1-p)*
      sigma_B*E_B[i]-(alpha+gamma_B+
      mu_B)*A_B[i]+
      DA_B*2*A_Brr[i];
    I_Bt[i]=q_I*pi_B*I_W[i]+p*sigma_B*
      E_B[i]-(alpha+gamma_B+mu_B)*
      I_B[i]+DI_B*2*I_Brr[i];
    I_BMt[i]=rg*q_R*pi_B*R_W[i]-
      (alpha+mu_B)*I_BM[i]+DI_BM*
      2*I_BMrr[i];
    R_Bt[i]=(1-rg)*q_R*pi_B*R_W[i]+
      gamma_B*A_B[i]+gamma_B*I_B[i]-
      (alpha+mu_B)*R_B[i]+DR_B*
      2*R_Brr[i];
    S_Wt[i]=alpha*S_B[i]-lambda_W[i]*
      S_W[i]-mu_W*S_W[i]+DS_W*2*S_Wrr[i];
```

```
E_Wt[i]=lambda_W[i]*S_W[i]-(sigma_W+
   mu_W)*E_W[i]+DE_W*2*E_Wrr[i]+
   DE_WI_V*2*E_WI_Vrr[i];
A_Wt[i]=(1-p)*sigma_W*E_W[i]-
   (gamma_W+mu_W)*A_W[i]+DA_W*
   2*A_Wrr[i];
I_Wt[i]=p*sigma_W*E_W[i]-(gamma_W+
   mu_W)*I_W[i]+DI_W*2*I_Wrr[i];
I_WMt[i]=alpha*I_BM[i]-mu_W*I_WM[i]+
   DI_WM*2*I_WMrr[i];
R_Wt[i]=alpha*R_B[i]+gamma_W*A_W[i]+
   gamma_W*I_W[i]-mu_W*R_W[i]+
   DR_W*2*R_Wrr[i];
S_Vt[i]=pi_V-lambda_V[i]*S_V[i]-
   mu_V*S_V[i]+DS_V*2*S_Vrr[i];
E_Vt[i]=lambda_V[i]*S_V[i]-
   (mu_V+sigma_V)*E_V[i]+
   DE_V*2*E_Vrr[i];
I_Vt[i]=sigma_V*E_V[i]-
   mu_V*I_V[i]+
   DI_V*2*I_Vrr[i]+DE_BI_V*
   2*E_BI_Vrr[i]+DE_WI_V*
   2*E_WI_Vrr[i];
}
```

The final } concludes the programming for i=1 with the
programming of 15 sets of ODEs, each set with 21 ODEs,
for $r = 0$.

- Eqs. (6.3-1) to (6.3-15) are programmed at $r > 0$. For
  example, eq. (6.3-1) is programmed as

```
S_Bt[i]=pi_B-q_A*pi_B*A_W[i]-
   q_I*pi_B*I_W[i]-q_R*pi_B*R_W[i]-
   lambda_B[i]*S_B[i]-(alpha+mu_B)*
   S_B[i]+DS_B*(S_Brr[i]+ri*S_Br[i]);
```

with $DS_B \left(\dfrac{\partial^2 S_B}{\partial r^2} + \dfrac{1}{r}\dfrac{\partial S_B}{\partial r} \right)$ = DS_B*(S_Brr[i]+ri*S_Br[i]) (with ri=1/r[i]).

The cross diffusion term in eq. (6.3-2),

$$DE_B I_V \left(\frac{\partial^2 E_B I_V}{\partial r^2} + \frac{1}{r}\frac{\partial E_B I_V}{\partial r} \right)$$

is programmed as DE_B*(E_Brr[i]+ri*E_Br[i]) (in the eq. for E_Bt[i]).

```
#
# r > 0
    if(i>1){
    ri=1/r[i];
    S_Bt[i]=pi_B-q_A*pi_B*A_W[i]-
        q_I*pi_B*I_W[i]-q_R*pi_B*R_W[i]-
        lambda_B[i]*S_B[i]-(alpha+mu_B)*
        S_B[i]+DS_B*(S_Brr[i]+ri*S_Br[i]);
    E_Bt[i]=lambda_B[i]*S_B[i]-(alpha+
        sigma_B+mu_B)*E_B[i]+DE_B*
        (E_Brr[i]+ri*E_Br[i])+
        DE_BI_V*(E_BI_Vrr[i]+
        ri*E_BI_Vr[i]);
    A_Bt[i]=q_A*pi_B*A_W[i]+(1-p)*
        sigma_B*E_B[i]-(alpha+gamma_B+
        mu_B)*A_B[i]+DA_B*(A_Brr[i]+
        ri*A_Br[i]);
    I_Bt[i]=q_I*pi_B*I_W[i]+p*sigma_B*
        E_B[i]-(alpha+gamma_B+mu_B)*
        I_B[i]+DI_B*(I_Brr[i]+ri*I_Br[i]);
    I_BMt[i]=rg*q_R*pi_B*R_W[i]-(alpha+
        mu_B)*I_BM[i]+DI_BM*(I_BMrr[i]+
        ri*I_BMr[i]);
    R_Bt[i]=(1-rg)*q_R*pi_B*R_W[i]+
        gamma_B*A_B[i]+gamma_B*I_B[i]-
```

```
        (alpha+mu_B)*R_B[i]+DR_B*
        (R_Brr[i]+ri*R_Br[i]);
    S_Wt[i]=alpha*S_B[i]-lambda_W[i]*
        S_W[i]-mu_W*S_W[i]+DS_W*(S_Wrr[i]+
        ri*S_Wr[i]);
    E_Wt[i]=lambda_W[i]*S_W[i]-(sigma_W+
        mu_W)*E_W[i]+DE_W*(E_Wrr[i]+
        ri*E_Wr[i])+DE_WI_V*(E_WI_Vrr[i]+
        ri*E_WI_Vr[i]);
    A_Wt[i]=(1-p)*sigma_W*E_W[i]-
        (gamma_W+mu_W)*A_W[i]+DA_W*
        (A_Wrr[i]+ri*A_Wr[i]);
    I_Wt[i]=p*sigma_W*E_W[i]-
        (gamma_W+mu_W)*I_W[i]+
        DI_W*(I_Wrr[i]+ri*I_Wr[i]);
I_WMt[i]=alpha*I_BM[i]-mu_W*I_WM[i]+
        DI_WM*(I_WMrr[i]+ri*I_WMr[i]);
    R_Wt[i]=alpha*R_B[i]+gamma_W*A_W[i]+
        gamma_W*I_W[i]-mu_W*R_W[i]+
        DR_W*(R_Wrr[i]+ri*R_Wr[i]);
    S_Vt[i]=pi_V-lambda_V[i]*S_V[i]-
        mu_V*S_V[i]+DS_V*(S_Vrr[i]+
        ri*S_Vr[i]);
    E_Vt[i]=lambda_V[i]*S_V[i]-
        (mu_V+sigma_V)*E_V[i]+
        DE_V*(E_Vrr[i]+ri*E_Vr[i]);
    I_Vt[i]=sigma_V*E_V[i]-mu_V*
        I_V[i]+DI_V*(I_Vrr[i]+ri*
        I_Vr[i])+DE_BI_V*(E_BI_Vrr[i]+
        ri*E_BI_Vr[i])+DE_WI_V*
        (E_WI_Vrr[i]+ri*E_WI_Vr[i]);
    }
}
```

The first } concludes the programming for i>1 with the programming of 15 sets of ODEs, each set with 21 ODEs, for $r > 0$. The second } concludes the programming of the for with index i for $r_l \leq r \leq r_u$.

- The 15 ODE vectors are placed in a single 315-vector, ut, for return to lsodes.

```
#
# Fifteen vectors to one vector
  ut=rep(0,15*nr);
  for (i in 1:nr){
    ut[i]      =S_Bt[i];
    ut[i+nr]   =E_Bt[i];
    ut[i+2*nr]=A_Bt[i];
    ut[i+3*nr]=I_Bt[i];
    ut[i+4*nr]=I_BMt[i];
    ut[i+5*nr]=R_Bt[i];
    ut[i+6*nr]=S_Wt[i];
    ut[i+7*nr]=E_Wt[i];
    ut[i+8*nr]=A_Wt[i];
    ut[i+9*nr]=I_Wt[i];
    ut[i+10*nr]=I_WMt[i];
    ut[i+11*nr]=R_Wt[i];
    ut[i+12*nr]=S_Vt[i];
    ut[i+13*nr]=E_Vt[i];
    ut[i+14*nr]=I_Vt[i];
  }
```

- The counter for the calls to pde1a is incremented and returned to the main program of Listing 6.3 with <<-.

```
#
# Increment calls to pde1a
  ncall <<- ncall+1;
```

- The derivative vector ut is returned to lsodes as a list. c is the R vector utility.

```
    #
    # Return derivative vector
    return(list(c(ut)));
    }
```

This concludes the discussion of the program of eqs. (6.3), (6.4) and (6.5). The output from the routines is considered next.

(6.3.3) Model output

The numerical output from the preceding coding is in Table 6.5.

[1] 6

[1] 316

t	r
0	0
S_B(t)	E_B(t)
A_B(t)	I_B(t)
I_BM(t)	R_B(t)
S_W(t)	E_W(t)
A_W(t)	I_W(t)
I_WM(t)	R_W(t)
S_V(t)	E_V(t)
I_V(t)	N_B(t)
N_W(t)	N_V(t)
5000	200
200	50
20	10
10000	220
400	100
120	200
500	100
100	5480

11040   700

t	r
0	1
S_B(t)	E_B(t)
A_B(t)	I_B(t)
I_BM(t)	R_B(t)
S_W(t)	E_W(t)
A_W(t)	I_W(t)
I_WM(t)	R_W(t)
S_V(t)	E_V(t)
I_V(t)	N_B(t)
N_W(t)	N_V(t)
0	200
200	50
20	10
0	220
400	100
120	200
0	100
100	480
1040	200

t	r
25	0
S_B(t)	E_B(t)
A_B(t)	I_B(t)
I_BM(t)	R_B(t)
S_W(t)	E_W(t)
A_W(t)	I_W(t)
I_WM(t)	R_W(t)
S_V(t)	E_V(t)
I_V(t)	N_B(t)
N_W(t)	N_V(t)

112	139
89	81
21	574
519	224
125	109
120	1049
6288	270
815	1016
2146	7373

t	r
25	1
S_B(t)	E_B(t)
A_B(t)	I_B(t)
I_BM(t)	R_B(t)
S_W(t)	E_W(t)
A_W(t)	I_W(t)
I_WM(t)	R_W(t)
S_V(t)	E_V(t)
I_V(t)	N_B(t)
N_W(t)	N_V(t)
79	129
85	77
21	564
406	211
120	104
120	1038
6249	276
862	955
1999	7388

ncall =   712

Table 6.5: Numerical output for eqs. (6.3), (6.4), (6.5)

We can note the following details about this output.

- The dimensions of the solution matrix out are 6×316 for 6 output points (programmed in Listing 6.3) and $(15)(21) + 1 = 316$ for 15 PDEs approximated with 21 ODEs, and one place at the beginning of each solution vector for t.

```
[1] 6
```

```
[1] 316
```

- The ICs of eqs. (6.4) are confirmed. This check is important since if the ICs are not correct, the subsequent solution will not be correct.
- The output is for $r = 0, 1$, $t = 0, 25$ as programmed in Listing 6.3.
- The 15 PDE numerical solutions appear to be nonnegative.
- The computational effort for a complete solution is modest, ncall = 712.

The graphical output includes 18 plots. A subset follows.

The Gaussian at $t = 0$, $S_B(r, t = 0) = 5000e^{-10r^2}$ programmed in Listing 6.3 identifies the beginning of the solution. The solution curves vary with r through the linear (Fickian) diffusion of eq. (6.3-1).

The infected babies increase from 50, and appear to reach a higher, stable equilibrium.

The infected humans remain at approximately the initial value of 100 (see Table 6.5 at $t = 25$).

The infected mosquito population, $I_V(r, t)$, continues to increase with t, as well as the susceptible and exposed mosquito populations, $S_V(r, t), E_V(r, t)$, so that mosquito control is required.

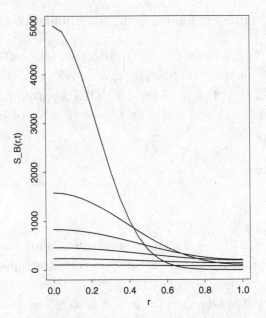

Figure 6.2-1: Numerical solution $S_B(t)$ from eq. (6.3-1)

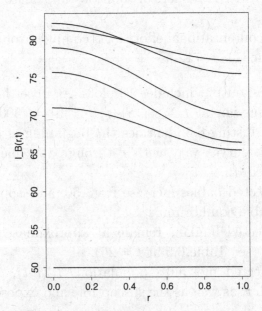

Figure 6.2-4: Numerical solution $I_B(r, t)$ from eq. (6.3-4)

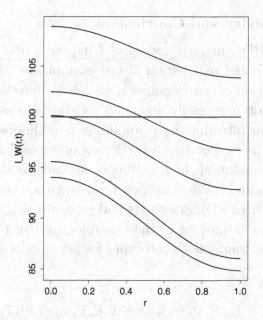

Figure 6.2-10: Numerical solution $I_W(r,t)$ from eq. (6.3-10)

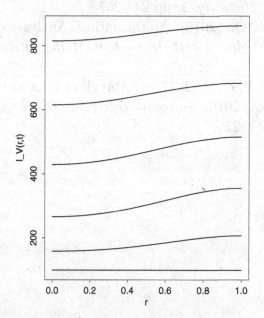

Figure 6.2-15: Numerical solution $I_V(r,t)$ from eq. (6.3-15)

(6.4) Summary and Conclusions

The 7×7 PDE malaria model of Chapter 5 and the 15×15 PDE Zika model of Chapter 6 are examples of the computer implementation of spatiotemporal models for infectious diseases. They are not necessarily intended as state-of-the-art models, but rather, as introductory examples of a methodology that can be applied to a spectrum of 1D spatiotemporal models. The detailed discussion of the R coding is intended to assist readers/analysts/researchers develop new models without having to first study numerical PDEs methods and programming. This can be facilitated by extensions of the examples, and/or the use of the R routines as templates/prototypes for new model development.

References

[1]   Agusto, F.B., S. Bewick and W.F. Fagan (2017), Mathematical model of Zika virus with vertical transmission, *Infectious Disease Modeling*, **2**, pp 244-267

[2]   Oluyo, T.O. (2016), Mathematical Analysis of Zika Epidemic Model, *IOSR Journal of Mathematics*, **12**, no. 6, pp 21-33

[3]   Ryan, S.J., et al (2017), Outbreak of Zika virus infections, Dominica, 2016, *Emerging Infectious Diseases*, **23**, no. 11, pp 1926-1927

Appendix A1: Function dss004

A listing of function dss004 follows.

```
    dss004=function(xl,xu,n,u) {
#
# An extensive set of documentation comments
# detailing the derivation of the following
# fourth order finite differences (FDs) is
# not given here to conserve space. The
# derivation is detailed in Schiesser, W. E.,
# The Numerical Method of Lines Integration
# of Partial Differential Equations, Academic
# Press, San Diego, 1991.
#
# Preallocate arrays
    ux=rep(0,n);
#
# Grid spacing
    dx=(xu-xl)/(n-1);
#
# 1/(12*dx) for subsequent use
    r12dx=1/(12*dx);
#
# ux vector
#
# Boundaries (x=xl,x=xu)
```

```
  ux[1]=r12dx*(-25*u[1]+48*u[  2]-36*u[  3]+
           16*u[  4] -3*u[  5]);
  ux[n]=r12dx*(  25*u[n]-48*u[n-1]+36*u[n-2]-
           16*u[n-3 ] +3*u[n-4]);
#
# dx in from boundaries (x=xl+dx,x=xu-dx)
  ux[  2]=r12dx*(-3*u[1]-10*u[  2]+18*u[  3]-
            6*u[  4]    +u[  5]);
  ux[n-1]=r12dx*(  3*u[n]+10*u[n-1]-18*u[n-2]+
            6*u[n-3]    -u[n-4]);
#
# Interior points (x=xl+2*dx,...,x=xu-2*dx)
  for(i in 3:(n-2)){
    ux[i]=r12dx*(-u[i+2]+8*u[i+1]-
            8*u[i-1]   +u[i-2]);}
#
# All points concluded (x=xl,...,x=xu)
  return(c(ux));
}
```

The input arguments are

xl   lower boundary value of x

xu   upper boundary value of x

n   number of points in the grid in x,
      including the end points

u   dependent variable to be differentiated,
      an n-vector

The output, ux, is an n-vector of numerical values of the first derivative of u.

The finite difference (FD) approximations are a weighted sum of the dependent variable values. For example, at point i

```
#
# Interior points (x=xl+2*dx,...,x=xu-2*dx)
  for(i in 3:(n-2)){
    ux[i]=r12dx*(-u[i+2]+8*u[i+1]-
              8*u[i-1]  +u[i-2]);}
```

The weighting coefficients are -1, 8, 0, -8, 1 at points i-2, i-1, i, i+1, i+2, respectively. These weighting coefficients are antisymmetic (opposite sign) around the center point i because the computed first derivative is of odd order. If the derivative is of even order, the weighting coefficients would be symmetric (same sign) around the center point.

For i=1. the dependent variable at points i=1,2,3,4,5 is used in the FD approximation for ux[1] to remain within the x domain (fictitious points outside the x domain are not used).

```
ux[1]=r12dx*(-25*u[1]+48*u[  2]-36*u[  3]+
             16*u[  4] -3*u[  5]);
```

Similarly, for i=2, points i=1,2,3,4,5 are used in the FD approximation for ux[2] to remain within the x domain (fictitious points outside the x domain are avoided).

```
ux[  2]=r12dx*(-3*u[1]-10*u[  2]+18*u[  3]-
                6*u[  4]  +u[  5]);
```

At the right boundary $x = x_u$, points at i=n,n-1,n-2,n-3,n-4 are used for ux[n],ux[n-1] to avoid points outside the x domain.

In all cases, the FD approximations are fourth order correct in x.

Appendix A2: Function dss044

A listing of function dss044 follows.

```
dss044=function(xl,xu,n,u,ux,nl,nu){
#
# The derivation of the finite difference
# approximations for a second derivative are
# in Schiesser, W. E., The Numerical Method
# of Lines Integration of Partial Differential
# Equations, Academic Press, San Diego, 1991.
#
# Preallocate arrays
  uxx=rep(0,n);
#
# Grid spacing
  dx=(xu-xl)/(n-1);
#
# 1/(12*dx**2) for subsequent use
  r12dxs=1/(12*dx^2);
#
# uxx vector
#
# Boundaries (x=xl,x=xu)
  if(nl==1){
    uxx[1]=r12dxs*
            (45*u[  1]-154*u[  2]+214*u[   3]-
```

```
                156*u[  4] +61*u[  5] -10*u[  6]);}
  if(nu==1){
    uxx[n]=r12dxs*
            (45*u[  n]-154*u[n-1]+214*u[n-2]-
            156*u[n-3] +61*u[n-4] -10*u[n-5]);}
  if(nl==2){
    uxx[1]=r12dxs*
            (-415/6*u[  1] +96*u[  2]-36*u[  3]+
            32/3*u[  4]-3/2*u[  5]-50*ux[1]*dx);}
  if(nu==2){
    uxx[n]=r12dxs*
            (-415/6*u[  n] +96*u[n-1]-36*u[n-2]+
            32/3*u[n-3]-3/2*u[n-4]+50*ux[n]*dx);}
#
# dx in from boundaries (x=xl+dx,x=xu-dx)
    uxx[  2]=r12dxs*
            (10*u[  1]-15*u[  2]-4*u[  3]+
            14*u[  4]- 6*u[  5]  +u[  6]);
    uxx[n-1]=r12dxs*
            (10*u[  n]-15*u[n-1]-4*u[n-2]+
            14*u[n-3]- 6*u[n-4]  +u[n-5]);
#
# Remaining interior points (x=xl+2*dx,...,
# x=xu-2*dx)
  for(i in 3:(n-2)){
    uxx[i]=r12dxs*
            (-u[i-2]+16*u[i-1]-30*u[i]+
            16*u[i+1]    -u[i+2]);}
#
# All points concluded (x=xl,...,x=xu)
  return(c(uxx));
}
```

The input arguments are

xl   lower boundary value of x

xu   upper boundary value of x

n   number of points in the grid in x,
     including the end points

u   dependent variable to be differentiated,
     an n-vector

ux   first derivative of u with boundary
     condition values, an n-vector

nl   type of boundary condition at x=xl
     1: Dirichlet BC
     2: Neumann BC

nu   type of boundary condition at x=xu
     1: Dirichlet BC
     2: Neumann BC

The output, uxx, is an n-vector of numerical values of the second derivative of u.

The finite difference (FD) approximations are a weighted sum of the dependent variable values. For example, at point i

```
for(i in 3:(n-2)){
  uxx[i]=r12dxs*
        (-u[i-2]+16*u[i-1]-30*u[i]+
    16*u[i+1]    -u[i+2]);}
```

The weighting coefficients are -1, 16, -30, 16, -1 at points i-2, i-1, i, i+1, i+2, respectively. These weighting coefficients are symmetric around the center point i because the computed second derivative is of even order. If the derivative is of odd order, the weighting coefficients would be antisymmetric (opposite sign) around the center point.

For nl=2 and/or nu=2 the boundary values of the first derivative are included in the FD approximation for the second derivative, uxx. For example, at x=xl (with nl=2),

```
if(nl==2){
uxx[1]=r12dxs*
        (-415/6*u[  1] +96*u[  2]-36*u[  3]+
         32/3*u[  4]-3/2*u[  5]-50*ux[1]*dx);}
```

In computing the second derivative at the left boundary, uxx[1], the first derivative at the left boundary is included, that is, ux[1]. In this way, a Neumann BC is accommodated (ux[1] is included in the input argument ux).

For nl=1, only values of the dependent variable (and not the first derivative) are included in the weighted sum.

```
if(nl==1){
uxx[1]=r12dxs*
        (45*u[  1]-154*u[  2]+214*u[  3]-
         156*u[  4] +61*u[  5] -10*u[  6]);}
```

The dependent variable at points i=1,2,3,4,5,6 is used in the FD approximation for uxx[1] to remain within the x domain (fictitious points outside the x domain are not used).

Six points are used rather than five (as in the centered approximation for uxx[i]) since the FD applies at the left boundary and is not centered (around i). Six points provide a fourth order FD approximation which is the same order as the FDs at the interior points in x.

Similar considerations apply at the upper boundary value of x with nu=1,2.

Index

A

alternate coordinate systems 183
  see also cylindrical, polar, radial
    coordinates
  coordinate free PDE 184
  fit to physical system 183

B

birth rate 3–4, 83
boundary condition (BC) 6, 17
  BC approximation 65, 67–68
  consistency with IC 20–21, 25,
    118, 123, 317
  fit to physical system 183
  radial coordinates
  successive differentiation 17, 48
  stagewise differentiation 17, 48
  symmetry 93, 96

C

Cartesian coordinates 2–3, 77,
  183–184
chemotaxis 179–180
composite plot 251
conservation principle 2
coordinate systems 183
  coordinate free PDE 184
cross diffusion 2, 135 *see also*
  malaria model, Zika model
  basic concepts 136, 180

chemotaxis 179–180
coding 147, 149–150
detailed analysis of terms 160,
  162–163, 168, 170, 173, 175,
  180
nonlinear diffusion 179–180
pattern formation 136
PDE statement 135–136
  boundary conditions 137,
    163, 168
  diffusivities 142, 150–151,
    161
  initial conditions 137–138
  model 136
  nonlinearity 146–147,
    149–150
  simultaneous linear, cross
    diffusion 143, 156, 288
  SIRC 136, 180
  main program 137, 211
  ODE/MOL routine 146, 170
  numerical output 151, 170
  3D plotting 211, 214, 218,
    226, 230
  main program 211
  ODE/MOL routine 219
  output 219, 230
  symmetry 221, 225, 229
solution features 154, 158, 206,
  209
stability 177

spatial derivatives 160, 162–163,
    167–168, 170, 173, 180
  main program 160
spatial scaling 180
steady state 177
temporal derivatives 175–176
cylindrical coordinates 184

D

DAE 113
  index 113
death rate 3–4, 83
derivative 5
differential-algebraic system *see*
    DAE
diffusion 2
diffusion equation 100
diffusivity 3–4, 100, 106
direct differentiation 57, 60, 63, 65
  comparison with stagewise
      72–73, 198
Dirichlet boundary condition 6,
    198, 317, 439–440
  homogeneous 6
dss004, dss044 *see R, utilities*
  dss004, dss044
discontinuity 20–21

E

editor *see R, utilities* Rstudio
epidemics 1
  evolution 1
error tolerances *see R, utilities*
  lsodes
exposed *see* SEIRS

F

Fick's first law 4, 142
finite differences 10 *see also*
    Appendices A1, A2
  BC approximation 65, 67–68

comparison with splines 52, 55
first derivative 433
  centered 435
  noncentered 435
second derivative 437
  centered 439
  Dirichlet BC 439–440
  Neumann BC 440
  noncentered 440
order 33, 198
Taylor series basis 32–33
finite elements 10

G

Gaussian function 26, 28, 31, 41,
    50, 61, 71, 79, 82, 101, 106, 123,
    137, 186, 189, 212, 215, 292,
    299, 322, 329, 402
geographical regions 1
graphical output 2

H

h refinement 32–33, 37, 63, 156
  order 37

I

infecteds 93 *see also* SIR, SEIR,
    SIRC
interaction with susceptibles 41,
    43, 58, 65, 77
initial condition (IC) 6–8, 11,
    78–79
  consistency with BC 20–21, 25,
      118, 123, 317
  Gaussian 26, 28, 31, 41, 50, 61,
      71, 79, 82, 101, 106, 123, 137,
      186, 189, 212, 215, 292, 299,
      322, 329, 402

J

Jacobian matrix 12, 300

L

l'Hospital's rule 199

M

main program 6

malaria model 235

  vector-borne 235

  mosquito dynamics 235–236, 251, 277, 288, 339, 343

  ODE model 235–236

    algebra 237, 252, 254, 277

    graphical output 258–260, 281–283

    high transmission 237–238, 269, 277

    initial conditions 237

    low transmission 235, 238, 253

    main program 239, 269

    numerical output 256, 278

    ODE/PDE routine 252, 276

    parameters 238, 240, 245–246, 269–270, 275, 285

    reproduction number 238, 262–269, 285–287

    SEIR 235

    sensitivity 239

    steady state 241, 246–247, 260–264, 284–285

    time scale 247, 257, 262, 270, 275

    total population 235, 248

  PDE linear model 288

    algebra 304, 309

    boundary conditions 289, 305, 310

    check solution 317

    diffusivities 288, 291, 297

    Fickian diffusion 288

    graphical output 303, 318, 322

    high transmission 292

    initial condition 289, 292, 316, 321

    Jacobian matrix 300

    main program 290

    numerical output 301, 313, 319

    ODE/MOl routine 303

    parameters 290, 296

    singularity 306, 311

    spatial grid 298

    time scale 298

    total population 293

  PDE nonlinear model 325

    algebra 337

    boundary conditions 326, 337–338

    cross diffusion 325, 352

    diffusivities 327–328, 334

    graphical output 332, 347

    high transmission 327

    initial conditions 328–329

    main program 326

    numerical output 330

    ODE/MOL routine 336, 341

    numerical output 344

    parameters 327, 352

    population products 325, 335, 339, 342–343, 350, 352

    p refinement 351

    r refinement 351

    Robin boundary condition 350

    singularity 339

    spatial grid 328, 351

    time scale 328

    total population 330, 346–347

  spatiotemporal 235

mathematical models 1–2 *see also* *ODE, PDE*

boundary condition (BC) 6
    Dirichlet 6
    Neumann 6
Cartesian coordinates 2
conservation principle 2
cross diffusion *see cross*
    diffusion, SIRC
derivation 3–6
    accumulation 3
    depletion 3
    limits 5
    rates 3
diffusion 2
initial condition (IC) 6–8
main program 6
nonlinear 2
method of lines *see MOL*
MOL 10, 76
    boundary conditions 17 *see also*
      Dirichlet, Neumann
    direct differentiation 57
    finite differences 10
    graphical output 20 *see also R,*
      utilities, matplot
    h refinement 32, 37, 62
      order 37
    initial condition 6–8, 11, 78, 99
    main program 78
    Neumann BC 6, 20, 65, 75, 78,
      99
    nonlinear terms 41, 43, 59, 65,
      78, 87
    numerical output 19
    ODE/MOL routine 10–11, 14,
      16, 45, 57–58, 66–67, 86–88
    ODE vector 15, 18
    p refinement 37–38
      order 37

radial coordinates 183
r refinement 43
simultaneous PDE 78
solution check 25
spatial resolution 28, 33
splines 43–45, 65–67
subordinate routine 18
spatial grid 11, 20, 79, 83
    variation 28–34
time scale 11, 20, 83
mosquito dynamics *see malaria*
    model, Zika model

N

Neumann boundary condition 6,
    20, 65, 75, 78, 99, 113, 198, 289,
    390, 440
    homogeneous 6, 78, 99, 113,
      137, 189, 310
    symmetry 93, 96
Newton's method 113
nonlinear 2, 14, 41, 43, 59, 65, 77,
    87, 146–147, 194
    diffusion 179 *see also cross*
      diffusion

O

ODE 1
    Jacobian matix 12
    numerical integration 10 *see*
      also R, utilities, lsodes
      error tolerances 8
      library integrators 10, 12
      order 8
      sparse matrix 8
    routine 8
    stiffness 12
ordinary differential equation *see*
    ODE

P

parameter estimation 352
parameter sensitivity 239
partial derivative 3
partial differential equation *see
also PDE*
  conservation principle 2, 77
  coordinate free PDE 184
  cross diffusion *see cross
    diffusion*
  derivation 3–6
  detailed analysis of terms 160
  nonlinear 2, 14, 41, 43, 59, 65,
    77 *see also
    malaria model, Zika model*
  simultaneous 78
pattern formation *see cross
  diffusion*
PDE 1,77
  boundary condiion (BC) 6
  initial condition (IC) 6–8, 11, 78
  MOL solution 10
polar coordinates 210–211, 233
p refinement 37–38, 156, 351
  order 37, 351

R

R programming system 1
  differential equation solution 76
  download 1
    Internet 1
  editor *see R, utilities* Rstudio
  graphics 2
  ODE/DAE utilities 1
  open source 1
  utilities
    <<- return 15, 18
    {} brackets 7
    ; statement end 7
    c vector 15
    cat 8, 13
    deSolve 1, 7, 12, 81

dss004 7, 10, 14, 17, 33, 79,
    86, 89–90, 101, 110–111,
    147, 150, 163, 167–168,
    296, 304, 309, 326, 333,
    337–338, 342, 391, 400,
    408–409, 417, 433 *see also
    Appendix A1*
dss006 37–38, 351
dss044 7, 57, 186, 189, 194,
    215, 227, 296, 304, 310,
    327, 333, 338–339, 342,
    392, 400, 410, 418–419,
    437 *see also Appendix A2*
for 7
  limits 8
function 7, 10, 13, 16
if 7, 9
library 7, 10
lines 244, 250, 273
list 15, 18
lsodes 8–9, 11–12, 16, 62,
    80, 84, 102, 139, 144, 161,
    187, 191, 213, 216, 224,
    227, 241, 248, 271, 292,
    300, 335, 360, 403
  *see also ODE numerical
    integration*
matplot 9, 13
matrix 8
ncol 8, 12, 19–20
nrow 8, 12, 19–20
par 9, 13
persp 214, 218, 226, 230
plot 243, 250, 273
points 244, 250, 273
print 246
rep replicate 7
return 15, 18
rm remove workspaces 6, 9
Rstudio R editor 2
seq sequence 7

`setwd` set working directory 7, 9

`source` access files 7, 10

`splinefun` splines 47, 65, 69

`sprintf` 8, 13

polar coordinates 210–211

radial coordinates 183
  boundary conditions 185, 194, 197
  diffusivities 186, 189
  initial conditions 185
  l'Hospital's rule 199
  main program 185
  ODE/MOL routine 194
  output 201
  singularity 195, 198
  variable coefficient 199

recovereds *see also* SIR, SEIR, SIRC 41, 77, 93

r refinement 43

reproduction number *see malaria model, Zika model*

Robin boundary condition 350

S

scientific programming system *see R*

SEIRS 2, 97, 133
  main program 101
  numerical solution 116
  ODE/MOL routine 110
  time solution 126–133
  total population 99–100, 104, 112, 118, 123

singularity 195, 198

SIR 1–2, 77 *see also PDE*
  cylindrical coordinates 184
  main program 78
  numerical solution 91
  ODE/MOL routine, 86–87
  radial coordinates 183

boundary conditions 185, 194, 197

diffusivities 186, 189

initial conditions 185

l'Hospital's rule 199

main program 185

ODE/MOL routine 194

output 201

singularity 195, 198

variable coefficient 199

SIRC *see cross diffusion*

spatial grid 11
  symmetry 93, 96

spatial scales 1, 20, 180

sparse matrix 8, 12 *see also R, utilities,* `lsodes`

spatial resolution 28, 34

spatiotemporal models 1, 76–77, 135

spectral methods 10

splines 43–45, 48, 65–67
  comparison with finite differences 52, 55
  differentiating constant 51
  errors 54

stagewise differentiation 17, 48, 60, 63, 113
  comparison with direct 72–73, 198

stiff ODEs 12

subordinate routine 18

successive differentiation 17, 48, 60, 63, 113

susceptibles *see also* SIR, SEIR, SIRC
  interaction with infecteds 41, 43, 59, 65, 77

symmetry 93, 96, 221, 225, 229

T

Taylor series 32

three dimensional plotting 211,
214, 218, 226, 230
main program 211
ODE/MOL routine 219
output 219, 230
symmetry 221, 225, 229
time scale 11, 20, 352
truncation error 33

U

unit roundoff 51

V

variable coefficient 199
vector-borne diseases 235
*see also malaria model, Zika
model*

W

weighted residuals 10
world health problem 1

Z

Zika model 353
vector-borne 353
mosquito dynamics 353–356,
374, 378, 412, 414, 422, 424
ODE model 353–354
algebra 355, 373, 376
dependent variables 355–356
graphical output 363–366,
371–372, 383–385
initial conditions 358,
360–368
main program 359
non-negativity constraint
374, 378, 382

numerical output 361–362,
370–371, 380–382
ODE/PDE routine 372
ODE order 353
parameters 356–357, 359,
367
time scale 359, 367
total population 369
PDE 385–386
algebra 408, 416–417
boundary conditions
390–391, 409, 418–419
check solution 429
cross diffusion 386–387,
411–414, 423
diffusivities 392, 401
extensions 432
Fickian diffusion 389
graphical output 396–399,
406–407, 430–431
initial condition 389,
392–393, 402
main program 391
numerical output 395–396,
405–406, 426–428
ODE/MOl routine 407
parameters 392, 400–401
population products
386–388, 419
singularity 411, 421
spatial grid 392
spatiotemporal 432
stability 429
time scale 392
total populations 394–395,
404

Printed in the United States
By Bookmasters